Evidence-Based Counseling and Psychotherapy for an Aging Population

Evidence-Based Counseling and Psychotherapy for an Aging Population

Morley D. Glicken, DSW

ELSEVIER

AMSTERDAM · BOSTON · HEIDELBERG · LONDON
NEW YORK · OXFORD · PARIS · SAN DIEGO
SAN FRANCISCO · SINGAPORE · SYDNEY · TOKYO

Academic Press is an imprint of Elsevier

Academic Press is an imprint of Elsevier
30 Corporate Drive, Suite 400, Burlington, MA 01803, USA
525 B Street, Suite 1900, San Diego, CA 92101-4495, USA
32 Jamestown Road, London NW1 7BY, UK

First edition 2009

Library of Congress Cataloging-in-Publication Data
A catalog record for this book is available from the Library of Congress

British Library Cataloguing in Publication Data
A catalogue record for this book is available from the British Library

ISBN: 978-0-12-374937-6

For information on all Academic Press publications
visit our website at elsevierdirect.com

Typeset by Macmillan Publishing Solutions
www.macmillansolutions.com

Printed and bound in the United States of America

09 10 11 12   10 9 8 7 6 5 4 3 2 1

Contents

Dedication

This book is dedicated to my father, Sam Glicken, who fought for the rights of working men and women, and who was among the vanguard of the forward thinking who promoted the health care and pension benefits for older people we so take for granted. I miss you dad, and I wish you were here with me now to share this book.

About the Author

Dr Morley D. Glicken is the former Dean of the Worden School of Social Service in San Antonio; the founding director of the Master of Social Work Department at California State University, San Bernardino; the past Director of the Master of Social Work Program at the University of Alabama; and the former Executive Director of Jewish Family Service of Greater Tucson. He has also held faculty positions in social work at the University of Kansas and Arizona State University. He currently teaches in the Department of Social Work at Arizona State University West in Phoenix, Arizona.

Dr Glicken received his BA degree in social work with a minor in psychology from the University of North Dakota and holds an MSW degree from the University of Washington and the MPA and DSW degrees from the University of Utah. He is a member of Phi Kappa Phi Honorary Fraternity.

In 2009 Elsevier published his book *Evidence-Based Practice with Emotionally Troubled Children and Adolescents: A Psychosocial Perspective*. Praeger published his book *A Simple Guide to Retirement*: How to Make Retirement Work for you was published in 2009. (with Brian Haas) In 2008 he published *A Guide to Writing for Human Service Professionals* for Rowman and Littlefield Publishers. In 2006 he published *Life Lessons from Resilient People*, published by Sage Publications. He published *Working with Troubled Men: A Practitioner's Guide for Lawrence Erlbaum Publishers* in Spring 2005 and *Improving the Effectiveness of the Helping Professions: An Evidence-Based Approach to Practice* in 2004 for Sage Publications. In 2003 he published *Violent Young Children*, and *Understanding and Using the Strengths Perspective* for Allyn and Bacon/Longman Publishers. Dr Glicken published two books for Allyn and Bacon/Longman Publishers in 2002: *The Role of the Helping Professions in the Treatment of Victims and Perpetrators of Crime* (with Dale Sechrest), and *A Simple Guide to Social Research*.

Dr Glicken has published over 50 articles in professional journals and has written extensively on personnel issues for Dow Jones, the publisher of the *Wall Street Journal*. He has held clinical social work licenses in Alabama and Kansas and is a member of the Academy of Certified Social Workers. He is currently Professor Emeritus in Social Work at California State University, San Bernardino and Director of the Institute for Personal Growth: A Research, Treatment, and Training Institute in Prescott Arizona offering management, consulting, and research services to public and private agencies. More information about Dr Glicken may be obtained on his website: www.morleyglicken.com, and he may be contacted by email at: mglicken@msn.com.

Preface

Let me begin this preface by informing the reader that I *am* an older adult (68 when the book was written) but that much of what I read about aging, work, retirement, and life after 65 seems to inaccurately describe me and many of the older adults around me. We seem like a healthy and engaged lot, many of us playing tennis and hiking well into our eighties, and even our nineties. We stay healthy, continue to work or volunteer, and maintain active, stimulating lifestyles. Yes, we hurt in the morning, and pain and certain signs of aging like forgetfulness are annoying, but in most ways we are as physically and emotionally healthy as ever, perhaps even more so. We planned for retirement and never saw it as a permanent state of inactivity and leisure, but as an opportunity to grow and expand as people.

And yet, many older adults haven't had these experiences. They come from employment that has taken its toll on their minds and bodies. They failed to develop and maintain healthy lifestyles throughout many of the years approaching old age. They lacked support groups and had troubled interpersonal experiences that often left them feeling lonely, depressed, or prone to abusing substances. Rather than planning for the economic realities of life without work, because they had so little to begin with, they live on the small subsidies provided by Social Security.

This book is written for them, but it is also written for the "healthy" older adults who begin to experience depression, anxiety, prolonged bereavement, and every emotional problem that younger clients experience, because emotional problems are part of the human condition at any age. It is also written to urge clinicians to begin helping older adults when they hurt emotionally, something the reader will discover often fails to happen. Finally, it is written to encourage clinicians to use best evidence in their work with older adults and to understand the use of evidence-based practice, an approach that offers great hope for effective work with many clients.

This is my third book on evidence-based practice and my 12th book in six years. I trust that this track record and the fact that I continue to teach and consult are strong arguments against the notion that older adults experience diminished abilities. You wouldn't know that, however, from the experiences many of us begin to have with organizations that no longer want us even though we've given our all to the health and vitality of those very organizations. Many of us have felt the subtle and not so subtle signs that once we are past 50 (and maybe even younger), our worth in society and in the workplace diminishes with each year we grow older.

Ageism, like any other stereotype or bias, is filled with misinformation and inaccuracies that lead otherwise healthy people to experience problems as they age that would never exist in a society that values the skills, wisdom, and work ethic of older people. In no small part many of the problems discussed in this book result from healthy people being treated badly in the workplace and by a society that devalues older people. Although this book is mainly clinical in nature, I'm including a chapter on needed social policies because they are so important to healthy aging.

People who have worked their entire lives deserve the best mental health service available. One solution to the increasing number of older adults who may not be aging well is to provide a competency-based service that focuses on what works best. By using best evidence from the rapidly increasing knowledge-base in psychotherapy, social work, counseling, and gerontology, human service workers can provide a research-oriented service whose objective is to keep aging clients engaged, independent, and healthy, even those clients who are not aging well because of poverty, poor nutrition, substandard housing, limited educational opportunities, lack of financial planning, elder abuse, or catastrophic losses that have reduced life chances and limit access to an "aging well lifestyle."

Workers providing services to older adults need to understand that psychosocial perspectives on aging have changed in the past 40 years from notions of disengagement, which argue that older adults will gradually withdraw or disengage from social roles as a natural response to lessened capabilities, diminished interest, and to societal disincentives for participation, to current beliefs that people who age successfully are those who carry forward the positive habits, preferences, lifestyles, and relationships of midlife into late life.

Evidence-based practice is an approach that offers reason and rationality to a population of people who are often ignored by the mental health and medical professions when they experience emotional distress. The book provides practice-oriented information that will help workers improve their work with older adults, as well as case studies followed by an analysis of the work done with clients over a range of problems experienced by older adults. The problems interfering with successful aging include depression, anxiety, reduction in functioning, prolonged grief, loss of friends and loved ones, feelings of isolation and aloneness, financial difficulties, problems with self-care and appropriate housing, health-related problems, difficulties receiving needed medical care, addictions and substance abuse, elder abuse, and many other problems described in more detail in the table of contents. Special features in the book include case studies in every chapter, personal stories on successful aging from older adults, and integrative questions at the end of each chapter.

Finally, I want to make clear that the most compelling purpose of this book is to remember the many older adults among us who suffer in silence and isolation, and grow old without the comfort of a loving family or a caring community. Their anguish should motivate us to open our hearts and minds to new ideas, to new treatment approaches, and, in Bertrand Russell's words, to have "unbearable sympathy for the suffering of others."

Morley D. Glicken, DSW

Acknowledgements

This is the second book I've written with Mica Haley and Renske van Dijk, my editors at Elsevier. It's rare in academic writing that you find two people so easy to work with or so supportive of your ideas. Thanks Mica and Renske, and thanks to Elsevier for accepting this book idea and letting me develop it as I saw best. Writing about aging is a gift, and having a publishing house that appreciates the need for a rational system of helping older adults experiencing late life emotional difficulties made this book a pleasure to write.

Because everyone needs someone to look at their work as it evolves who will give sincere and helpful feedback, I feel very fortunate that my significant other, Patricia Fox, was kind enough to perform this task and to do it in a way that left me endlessly aware that anyone who writes requires a sane and supportive mate. Thanks, Pat. You are a gift to me in my later years.

Thanks to Dr Suzanne Bushfield, my former colleague at the Arizona State University Department of Social Work for the discussions we had about evidence-based practice and her willingness to include that discussion in this book, and to provide additional information on issues in several chapters of the book, particularly the chapters on Alzheimer's and disabilities and terminal illness. Thanks, Suzanne, and best wishes for a long and successful career. You were a joy to work with.

Thanks also to Rebecca Hampton, MSW for her much appreciated contribution to the chapter on hospice care.

I also want to thank the many older adults who contributed to this book with personal stories. Their lives and the positive ways they approach aging should offer all of us a model of the benefits of healthy living and a positive and optimistic way of approaching life.

Finally, I want to thank the far-sighted people, among them my father, Sam Glicken, who envisioned the future as a time when older adults could enjoy the fruits of long years of labor by enacting the Social Security and Medicare Programs, and the various state and private pension plans that allow many of us to fulfill dreams and enjoy life in ways those before us never could. In no small part this book was written as a way of thanking them for their persistent belief that aging is a time for continued growth and creative opportunity, and that as good as our later years are for many of us, many older men and women suffer in silence and despair, making it absolutely necessary that we work to make life better for everyone, old and young.

Part one

Psychosocial Perspectives of Aging

Chapter one

Aging in America: Psychosocial Treatment Issues

1.1 INTRODUCTION

This is a book about best evidence in our work with a growing population of older adults, some of whom are aging badly and require services they often fail to get. It is a book for human service professionals who provide clinical services and who will see an increasing number of people in practice we traditionally see at younger ages. Although the book is based on best evidence in the research literature and will, by design, focus on clinical practice, I encourage the reader to remember that clinical practice is an intimate experience between us and the sometimes troubled and bewildered older adults who may wonder why, after a lifetime of feeling strong, secure, and healthy, that emotional problems are affecting them just as life seems to be going so well.

Like many of us who begin to feel the weight of a serious depression or an unwanted anxiety, older adults are often reluctant to seek help because they may feel that it shouldn't be happening to them after so many years of good mental health, and that it's some sort of bad joke that someone is playing on them to feel the heavy weight of emotional pain. When that feeling hits, we should be there for them and we should know what works.

Having said that, I don't want to lose the reality of what therapy is from the point of view of both the practitioner and the client. For us it is often hard to sit in a room and talk to another person in the way that therapy calls upon you to do. The inevitable silences, the halting admissions, the difficulty finding the right word, the struggles with that enraging, adored person facing you, the secret pleasures of the embarrassing focus on you – just you, and nobody but you – may look dull from the outside, but to the people involved it's a highly charged, tense and active situation. (Franklin, 2008, p. 78)

For the older client it is the abject confusion of facing someone so much younger and wondering if they can trust that person to provide wise and competent help when after a lifetime of solving problems on their own, they've suddenly lost their way and wonder if they will ever find it again. No one says aging is easy and to think otherwise ignores the very real problems older adults face: that what was once so easy for them has now become increasingly difficult.

So have some empathy, dear reader, and begin this book with the knowledge that older people make up an ever-increasing number of Americans. They have the same right to have their pain, their fears, and their sorrows listened to, and you can't help them until you move from thinking of aging as a time of death to remembering that we're talking about 30 or more years of life during which time older people have the same need to resolve problems that affect them as do younger groups. We reject ageism in this book, and hopefully you will too.

That's what I have to say to you before we begin this journey together. I hope that when the journey is over you will be able to say that you've moved to not imagining older people in your workload to now feeling anticipation and excitement at the prospect.

1.2 SOME DEMOGRAPHICS OF AGING

Older adults increasingly make up a larger percentage of the population of the USA. In growing numbers, their issues and life experiences influence social policies and health and social welfare services. For the year 2006, the Department on Aging (2007) reported that adults 65-years or older numbered 37.3 million. This represented 12.4% of the US population, or one in every eight Americans. By 2030, the Department on Aging predicts there will be about 71.5 million older persons, more than twice the number in 2000, and more than 20% of the total population.

The population of Americans is getting older, with the number of Americans over age 85 increasing faster than any other group. Since 1900 the proportion of Americans age 65 and older has more than tripled, with current life expectancy for men at 73 years and for women at 80 years. Not only are more people living into the second 50 years of life, but 70,000 centenarians have entered their third 50 years. By 2050, the US Census Bureau estimates the number of centenarians at 834,000 – although the bureau's "high-end" calculation predicts that this figure could climb as high as 4.2 million, with 35% of the American population over the age of 65 and rising.

Arrison (2007) believes that 80 is the new 65. Because of the use of nano-technology and stem cell research, Arrison believes that older adults may live well beyond 120 years of age, while researchers in England are working on "engineered negligible senescence – which would in theory eliminate most of the physical damage of aging and lead to indefinite life spans" (Arrison, 2007, p. A17).

Many Americans over 65 suffer from disabilities that affect their daily functioning. Ten percent of the total number of people in the population living below the poverty line are over the age of 65, with many living on an average social security pension of $12,500 a year with no other source of income. Forty-two percent of all Americans 65 and older suffer from disabilities that affect their daily functioning. As the number of older Americans grows, so does the recognition that many older Americans have serious social, emotional, health and financial problems that make aging a joyless and sometimes anxious and depressing experience. Many older adults with social and emotional problems have conditions that go undiagnosed and untreated because underlying symptoms of anxiety and depression are thought to be physical in nature, and health and mental health professionals frequently believe that older adults are neither motivated for therapy nor find it an appropriate treatment. This often leaves many older adults trying to cope with serious emotional problems without adequate help.

Persky (2008) notes that although older adults make up 13% of the US population, their use of inpatient and outpatient mental health services falls far below expectations. Elders account for only 7% of all inpatient psychiatric services, 6% of community mental health services, and 9% of private psychiatric care. Less than 3% of all Medicare reimbursements are for the psychiatric treatment of older patients although 18% to 25% of elders are in need of mental health care for depression, anxiety, psychosomatic disorders, adjustment to aging, and schizophrenia. Yet, according to Persky, few seem to receive proper care and treatment for these illnesses even though it is a distressing reality that the suicide rate of the elderly is an alarming 21%, the highest of all age groups in the USA. Every day, 17 older individuals kill themselves.

As this chapter will describe, the numbers of older adults dealing with anxiety and depression are considerable and growing as the numbers of older adults increase in the USA. Health problems, loss of loved ones, financial insecurities, lack of a support group, a growing sense of isolation, and a lack of self-worth are common problems among the elderly that lead to serious symptoms of anxiety and depression, problems that often co-exist among many older adults. A case study presented in this chapter provides added information about the cause and treatment of depression and anxiety in the elderly.

What does this mean for the institutions providing services to older adults, and how can human service professionals provide competent and effective service? One answer to the increasing number of older adults in need is to provide an evidence-based service that focuses on what works best. By using best evidence from the rapidly increasing knowledge base in gerontology, human service workers can provide a research-oriented service whose objective is to keep aging clients engaged, independent, and healthy, even those clients who are not aging well because of poverty, poor nutrition, substandard housing, limited educational opportunities, lack of financial planning, abuse, or catastrophic losses that have reduced life chances and limited access to an "aging well lifestyle."

In addition to the need to provide new approaches to older adults that will prolong health and retain cognitive functioning and life satisfaction, theories of aging have been rapidly changing. Workers providing services to older adults need to understand that psychosocial perspectives on aging have changed in the past 40 years from notions of disengagement, which argue that older adults will gradually withdraw or disengage from social roles as a natural response to lessened capabilities, diminished interest, and societal disincentives for participation, to current beliefs that people who age successfully are those who carry forward the positive habits, preferences, lifestyles, and relationships from midlife into late life.

1.3 FUTURE GROWTH OF OLDER ADULTS

The older population will continue to grow in the future. This growth slowed somewhat during the 1990s because of the relatively small number of babies born during the Great Depression of the 1930s. The most rapid increase is expected between the years 2010 and 2030 when the "baby boom" generation reaches age 65.

By 2030, there will be about 70 million older persons, more than twice their number in 1996. People over 65 are projected to represent 13% of the population in the year 2000 but will be 20% of the population by 2030.

Minority populations are projected to represent 25% of the elderly population in 2030, up from 13% in 1990. Between 1990 and 2030, the white non-Hispanic population over 65 is projected to increase by 91% compared with 328% for older minorities, including Hispanics (570%) and non-Hispanic blacks (159%), American Indians, Eskimos, and Aleuts (294%), and Asians and Pacific Islanders (643%) (AARP, 1997).

1.4 COMMON EMOTIONAL PROBLEMS EXPERIENCED BY OLDER ADULTS

The following data about common emotional problems experienced by older adults are summarized from the American Psychological Association website (2003):

1. Five to seven percent of older adults between the ages of 65 and 85 and 30% of those over the age of 85 suffer from dementia, an irreversible deterioration of cognitive abilities accompanied by emotional problems including depression, anxiety, paranoia and serious problems in social functioning.
2. Six percent of older adults experience problems with anxiety for a period of six months or more.
3. Older adults have much higher suicide rates than other age groups, with Caucasian men who live alone suffering the highest suicide rates.
4. Sleep problems often increase with age, and roughly half of all older adults over the age of 80 have problems sleeping.
5. While rates of alcohol problems are lower than other age groups, 2–5% of all men over the age of 65 and 1% of all women in this age group experience alcohol problems.
6. Drug abuse is a common problem among older adults, who use 25% of the medication taken in the USA. The drug addiction problem is complicated by the fact that older adults are often pre-scribed too many medications.

7. Older adults experience high rates of depression, which is often characterized by feelings of sadness and helplessness. Depression may come on quickly in older adults who are experiencing physical problems or have had prior emotional problems that may result in complaints about memory loss.

8. Older adults often experience the onset of Alzheimer's disease, which affects memory and produces symptoms of disorientation. The symptoms of Alzheimer's are often gradual and may take eight to 20 years from onset to complete deterioration and memory loss. The symptoms are profound, and memory loss may be so severe that victims of the disease may not recognize family members and are often unable to function without help from others whom they may not even recognize (American Psychological Association website, 2004).

1.5 STUDIES OF COUNSELING AND PSYCHOTHERAPY USE BY OLDER ADULTS

Although people over the age of 60 make up almost 13% of the total US population (AARP, 2000), they represent only 6–8% of persons seen in community mental health clinics and outpatient mental health settings, and an even smaller percentage of clients seen by private counseling practitioners (Smyer and Qualls, 1999). Morgan (2003) reports that, "Even though the percentage of the population older than 65 years is growing and will continue to do so, elderly persons are underrepresented in all forms of psychotherapy" (p. 1592).

Barriers to the use of these services by an older population include bias toward older persons among service providers and reluctance of older persons to seek counseling, as well as a lack of adequate training and supervised clinical practice with older adults that allow human service professionals to be comfortable and effective with older clients (Nordhus and VandenBos, 1998). Such training requires an understanding of effective intervention practices. Blake (1975) described older persons as "the forgotten and ignored" (p. 733) by the counseling profession.

The Council for Accreditation of Counseling and Related Educational Programs (CACREP; 2003) reports that only two counselor training programs are accredited in gerontological counseling, and suggests that the lack of training for work with older clients may dissuade counselor practitioners from offering services to older adults. Similarly in social work, the Hartford Foundation (2003) reports that most social work education programs "provide only limited gerontology content in their foundation curricula, and many graduate schools do not offer geriatrics as a specialty option" (p. 1). The report continues on by saying that "[a]s a result, most social work students graduate without the aging-related information and training which they will need to assist the growing number of older adults and their caregivers" (p. 1).

Studies of the use of mental health services by older adults indicate an under usage (Smyer and Qualls, 1999). For example, a survey of Los Angeles County psychologists cited by Myers and Schwiebert (1996) concerning services they offered to older adults revealed that, among 114 respondents, only 3.1–4.4% specialized in serving older adults. Although this study was limited to services available in one urban county and cannot be generalized to the older population as a whole, the results are consistent with earlier studies demonstrating a lack of needed mental health services for the older population nationally (Myers and Schwiebert, 1996).

Black et al. (1997) believe that the underutilization of psychological services in older adults might be explained by either a lack of recognition of mental health problems, or denial, and that many older adults do not have medical coverage for emotional problems. In their study, the authors found in their research population of 371 older residents living in six public housing developments in Baltimore, Maryland, with the majority living alone (95%), African-American (95%), and female (84%), that although a third of the participants had used mental health services, only 4% received those services from a mental health specialist. Most received mental health services from a primary medical care provider. More than half the participants who were identified through interviews and mental health instruments and were found to in need of mental health services indicated that they had not received mental health services of any kind in the previous six months.

Roth and Fonagy (2004, p. 323) identified the following reasons for underutilization of psychological services in older adults: "Reluctance by therapists to treat older adults; lack of identification of older adult psychological problems by primary care physicians; and incorrect diagnosis of depression as dementia, which results in a low rate of referral for psychological treatment."

1.6 OLDER ADULTS BENEFIT FROM HUMAN SERVICE INTERVENTIONS

A number of chapters in the book show how older adults benefit from a variety of approaches for problems ranging from depression and anxiety to sleep disturbances and pain management. In a review of a small amount of that evidence, Pinquart and Soerensen (2001) document that older adults respond well to a variety of forms of psychotherapy and counseling and benefit to the same extent as younger adults. Gatz et al. (1998) and Teri and McCurry (1994) have shown that cognitive-behavioral, psycho-dynamic, interpersonal and other approaches have been effective with a variety of problems experienced by older adults. Those problems include depression (Areán and Cook, 2002), anxiety (Stanley et al., 1996), sleep disturbance (Morin et al., 1999), and alcohol abuse (Blow, 2000).

Burgio (1996) has shown that cognitive training techniques, behavior modification strategies, and socio-environmental modification help in treating depression and improving functional abilities in cognitively impaired older adults. Areán et al. (1993) report that life review therapy is helpful in the treatment of depression, while Maercker (2002) found that life review therapy can be helpful in treating post-traumatic stress disorder in older adults, although Areán (2002) notes that the research evidence is inadequate when it comes to ethnic minority older adults. Watkins et al. (1999) have shown that treatment interventions are effective in managing pain and with changing social circumstances including housing issues, moving to assisted care and improving interpersonal relationships, particularly with family members. Much more evidence of treatment effectiveness with older adults experiencing a wide range of social and emotional problems will be offered in the following chapters.

Bonhote et al. (1998, p. 606) have had anecdotal success in working with groups where the specific theoretical model was using altruism and the creative expression of feelings. The specific goals of their group work were to:

1. decrease feelings of powerlessness and helplessness accompanying life changes;
2. develop insight into feelings experienced in the group, which can facilitate adaptation to loss and change;
3. explore coping and preventative strategies to facilitate adaptation to change and/or loss;
4. combat stereotypes, false labels, and myths imposed by a youth-oriented society.

In this form of group therapy, altruism is a primary technique based on Yalom's (1995) belief that altruism is one of the curative factors in group therapy. Bonhote et al. (1998, p. 606) note that in their groups with older adults, "[t]he notion that one can benefit from helping others can be a motivator for engaging in the group process and a reinforcer for continued involvement, particularly for more isolated or regressed older adults." The authors believe that groups can be particularly helpful because they allow for expression of feelings and helping others, and therefore make more isolated and lonely people feel more engaged and involved with others.

Reason for Grp.

Sadavoy et al. (1991) report that common group themes that repeatedly emerge in group work with older adults are "changes in significant relationships, decline in physical health, diminished self-worth and self-esteem, loneliness and social isolation, depression, issues of dependency versus autonomy, interpersonal discord, hopelessness, existential crises, and 'a wish to restore a sense of competence and mastery'." Bonhote et al. (1998, p. 606) believe that groups can be very effective in the "facilitation of member expression of feelings, use of group process to address themes directly and symbolically and to address psychodynamic conflicts, and life review and assisted recollection of past accomplishments."

Morgan (2003) believes that psychotherapy fits well with the developmental processes of late life. For Erikson (1963), late life is about:

> [P]utting one's life into perspective and negotiating between ego integrity and despair. The expectable events of aging, such as retirement or relationships with adult children and grandchildren, often serve as an impetus for self-reflection and psychotherapy. (p. 117)

Morgan (2003) notes that in late life, "[t]herapists can help older persons understand how their mode of managing difficulties earlier in life may be used appropriately for current late-life problems" (p. 1592).

Evidence that cognitive-behavioral therapy works with older adults can be found in the works of a number of researchers. In a meta-analyisis of cognitive treatment with older adults, Scogin and McElreath (1994) found that cognitive therapy with depressed older adults was as effective as using anti-depressants and that therapy with older adults had positive effectiveness results similar to that of younger adults. Areán and Miranda (1996) found that cognitive therapy helped relieve symptoms of depression in medically ill outpatients. Lopez and Mermelstein (1995) found cognitive and behavioral interventions successful in treating depression with inpatients in a hospital geriatric unit. Gallagher and Thompson (1983) compared cognitive, behavioral, and brief insight-oriented therapy with a total of 38 adults over the age of 55. All three groups showed reduction in symptoms of depression, but the cognitive and behavioral groups maintained gains better at follow-up. A similar study with 115 subjects over the age of 60, with the same three treatment conditions and a wait-list control, found all three treatment approaches superior to the control group, with each mode of psychotherapy equally effective. At follow up, all three treatment groups maintained gains equally (Thompson et al., 1987).

In a study sponsored by NIMH (2006), depressed patients 70 and older who achieved full remission of symptoms after treatment using Paroxetine (a selective serotonin reuptake inhibitor) and interpersonal psychotherapy (IPT: psychotherapy that focuses on interpersonal relationships) were randomly assigned to one of four maintenance treatment groups: (1) Paroxetine; (2) placebo; (3) Paroxetine and monthly interpersonal psychotherapy; and (4) placebo and IPT. Across all four treatment groups, rates of remission significantly differed. Among patients who received Paroxetine in the maintenance phase, 63% remained in remission; 42% of those who received placebo remained in remission; 65% of patients who received paroxetine and IPT remained in remission; and only 32% of patients who received placebo and IPT remained in remission. The researchers had hypothesized that IPT would significantly reduce rates of recurrence. In trying to determine why their hypothesis was proven wrong, the researchers concluded that older depressed adults need a more structured and focused type of psychotherapy – one that works better with cognitive impairment and greater disability than does IPT. Therapies such as cognitive behavioral and problem-solving psychotherapies were thought to be good approaches to use when they increasingly involved caregivers.

Chambless et al. (1998) report that behavioral and environmental interventions for older adults with dementia meet the standards for well-established empirically supported therapy. According to Knight and Satre (1999), therapies for older adults with good success include cognitive behavioral treatment of sleep disorders and behavioral treatments for clinical depression. For problems of memory and cognitive training, cognitive behavioral approaches are probably effective in slowing cognitive decline. The authors also found life review approaches "probably efficacious in improvement of depressive symptoms or in producing higher life satisfaction" (p. 196).

CASE STUDY: EVIDENCE-BASED PRACTICE WITH A DEPRESSED OLDER FEMALE CLIENT

Linda Johnson is a 68-year-old retired executive assistant for a large corporation. Ms Johnson had a long, successful, and happy career moving up the ladder in her company to one of its most important and highly paid positions. She retired at age 65 in good health and wanted to travel and spend more time with her grown children and her grandchildren. A year earlier, still in good health and happy with her decision to travel, Linda experienced the beginning signs of depression. Alarmed, since she had never experienced prolonged depression before, she saw her gynecologist during her annual physical examination and shared her symptoms with him. He immediately referred her to a psychiatrist who placed her on an anti-depressant medication and urged her to consider therapy. Since she had no idea what was causing the depression and thought that it might be something bio-chemical related to aging and the discontinuation of hormone therapy for symptoms of menopause some years earlier, she decided against therapy and stayed with the anti-depressant. There was little relief with the medication and a second visit with the psychiatrist confirmed the need for therapy and a change in medication. The second medication made her fatigued and lethargic. After an additional month of feeling depressed, she saw a clinical social worker who worked with a group of physicians recommended by her psychiatrist.

Linda was very pessimistic about seeing a social worker. She had known many people in her company who had gone for therapy and who had come back, in her opinion, worse than before they'd entered treatment. She also thought therapy was for weak people and refused to see herself that way. When she began seeing the social worker, she was very defensive and kept much of the problem she was having to herself. The social worker was kind and warm and didn't seem to mind at all. This went on for four sessions. In the fifth session, Linda broke down and cried and described the awful feeling of depression and her confusion about why someone who had never been depressed before would experience such feelings. The social worker asked her if she had any ideas about why she was experiencing depression now. She didn't. All she could think that might be relevant was that she had been an active woman all of her life and since her divorce at age 55, she had put all of her energies into her work and her children but now felt as if she was of little use to anyone. She was bored and thought it had been a mistake to retire.

The worker thought this was a very good theory and suggested that she might want to explore the possibility of going back to work, perhaps part-time, at first, to see if she liked it. She also suggested that Linda read some articles about aging and depression and suggested several articles and websites. The worker also explained the research about effective treatment of elder depression and recommended that Linda read several articles on treatment effectiveness, which, the worker told Linda, indicated promising results.

Linda returned to her old company, worked part-time in a very accepting and loving department where people were genuinely happy to have her back, and found that, if anything, the depression was increasing. Alarmed, she contacted the social worker and they began the work that ultimately led to an improvement in her depression.

The social worker felt that Linda had put many of her intimacy needs aside when she divorced her husband. She had not had a relationship since her divorce and felt bitter and angry with her ex-husband for leaving her for a younger woman. She had no desire to date or to form intimate relationships and repeatedly said that her good female friends were all she needed in her life. It turned out, as the clinical social worker helped Linda explore her past, that Linda was given large responsibilities to managing her dysfunctional family when she was a child. Never having learned about her own needs, Linda took care of people and now wondered who would take care of her as she tried to deal with depression and aging. Her very good friends found it difficult to be around her when she spoke about her depression. Increasingly, she felt alone and unloved. Her children were busy with their own lives and she didn't feel it was right to ask for their help. The social worker arranged for several family meetings and her children were, as Linda predicted, sympathetic but unwilling to help in more than superficial ways. The recognition that her family didn't care about her as fully as she cared about them validated feelings she had not expressed to the therapist that her family and friends were not the supports she imagined them to be and that, in reality, she was alone in life.

This recognition of being alone led to a discussion of what Linda wanted to do in treatment. Improving the depression was foremost in her mind, but she also wanted to make some changes in her life. She expressed interest in social activities and accepted the social worker's suggestion that she join a self-help group for depressed older people going through an adjustment to retirement. Going to the group made Linda realize that she was a much more healthy and optimistic person than many of the severely depressed people in the group. She also made several friends who turned out to be true friends, one of whom was male. While the relationship didn't become intimate, they were able to have companionship, travel together, and attend social events. Linda found his company very comforting and supportive. She joined a dance group and, through the group, also made several friends. She began to date and experienced a type of intimacy with the man she was dating that she hadn't known in her marriage. In treatment, she focused on what she wanted in her life and how to use her highly advanced skills to achieve those goals. The depression began to lift as her social and personal life improved.

There are moments when she is still depressed and the therapist believes these are more bio-chemical and situational than serious signs of depression. She continues to work with the psychiatrist on finding a better way to manage her depression bio-chemically. After six months of trial and error, they found a medication and dosage that worked well for her. She continues to work part-time, recognizes the primary reasons for her depression, and continues to work on those reasons with her therapist.

Discussion

Linda is like many older adults who find that retirement brings with it the painful realization that they are often alone in life. Depression isn't an unusual end result of this realization. Linda is a highly successful woman with many strengths. The one thing she could not easily do is to seek help, a common condition in people who have cared for others throughout their lives with little thought of being cared for themselves. The social worker stayed with Linda during her moments of denial and rejection of help and allowed Linda to go at her own pace. Once Linda confirmed her painful depression and explained why she thought it was happening, the social worker supported her theory, which led to a helping agenda Linda could accept. Like many parents, the recognition that her children were only marginally involved in her life was a difficult one for Linda to accept, and it felt hurtful to her in the extreme. However, Linda now recognizes that her children have resented her intrusiveness into their lives since her divorce. The reaction of the children made Linda realize that she was using her children for intimacy needs before and after her divorce, and that they resented it.

Once again, Linda feels in control of her life and, highly intelligent and insightful woman that she is, sees the rebuilding of her life as a primary goal to ensure health and happiness. She has moved to another self-help group of more highly functioning people and feels a kinship with them. Her relationships with her male friends have blossomed and she realizes that the anger she had for her husband limited her ability to allow men into her life. The new feeling of comfort with her male friends has made her aware that many men find her interesting and attractive, and she is experiencing the pleasant sense of being in demand as a friend and companion. She values her male friends and sees in them the true friendships she wasn't always able to have before therapy began.

The author spoke to Linda about her experiences in treatment. "I think I'd been a bit depressed since my marriage started to fail," she told me. "To cover it up, I was busy every second of the day. I'd work all day and then went to every play, musical event, and function I could find, usually with friends. My relationships were very superficial and it came as no real surprise that my friends weren't there for me when I became really depressed. The first thing I realized after retirement was that I had free time that I'd never had before. I filled it with everything I could find but still, I had time on my hands and at some point, I didn't know what to do with myself. It was clear to me that my children felt confused about having me around so much but I talked myself into thinking they needed me. I certainly didn't pick up on the signs of their unhappiness over my frequent calls and visits. When the depression hit, I knew I needed help but I talked myself into believing it was hormonal. I knew better, of course, but I just didn't want to accept that I was depressed because I was living a depressing life.

"My social worker was pretty amazing. She let me babble on and not ever get to the point until I finally had nowhere to go with my feelings and just fell apart in her office. She involved me in determining the issues we would work on and was very clear that in a cooperative relationship it was necessary that I know a lot about the best treatment approach to use, so I read about different treatment approaches, and it was very helpful and empowering to me. My therapist was very supportive and encouraging and always seemed to be able to see things in a positive way. In time I guess I began to see things more positively. The groups I went to, run by other depressed people, really made a difference in my life. I've made some very good friends through the people I've met in group. They're not superficial people and they care about me. I've stopped bugging my family and I don't need to be busy every minute of the day. I have moments when I'm depressed but it's not like the depression I had when I began therapy. That depression felt like I was falling down a black hole and I'd never get out. My therapist made me realize that I had many skills to manage my depression, and the discussions about my life gave me an opportunity to see that I had never really asked anyone to give back to me emotionally. I think my husband got tired of my always giving even when he didn't need anything. He'd ask what he could do for me and I'd never know what to say. I think he started to feel irrelevant. I have a relationship in which both of us give equally, and while it sometimes feels wrong to even ask for anything, I'm getting a lot better at it. Would I have gotten better without therapy? I doubt it very much. Medication helps a little, but it's no magic cure. My social worker pretty much saved my life."

1.7 A PERSONAL STORY: THE REALITY OF RURAL HEALTH CARE

A sign in the back of a van in my hometown of Prescott, Arizona sums up the concerns many older Americans have about our health care system. It read: "If you're old and sick in Prescott, there aren't enough doctors, most of them aren't any good, they charge too much, and you come back from seeing them and you're still sick." I should add that like much of rural Arizona, the rural county I live in (just an hour from the opulence of Sedona) has half the national average of doctors recommended per 100,000 people and many of them are not primary care, mental health providers, or internal medicine physicians.

When I moved to Prescott and became violently ill during my move, we called all 60 primary care doctors on my insurance list and none of them would see me. The doctor I had arranged an appointment with as a new patient before my move wouldn't see me until our appointment a month later and said I should go to the emergency room. My bill in the emergency room was over $3,000. Prescott lacked a single acute care facility even though the combined communities in and around the city have a population of 150,000. Reality hits home about health care when it touches you personally.

I have excellent health insurance. I hate to think what a person in poverty would have gone through had they been as sick as I was and were unable to afford going to an emergency room. Even the most affluent and healthy among us can have our life satisfaction lowered by ineffective helping systems. Many of the people I know in Prescott have given up on local care and drive two hours each way to Phoenix where doctors are plentiful and health care is excellent, but try doing that in a health emergency and you begin to understand that the benefits of rural living that many retiring Americans look for are sometimes negated by the lack of quality services for older adults. You can't age well when you know that in a serious health emergency you may not make the two-hour drive and live.

1.8 SUMMARY

This chapter discusses the growing number of older adults and the psychosocial needs that are likely to occur as the population of elder adults dramatically increases over the next several decades. The chapter notes the importance of using best evidence when working with older adults and the social, emotional and health-related problems that are currently prevalent among older adults and are likely to increase in coming years. Future chapters will explain EBP in more detail and will note the use of EBP with a host of psychosocial problems.

1.9 QUESTIONS FROM THE CHAPTER

1. One often hears from women of a certain age that they'd rather be with their female friends than with a man because they've had so many bad experiences with men. They frequently say that their friends are more supportive than any man could ever be. Do you think this is true, and do you know older women who feel this way? Do you think their relationships with other women are true friendships or are they more like the superficial acquaintances described by Linda?

2. It's painful to think that Linda's children are unsupportive and even resentful of their mother and believe that she's been too involved in their lives as a way of not dealing with her own. Do you have any suggestions for the social worker to bring the family closer together, or do you think the situation should be left alone while Linda develops other areas of intimacy and friendship?

3. Do you think Linda retired too early, or is this a problem that would have occurred anyway?

4. Can you imagine at your age suddenly stopping school and work and not having anything to do during the day? Many people at 65 are in excellent health but are bored and burned out with their jobs. What would you tell them about retiring?

5. Linda may be co-dependent, which means that she was trained by her biological family to care for others and not to think about her own needs. How is it possible for co-dependent people to ever gain real happiness when they have no idea of what it takes to be happy? Do you know anyone like this? How do they deal with having their own needs met?

REFERENCES

American Association of Retired Persons. (1997). *Future growth*. Retrieved 5.12.2004 <http://research.aarp.org/general/profile97.html/>.

American Psychological Association Website. (2003). *Psychological problems of older adults*. Retrieved 8.5.2007 <http://www.apa.org/pi/aging/older/psychological.html/>.

An aging infusion: Gerontology finds its place in the social work curriculum. Programs innovate to prepare students for tomorrow's clients. The John A. Hartford Foundation, 55 East 59th Street, New York, NY 10022. 212 832–7788. Monograph 2003.

Areán, P. A., & Cook, B. L. (2002). Psychotherapy and combined psychotherapy/ pharmacotherapy for late life depression. *Biological Psychiatry, 52*, 293–303.

Areán, P., & Miranda, J. (1996). The treatment of depression in elderly primary care patients: A naturalistic study. *Journal of Clinical Geropsychology, 2*, 153–160.

Areán, P. A., Perri, M. G., Nezu, A. M., Schein, R. L., Christopher, F., & Joseph, T. X. (1993). Comparative effectiveness of social problem-solving therapy and reminiscence therapy as treatments for depression in older adults. *Journal of Consulting and Clinical Psychology, 61*, 1003–1010.

Arrison, S. (2007, March 12). 80 is the new 65. *Los Angeles Times, 126*(100), A17.

*Black, B. S., Rabins, P. V., German, P., McGuire, M., Roca, R. (1997, December). Need and unmet need for mental health care among elderly public housing residents. *The Gerontologist, 37*(6), 717–728.

Blake, R. (1975). Counseling in gerontology. *The Personnel and Guidance Journal, 53*, 733–737.

Blow, F. C. (2000). Treatment of older women with alcohol problems: Meeting the challenge for a special population. *Alcoholism Clinical and Experimental Research, 24*, 1257–1266.

Bonhote, K., & Romano-Egan, J. (1998). *Altruism and creative expression in a long-term older adult psychotherapy group*, Behavioral Health Older Adults Clinic, University of Rochester, Strong Memorial Hospital, Rochester, New York, USA.

Burgio, L. (1996). Interventions for the behavioral complications of Alzheimer's disease. *International Psychogeriatrics, 8*(Suppl. 1), 46–52.

Chambless, D. L., & Hollon, S. D. (1998). Defining empirically supported therapies. *Journal of Consulting and Clinical Psychology, 66*, 7–18.

Cornwell, D. (1999). Strong behavioral health nursing, Senior Associate, School of Nursing, University of Rochester. *Issues in Mental Health Nursing, 20*, 603–617.

Council for Accreditation of Counseling and Related Educational Programs (2003). *Directory of CACREP-accredited programs*. Alexandria, VA: CACREP.

Department on Aging. (2007). *Statistics on the aging population*. Retrieved 21.7.2007 <http://www.aoa.gov/prof/Statistics/statistics.asp/> .

Erikson, E. H. (1963). *Childhood and society* (2nd ed). New York: Norton and Company.

Franklin, N. (2008, February 4). Patients, patients. *The New Yorker, LXXXIII*(46), 78–79.

Gatz, M., Fiske, A., Fox, L. S., Kaskie, B., Kasl-Godley, J. E., McCallum, T. J., & Wetherell, J. L. (1998). Empirically validated psychological treatments for older adults. *Journal of Mental Health and Aging, 4*, 9–46.

Gallagher, D. E., & Thompson, L. W. (1983). Treatment of major depressive disorder in older adult outpatients with brief psychotherapies. *Psychotherapy: Theory, research, and practice, 19*, 482–490.

Gatz, M., Fiske, A., Fox, L. S., Kaskie, B., Kasl-Godley, J. E., McCallum, T. J., & Wetherell, J. L. (1998). Empirically validated psychological treatments for older adults. *Journal of Mental Health and Aging, 4*, 9–46.

Himmelfarb, S., & Murrell, S. A. (1984). Prevalence and correlates of anxiety symptoms in older adults. *Journal of Psychology, 116*, 159–167.

Knight, R. G., & Satre, D. (1999). Cognitive behavioral psychotherapy with older adults. *Clinical Psychology: Science and Practice, 6*(3), 188–203.

Maercker, A. (2002). Life-review technique in the treatment of PTSD in elderly patients: Rationale and three single case studies. *Journal of Clinical Geropsychology, 8*, 239–249.

Morgan, A. C. (2003). Psychodynamic psychotherapy with older adults. *Psychiatric Services, 54*, 1592–1594.

Morin, C. M., Kowatch, R. A., Barry, T., & Walton, E. (1993). Cognitive-behavior therapy for late-life insomnia. *Journal of Consulting and Clinical Psychology, 61*, 137–146.

Morin, C. M., Colecchi, C., Stone, J., Sood, R., & Brink, D. (1999). Behavioral and pharmacological treatments for late-life insomnia: A randomized controlled trial. *Journal of the American Medical Association, 281*, 991–999.

Myers, J. E., & Schwiebert, V. L. (1996). *Competencies for gerontological counseling.* Alexandria, VA: American Counseling Association.

NIMH. (2006). *Maintenance treatment prevents recurrence in older adults with Single-Episode depressions.* <http://www.nih.gov/news/pr/mar2006/nimh-15a.htm/>.

Nordhus, I. H., & VandenBos, G. R. (Eds.), (1998). *Clinical Gero-Psychology.* Washington, DC: American Psychological Association.

Persky, T. (2008) Overlooked and underserved: Elders in Need of Mental Health Care. Mental Health and Aging: Getting information. Retrieved 5.2.2008 <http://www.mhaging.org/info/olus.html/>.

Pinquart, M., & Soerensen, S. (2001). How effective are psychotherapeutic and other psychosocial interventions with older adults? A meta analysis. *Journal of Mental Health and Aging, 7*, 207–243.

*Roth and Fonagy (2004). Evidence-based effective practices with older adults. *Journal of Counseling and Development*, Spring 2004. Vol. 82, 209, 317–329.

Sadavoy, J., Lazarus, L., & Jarvik, L. (Eds.), (1991). *Comprehensive review of geriatric psychiatry.* Washington, DC: American Psychiatric Press.

Scogin, F., & McElreath, L. (1994). Efficacy of psychosocial treatments for geriatric depression: A quantitative review. *Journal of Consulting and Clinical Psychology, 62*, 69–74.

Smyer, M. A., & Qualls, S. H. (1999). Aging and mental health. Malden, MA: Blackwell.

Stanley, M. A., Beck, J. G., & Glassco, J. D. (1996). Treatment of generalized anxiety in older adults: A preliminary comparison of cognitive-behavioral and supportive approaches. *Behavior Therapy, 27*, 565–581.

Teri, L., & McCurry, S. M. (1994). Psychosocial therapies with older adults. In C. E. Coffey & J. L. Cummings (Eds.), *Textbook of geriatric neuropsychiatry* (pp. 662–682). Washington, DC: American Psychiatric Press.

Thompson, L. W., Gallagher, D., & Breckenridge, J. S. (1987). Comparative effectiveness of psychotherapies for depressed elders. *Journal of Consulting and Clinical Psychology, 55*, 385–390.

Watkins, K. W., Shifrin, K., Park, D. C., & Morrell, R. W. (1999). Age, pain, and coping with rheumatoid arthritis. *Pain, 82*, 217–228.

Yalom, I. (1995). The theory and practice of group psychotherapy (4th ed). New York: Basic Books.

Chapter | two

Successful Aging

2.1 INTRODUCTION

A considerable amount of literature in the past few years suggests that successful aging is the absence of physical and emotional disabilities, but new research suggests that perceptions of older adults about the aging process are more important than the influence of illness and physical disability and depend on attitude, resilience, optimism and coping style. When those issues are taken into consideration, an older person can often control successful aging. This chapter on successful aging will explore the various studies suggesting a wide range of definitions of successful aging.

2.2 DEFINITIONS OF SUCCESSFUL AGING

There is no single definition of successful aging that satisfies everyone. Havighurst (1961) says that successfully aging individuals add life to their years and get considerable satisfaction from life. Ryff (1989) defines successful aging as positive or ideal functioning related to developmental work over the life course. Fisher (1992) interviewed 19 senior center participants ages 62–85 and found that they tended to define successful aging in terms of strategies for coping. Gibson (1995) stated that successful aging "refers to reaching one's potential and arriving at a level of physical, social, and psychological well-being in old age that is pleasing to both self and others" (p. 279). In the *Encyclopedia of Aging*, Palmore (1995) writes that a comprehensive definition of successful aging "would combine survival (longevity), health (lack of disability), and life satisfaction (happiness)" (p. 914). Additionally, some gerontologists have discussed similar issues using different terms such as "adjustment" or "adaptation" to aging.

Even in the midst of illness and disabilities, older adults who are aging successfully have a zest for life, are engaged in personal relationships, have concern for the welfare of others, maintain a positive and optimistic view of life, and believe that their later years are a time to leave a legacy for others that is grounded in affirmation. Successful aging does not ignore the physical changes that take place as we age, but it does believe that those who have chosen a positive and optimistic approach to life will bring that approach with them as they age and, as a result, will be able to maintain creative, involving, and interesting activities throughout the life span. Illness and disability for the successfully aging person occur at much later junctures in life and successfully aging individuals can anticipate a longer and more productive life span.

2.3 ACHIEVING SUCCESSFUL AGING

In their research on successful aging, Vaillant and Mukamal (2001) believe that we can identify the predictors of longer and healthier lives before the age of 50 by using the following indicators: parental social class, family cohesion, major depression, ancestral longevity, childhood temperament, and physical health at age 50. Seven variables indicating personal control over physical and emotional health that are also related to longer and healthier lives include the absence of alcohol abuse and smoking, and the presence of marital/relationship stability, exercise, a normal body mass index, positive coping mechanisms, and involvement in continuing education. The authors conclude that we have much greater control over our post-retirement health than had been previously recognized in the literature.

For the purposes of understanding what is meant behaviorally by successful aging, the authors identify the following indicators:

1. Although elderly people taking 3–8 medications a day were seen as chronically ill by their physicians, the cohort deemed to be aging successfully saw themselves as healthier than their peers.
2. Elderly adults who age successfully have the ability to plan ahead and are still intellectually curious and in touch with their creative abilities.
3. Successfully aging adults, even those over 95, see life as being meaningful and are able to use humor in their daily lives.
4. Aging successfully includes remaining physically active and continuing activities (walking, for example) that were used at an earlier age to remain healthy.

5. Older adults who age successfully are more serene and spiritual in their outlook on life than those who age less well.

6. Successful aging includes concern for continued friendships, positive interpersonal relationships, satisfaction with spouses, children and family life, and social responsibility in the form of volunteer work and civic involvement.

In a study of the relationship between the ability to cope with stress and physical and emotional well-being in women ages 65–87 years of age, Barnas and Valaik (1991) found that women with insecure attachments to their adult children had poorer coping skills and lower levels of psychological well-being than women with positive attachments. Women with a mean age of 20 and a sample of women with a mean age of 38 with attachment problems with their mothers, suffered more anxiety and depression and were seen by friends as being more anxious than women in both groups with positive attachments. These findings led the authors to conclude that insecure attachments produce poorer coping skills, which lead to more vulnerability to stress across the life cycle. The authors define attachment as relationships of affection that are formed throughout the years and are not necessarily limited to a child's bond with his or her parents.

Vaillant and Mukamal (2001) report that the two most important "psychosocial predictors of successful aging were high level of education (which probably reflects traits of self-care and planfulness as much as social class) and having an extended family network" (p. 243). In his research on aging, Valliant (2002) found the following variables contributed to successful aging:

1. seeking and maintaining relationships and understanding that relationships that help us to heal and grow require gratitude, forgiveness, and intimacy;

2. having interest and concern about others and being able to give of oneself;

3. a sense of humor and the ability to laugh and play well into later life;

4. making new friends as we lose older ones, which has a more positive impact on aging well than retirement income;

5. the desire to learn and to be open to new ideas and points of view;

6. understanding and accepting limitations and accepting the help of others;

7. understanding the past and its effect on our lives while living in the present;
8. focusing on the positives and the good people in our lives rather than on the negative things that may happen to us.

Robert and Li (2001) argue that despite the commonly held belief in the relationship between socioeconomic status and health, research actually suggests a limited relationship between the two variables. Rather, there seems to be a relationship between community levels of health and individual health. Lawton (1977) suggests that older adults may experience communities as their primary source of support, recreation, and stimulation, unlike younger adults who find it easier to move about in search of support and recreation. Lawton and Nahemow (1977) believe that positive community environments are particularly important to older adults who have emotional, physical, or cognitive problems. The need for healthy and vital communities is particularly relevant for older adults who have health problems that limit their mobility. A tragic example of the impact of unhealthy communities is the Chicago heat wave of 1995, where 739 older and less mobile people died. The reason for the very large death rate turned out to be that many elderly and less mobile people were afraid to leave their homes and to be exposed to environments they felt were dangerous and unsafe (Gladwell, 2002). In explaining why she was afraid to leave her home, even though she was literally dying of heat prostration, one elderly lady said, "Chicago is just a shooting gallery" (Gladwell, 2002, p. 80). Furthermore, Chicago had no emergency system for helping elderly and less mobile people. So many people died during the heat wave that,

> Callers to 911 were put on hold. ... The police took bodies to the Cook County Medical Examiner's office, and a line of cruisers stretched outside the building. The morgue ran out of bays in which to put the bodies. The owner of a local meatpacking firm offered the city his refrigerated trucks to help store the bodies. The first set wasn't enough. He sent a second set. It wasn't enough. (Gladwell, 2002, p. 76)

Rather than thinking in terms of a relationship between individual SES and health among an aging population, Robert and Li (2001) suggest three indicators of healthy communities that relate directly to individual health:

1. a positive physical environment that provides an absence of noise and traffic and has adequate lighting;

2. a positive social environment that includes an absence of crime, the ability to find safe environments to walk in, and easy access to shopping;
3. a rich service environment that includes simple and safe access to rapid and inexpensive transportation, the availability of senior centers, and easy access to meal sites.

In studying the impact of natural disasters on a population of elderly adults demonstrating pre-disaster signs of depression, Tyler and Hoyt (2000) noted that elderly adults reporting high levels of social support had lower levels of depression before and after a natural disaster. They also report that "older people with little or no social support, perhaps due to death of a spouse and/or loss of friends, may have a more difficult time dealing with life changes and, as a result, are particularly vulnerable to increases in depression" (p. 155).

But overall, Pearlin and Skaff (1996) note how remarkable it is that so many older adults cope so well with life stressors. Solomon (1996) reports that specific personality characteristics are highly related to successful coping in older adults. The characteristics most likely to show a positive relationship between successful coping and aging are "flexibility, adaptability, and a sense of humor as well as financial, social, and organizational skills" (p. 48). Solomon also indicates that the ability to find meaning in crisis situations instead of just being able to manage them is a critical aspect of coping. Butler et al. (1991) suggest that coping is enhanced in older adults as they are able to shift their priorities to accommodate change, while Solomon (1996) believes that a person's sense of mastery is closely related to his or her ability to cope with stressors related to aging. She identifies two personality factors that are particularly related to coping in older adults: "1) the ability to interpret success in controlling past hardships as evidence of competence to master current hardship and, 2) the ability to shift priorities from areas where a measure of control has been lost to areas where control may still be maintained" (p. 48).

Rowe and Kahn (1998) believe successful aging includes the following three components:

1. good health with a low risk of disease and disability: good health includes regular exercise, a healthy diet, and regular check-ups;
2. high mental and physical functioning, which suggests that in healthy aging, people are intellectually active and stimulated;
3. an active engagement with life, and a strong system of social supports.

The authors believe social supports are very important in maintaining successful aging and provide the following reasons: isolation is a powerful risk factor for poor health; social support – such as emotional, physical, and personal contact – has direct positive effects on health; social support can buffer or reduce some health-related effects of aging, and; social support helps protect one against the stresses of life. The authors believe that it's never too late to reverse bad health habits. They provide the following examples of good health practices in older adults:

1. Physical activity is the crux of successful aging. Physical activity includes aerobic activity such as walking, dancing, and gardening and more strenuous activity like weight training (or weight lifting).
2. Diet and exercise help reduce weight, the chances for heart disease and colon and rectal cancer, reduce the effects of diabetes, arthritis, and osteoporosis, and help to increase strength and balance, which help to reduces falls.
3. Fitness cuts our risk of dying. Older women who exercise are 20% less likely to die than those who were sedentary.
4. The risk of heart disease falls as soon as one stops smoking. After five years of cessation, an ex-smoker is not much more likely to have heart disease than a non-smoker.
5. Smoking cessation results in reduced chances of heart disease, increased lung capacity, and a decrease in blood pressure.
6. Active mental stimulation and keeping up with social relationships with friends and family also help to promote physical ability.
7. Older people can sustain, perhaps even increase, their mental functioning by reading, through word games and mental exercises, and by engaging in stimulating conversation (Rowe and Kahn, 1998).

2.4 OPTIMISM AS AN ASPECT OF SUCCESSFUL AGING

A person's positive view of life can have a significant impact on physical and emotional health. Longitudinal studies of the many aspects of physical and emotional health among a Catholic order of women in the Midwest (Danner et al., 2001) suggested that the personal statements written by very young women when entering the religious order correlated positively with life span. The more positive and affirming the personal statement written when the applicant was in her late teens and early twenties, the longer her life span, sometimes as long as 10 years beyond the mean length of life for the religious order as a whole, and up to 20 years or more longer than the general population. Many of the women in the sample lived well into their nineties, and beyond. In a sample of 650, six nuns were over 100 years of age. While some of the women in the sample suffered from serious physical problems, including dementia and Alzheimer's, the numbers were much smaller than in the general population and the age of onset was usually much later in life. The reasons for increased life span in this population seem to be related to good health practices (the order doesn't permit liquor or smoking, and foods are often fresh with a focus on vegetables), and an environment that focuses on spiritual issues and helping others. The order also has a strong emphasis on maintaining a close, supportive relationship among its members so that when illness does arise, there is a network of positive and supportive help.

In discussing research on successful aging, Jeste (2005, p. 1) notes, "The commonly used criteria suggest that a person is aging well if he has a low level of disease and disability. However, this study shows that self-perception about aging can be more important than the traditional success markers." To determine successful aging, Jeste and colleagues studied over 500 older Americans, age 60 to 98, who lived independently within the community (i.e., did not live in a nursing home or assisted care facility). Participants were asked to complete a questionnaire including medical, psychological, and demographic information. The sample was representative of national averages regarding incidences of medical conditions (e.g., heart disease, cancer, diabetes, etc.). Similarly, 20% to 25% of the respondents had been diagnosed with and/or received treatment for a mental health problem. Despite the prevalence of physical illness and disabilities in the group, when study participants were asked to rate their own degree of successful aging on a 10-point scale (with 10 being "most successful"), their average rating was 8.4.

Most of the respondents who gave themselves high ratings would not be able to meet the standard used for successful aging, which includes the absence of disease and freedom from disability. Less than 10% of the participants would have been considered to be aging successfully using the standards proposed by Rowe and Kahn (1998). Jeste notes that "[w]hat is most interesting about this study is that people who think they are aging well are not necessarily the most healthy individuals. In fact, optimism and effective coping styles were found to be more important to aging successfully than traditional measures of health and wellness. These findings suggest that physical health is not the best indicator of successful aging – attitude is" (p. 1).

Jeste (2005) also found that participants of the study who spent time each day on hobbies, such as reading and writing, or socializing with other members of the community, consistently gave themselves higher scores on the scale measuring successful aging. Participants who had a paid job outside of the home were also more likely to give themselves higher scores. Interestingly, volunteer activities were not found to exert the same influence on participants' self-reports. Factors that were not correlated with high self-report ratings included age, gender, education, marital status, and income. Jeste (2005) concludes that "[f]or most people, worries about their future aging involve fear of physical infirmity, disease or disability. However, this study is encouraging because it shows that the best predictors of successful aging are well within an individual's control" (p. 1).

2.5 RESILIENCE AS AN ASPECT OF SUCCESSFUL AGING

Walsh (2003) defines resilience as "the ability to withstand and rebound from disruptive life challenges. Resilience involves key processes over time that foster the ability to struggle well, surmount obstacles, and go on to live and love fully" (p. 1). Gordon (1996) defines resilience as "the ability to thrive, mature, and increase competence in the face of adverse circumstances" (p. 1). Glick (1994) writes, "resilience is the ability to bounce back from adversity and to overcome the negative influences that often block achievement. Resilience research focuses on the traits, coping skills and supports that help people survive, and even thrive, in a challenging environment" (p. 1). Henry (1999) defines resilience as "the capacity for successful adaptation, positive functioning, or competence despite high risk, chronic stress, or prolonged or severe trauma" (p. 521). In a further definition of resilience, Abrams (2001) indicates that resilience may be seen as the ability to readily recover from illness, depression, and adversity. Walsh (2003) says that "The concept of family resilience extends our understanding of healthy family functioning to situations of adversity. Although some families are shattered by crisis or chronic stresses, what is remarkable is that many others emerge strengthened and more resourceful" (p. 1). Anderson (1997) notes that resilient people have been described as being

> Socially, behaviorally, and academically competent despite living in adverse circumstances and environments as a result of poverty

(Werner and Smith, 1992), parental mental illness (Beardslee and Podorefsky, 1988), interparental conflict (Neighbors, Forehand, and McVicar, 1993), inner-city living (Luthar, 1993), and child abuse and neglect (Farber and Egeland, 1987). (p. 594)

Mandleco and Peery (2000) are concerned with the inconsistent meaning of the term resilience and wonder if it has begun to mean whatever the author wishes it to. The authors point out that resilience has been described as a personality characteristic not related to stress; a characteristic of some people from at-risk environments; the absence of psychopathology when parents have serious emotional problems; success in meeting societal expectations or developmental tasks; characteristics which help people succeed, contrary to predictions; and the ability to restore equilibrium and adapt to life situations. The authors note that Polk (1997) tried to synthesize a model of resilience, suggesting that "resilience is a midrange theory with a four-dimensional construct, where dispositional, relational, situational, and philosophical patterns intermingle with the environment to form resilience" (Mandleco and Peery, 2000, p. 100). The result of these various definitions of resilience is that while a "commonsense universal definition is assumed, when one attempts to identify specifics affecting resilience, these definitions are inadequate and confusing" (Mandleco and Peery, 2000, p. 100).

2.6 ATTRIBUTES OF RESILIENT PEOPLE

A consistent finding over the last 20 years of resilience research is that most people from highly dysfunctional families or very poor communities do well as adults. This finding applies to almost all populations found to be at risk for later life problems, including those children whose parents divorce, children who live with step-parents, children who have lost a sibling, children who have attention deficit disorder or suffer from developmental delays, and children who become delinquent or run away. More of these children make it than don't. A review of the research literature found that 70–75% of children at risk do well as younger and older adults, including children born to teenaged mothers (Furstenberg, 1998), children who were sexually abused (Wilkes, 2002), children who grew up in substance-abusing or mentally ill families (Werner and Smith, 2001), and children who grew up in poverty (Vaillant, 2002). Even when children have experienced multiple risks, Rutter (2000) found that half of them overcame adversity and achieved good emotional and social development as adults.

Masten (2001) believes that resilience is part of the genetic makeup of humans and that it is the norm rather than the exception. "What began as a quest to understand the extraordinary has revealed the power of the ordinary. Resilience does not come from rare and special qualities, but from the everyday magic of ordinary, normative human resources in the minds, brains, and bodies of children, in their families and relationships, and in their communities" (Masten, 2001, p. 9).

We tend to think that traumas will generally lead to malfunctioning behavior in children and adults, but often this isn't the case. A good example of how well people actually cope with trauma may be seen in the response to the World Trade Center bombings. Gist and Devilly (2002) report that the estimates of PTSD after the 9-11 bombing dropped by almost two-thirds within four months of the tragedy and concluded that, "[t]hese findings underscore the counterproductive nature of offering a [treatment] with no demonstrable effect, but demonstrated potential to complicate natural resolution, in a population in which limited case-conversion can be anticipated, strong natural supports exist, and spontaneous resolution is prevalent" (p. 742). In other words, resilience to severe trauma exists when we accept the possibility that people will heal on their own and when strong social and emotional supports are present. Introducing treatment too early in the process may actually interfere with resilience.

Werner and Smith (1982, 1992) identified protective factors that tend to counteract the risk of stress. They categorized protective factors as genetic (e.g., an easygoing disposition), strong self-esteem and a sense of identity, intelligence, physical attractiveness, and supportive caregivers. Garmezy et al. (1964) note three protective factors in resilient people: dispositional attributes of the child, family cohesion and warmth, and the availability and use of external support systems when needed. Seligman (1992) says that resilience exists when people are optimistic, have a sense of adventure, courage, and self-understanding, use humor in their lives, have a capacity for hard work, and posses the ability to cope with and find outlets for emotions. Luthar and Zigler (1991) found that resilient people are active, humorous, confident, competent, prepared to take risks, flexible, and, as a result of repeated successful coping experiences, confident in both their inner and outer resources. Luthar (1993) suggests that resilient people have high levels of emotional intelligence.

Other factors associated with resilience include the finding by Arend et al. (1979) that very curious people are more resilient than those who are less curious. Radke-Yarrow and Brown (1993) associate resilience with those who have more positive self-perceptions. Egeland et al. (1993) and Baldwin et al. (1993) found a relationship between resilience and assertiveness, independence, and a support network of neighbors, peers, family, and elders. In their 32-year longitudinal study, Werner and Smith (1982) found a strong relationship between problem-solving abilities, communication skills, and an internal locus of control in resilient people. As Henry (1999) notes, "resilient people believe their lives have meaning and that they control their own fate" (p. 522).

Resiliency research originally tried to discover the characteristics of at-risk children who coped well with stress (Werner, 1989). Over time, however, resiliency research has focused less on the attributes of resilient children and more on the processes of resilience. As the research has attempted to understand the processes associated with resilience, one important finding suggests that rather than avoiding risks, resilient people take substantial risks to cope with stressors leading to what Cohler (1987) calls adaptation and competence.

In a review of the factors associated with resilience to stressful life events throughout the life span, Tiet et al. (1998) found that: (a) higher IQ; (b) quality of parenting; (c) connection to other competent adults; (d) an internal locus of control; and (e) excellent social skills have been identified as protective factors that allow people to cope with stressful events. Protective factors, according to Tiet et al. (1998), are primary buffers between the traumatic event and the person's response. When a person's response to stress has a positive effect on the person experiencing stress, whether the risk is low or high, the author's term this a resource factor. The authors believe that both protective and resource factors are crucial in understanding the way resilience protects people.

But resilience should not suggest that people are always resilient in every situation or that there are not problems related to stress, trauma and other forms of social and emotional difficulties. Tiet et al. (1998) indicate that even resilient children respond inconsistently to stressful events and that another way to look at resilience is to show the relationship between the specific traumatic event and the response. For example, in many of the maltreated children studied for resilience, school-based outcomes have been used that include grades, deportment, and the degree of involvement in school activities. Luthar and Zigler (1991) note that while resilient children do well in many school-based outcomes, many of these children suffer from depression. Interestingly, however, even though many of the maltreated children studied show signs of depression, they still did well on behavioral outcome measures such as grades and school conduct (Luthar and Zigler, 1991). Tiet et al. (1998) believe that the key reason resilient children cope well with adversity is that they:

> [T]end to live in higher-functioning families and receive more guidance and supervision by their parents and other adults in the family. Other adults in the family may complement the parents in providing guidance and support to the youth and in enhancing youth adjustment. Higher educational aspiration may also provide high-risk youth with a sense of direction and hope. (p. 1198)

This leads one to believe that resilience doesn't negate vulnerability to all outside stressors, but that it does provide primary coping mechanisms that permit high levels of functioning even in the midst of emotional side effects, including depression.

In conversations with older adult survivors of the Holocaust, Tech (2003) found characteristics of those who survived to include a desire for mutual cooperation to cope with survival. This included caring for ill concentration camp inmates, sharing rations that were minute to begin with, and forming "bonding groups" that kept inmates optimistic and positive. Tech also points out that inmates who were emotionally flexible were more likely to survive. Inmates who were very traditional in their outlook on life or who felt that they had lost a considerable amount of status were often unable to cope and frequently perished before other less healthy inmates died. However, many terribly unhealthy inmates who had a positive view of their lives survived against all medical odds. Tech reports that the older adult survivors she interviewed were filled with compassion and sadness, and that "conspicuously absent were expressions of hatred or hostility" (p. 345) toward their captors. Even though conditions in the camps were dreadful, "many inmates created for themselves make-believe worlds – a blend of dreams, fantasies, friendships and resistance – as an antidote" (p. 351). Prisoners found these fantasies very gratifying and "such escapes into fantasy may have improved the prisoners hold on life – prisoners created bonding groups which, however illusory, forged links with the past and the future" (p. 351).

There are many similarities between the recollections of the survivors Tech interviewed and more scientific studies of survivors of the Holocaust. Baron et al. (1996) report that many clinicians who first interviewed survivors of the Holocaust believed that they would be very troubled parents and that their children would suffer from a range of emotional difficulties. Children of survivors, however, have shown no pattern of maladjustment or psychopathology in most research studies other than the normal problems one might expect in any population of children. Children who have maintained the traditional religious beliefs of their parents have done particularly well socially, financially, and emotionally (Last, 1989).

In studies of the development of symptoms of PTSD following a traumatic event, Ozer et al. (2003) report that those most likely to develop PTSD have a lack of psychological resilience which can be seen as a cluster of prior social and emotional problems that include prior loss, depression, poor support from others, prior traumas, and a family history of pathology. The authors write, "It is tempting to make an analogy to the flu or infectious disease: Those whose immune systems are compromised are at greater risk of contracting a subsequent illness. Similarly, this cluster of variables may all be pointing to a single source of vulnerability for the development of PTSD or enduring symptoms of PTSD – a lack of psychological resilience" (p. 71). What the authors fail to answer is why some people who have had all of the earlier signs of coping poorly with a new trauma, in fact cope surprisingly well. Many resilient older adults have had prior traumas and loss, an absence of family support and episodes of depression, but still cope well enough with new traumas to avoid serous social and emotional malfunction.

One of the continuing beliefs in the helping professions is that the greater the social and emotional risk to an individual, the more likely we are to see pathology. But resilience research suggests that risk factors are predictive of some types of dysfunction for only about 20–49% of a given high-risk population, suggesting high levels of resilience in the majority of those at risk (Rutter, 2000; Werner, 2001). In contrast, "protective factors," the supports and opportunities that buffer the effect of adversity and enable development to proceed, appear to predict positive outcomes in anywhere from 50 to 80% of a high-risk population.

In summarizing our understanding of resilience, Mandleco and Peery (2000) argue that we still don't know which attribute of resilience is most significant for a particular person. "In addition, there is often marked variation in an individual's responses to stress, suggesting that the presence of any specific factor does not always produce *resilience* if the person is particularly vulnerable or the adversity too great to overcome" (Mandleco and Peery, 2000, p. 101). The authors continue by noting the confusion over the factors affecting resilience. While some researchers have taken a theoretical perspective, others have summarized the research literature. There is, however, confusion over the following factors: "(a) the age domain covered by the construct, (b) the circumstances where it occurs, (c) its definition, (d) its boundaries, or (e) the adaptive behaviors described" (Mandleco and Peery, 2000, p. 102).

We should be aware of a particular problem with resilience research: it isn't all inclusive of a broad population of people. Some studies consider certain age groups, most notably childhood and adolescence, and from those age groups project resilience to older populations. Another type of research considers specific problems such as mental illness or alcoholism and generalizes these findings to broader populations. This leads Mandleco and Peery to believe that the definition of resilience is still vague and continues to affect research results.

2.7 COPING WITH STRESS IMPROVES SUCCESSFUL AGING

Courbasson et al. (2002) define coping as "one's efforts to reduce the impact of a difficult or stressful situation. This transactional process involves both cognition and behavior" (p. 35). The authors indicate that there are three primary styles of coping with stress: task-oriented, emotion-oriented, and avoidance-oriented coping (Endler and Parker, 1999). Task-oriented coping attempts to solve or limit the impact of the stressful situation. Emotion-oriented coping tries to limit the emotional impact of stress rather than resolve the stressful situation. Avoidance-oriented coping uses distraction and diversion unrelated to the stressful situation to reduce stress. The authors found that research in coping with stress suggests that a task-oriented approach benefits people under great stress more than the use of other coping strategies. "That is, task-oriented coping is associated with problem resolution or amelioration more often than the use of other coping strategies. Alternatively, both emotion and avoidance-oriented coping strategies may exacerbate the problematic situation" (Courbasson et al., 2002, p. 37).

Miller and Smith (2005) suggested that there are different types of stress, each with its own attributes, symptoms, duration and treatment.

1. Acute stress is the common type of stress we all feel when something goes badly or makes life temporarily more complicated. This is time-limited stress and goes away when the situation rectifies itself.
2. Episodic stress is frequently experienced by some people because they often place themselves in stressful situations by being late or

by being in one crisis or another. These people are crisis prone and appear to lack the ability to order problems in logical ways or to deal with them in pragmatic and rational ways, allowing the crisis to be constant.

3. Chronic stress "is the grinding stress that wears people away day after day, year after year. Chronic stress destroys bodies, minds and lives. It wreaks havoc through long-term attrition. It's the stress of poverty, of dysfunctional families, of being trapped in an unhappy marriage or in a despised job or career" (Miller and Smith, 2005, p. 1). The authors go on to say, "Chronic stress kills through suicide, violence, heart attack, stroke, and, perhaps, even cancer. People wear down to a final, fatal breakdown" (p. 1).

Coping with stress has been thought to be a dimension of resilience, although there is disagreement in the literature about the definition of coping. Some researchers see coping as a dynamic process but measure its existence by considering a person's disposition or by viewing it as something triggered by a life situation (Parkes, 1984). In this definition of coping, it is a fluctuating or transitory state. Other researchers see the ability to cope with stress as a permanent and enduring personality trait (Carver et al., 1989; McCrae, 1984; Parkes, 1986), a definition that sounds much like the definition of resilience. Still other researchers view coping as a set of positive and negative modes of behavior. People with positive coping skills are described as using "more mature, flexible, purposive, future-oriented, reality-based, and metered approaches to combating stressful and anxiety-provoking situations, whereas those with negative coping skills are viewed as rigid, past-propelled, reality-distorting, and generally real adaptive processes" (Livneh et al., 1996, p. 503).

Lazarus (1966) believes that coping: (a) serves to reduce the impact of harmful events and to maintain positive self-concept; (b) includes situational factors such as the availability of resources coupled with individual factors including one's belief system and other physical and emotional skills; (c) includes an appraisal of a situation and how that situation may affect one's well-being, including the options and limitations of alternative approaches to the situation; and (d) that coping includes very basic options such as seeking more information, asking others how they might resolve a stressful situation, and direct action.

Billings and Moos (1981; 1984) and Barnas and Valaik (1991) believe that there are three alternative strategies individuals use to cope with stressful situations: (a) they may attempt to control the negative effect of the situation; (b) they may try to modify the seriousness and the meaning of the stressful event; or, (c) they may respond directly by trying to change the stressful event through the use of strategies that may have worked in the past.

Livneh et al. (1996) found three active styles of coping for older adults that resemble notions of resilience: (a) a style of coping that utilizes planning and seeking help from others; (b) a style of coping that seeks a support group to help with the stressor rather than passively putting it in the hands of fate; and, (c) a style of coping that utilizes direct techniques to deal with the stressor rather than such indirect techniques as denial or using other activities to temporarily try and forget about the stressor. The authors found that placing a problem in the hands of God or using prayer almost exclusively as a way of resolving a stressful situation was not a particularly effective way of coping and suggested an external locus of control. The more active the coping approach, the better subjects in their study were able to cope.

In determining whether treatment with substance abusing patients would improve the type of coping approach used, Courbasson et al. (2002) treated 71 substance abusing clients in an outpatient setting, three full days a week using anger management, relaxation, stress management, nutrition, leisure activities, assertiveness training, loss, drug education, goal setting, relationships and intimacy, and group psychotherapy (a client-centered orientation). The authors found that therapy had the following impact:

1. Following treatment, task-oriented coping increased significantly and with it, a large decrease in anxiety and other stress-related symptoms.
2. The use of emotion-oriented coping also decreased.
3. The use of avoidance-oriented coping didn't change with treatment.
4. Although the purpose of the treatment was to stop the substance abuse, better coping skills (those that tried to resolve stressful situations) resulted in sustained improvement in psychological distress.

Solomon believes that older people experience fewer life stressors than they experienced in earlier years. When older adults do experience difficulty in coping with stress, she writes, "Life changes per se do not create stress; rather, adverse effects result from events that are considered unexpected or for which people are unprepared. The individual's perception of this experience has much to do with whether or how much stress accompanies the life events" (p. 46). Solomon (1996) suggests that an older person's sense of mastery and competence influences the way he or she manages stress. According to Solomon, when older people maintain high levels of mastery in the face of difficult life circumstances, two personality factors emerge as key: (1) the ability to interpret success in controlling past hardships as evidence of competence to master current hardship and, (2) the ability to shift priorities from areas where a measure of control has been lost to areas where control may still be maintained (p. 48).

2.8 PERSONAL STORY: AN EXAMPLE OF SUCCESSFUL AGING: LIFE IN THE SLOW LANE

"My philosophy about life, now that I'm 73, has changed, and it continues to change as I age and all the ills of growing older become more apparent each day. I'm easier on myself now that I've accepted the fact that I can no longer function as I did five years ago. I know that what I felt was important at the age of 30, isn't. Wearing the right clothes with the right labels, flashing the diamond rings, living in area of town that is considered "right" and all those other restrictions we put on ourselves early in life, don't count for anything anymore. Family, friends, social activities, keeping one's mind active, volunteering, promoting a favorite charity, being grateful for every day you can keep functioning; that's what's important.

"I'm in reasonably good health, with cancer and a bilateral knee replacement behind me and a few chronic conditions I cope with on a daily basis. I feel better when the sun shines and I do everything reasonably possible to get up each morning and focus on what I want to accomplish that day.

"I still work part-time from home, and find the contact with the outside world through working very invigorating. Solving crossword puzzles, reading the newspaper every day, devouring the latest mystery books are all a source of enjoyment. I love music and sing in an all-women's group plus my church choir and fill the rest of my free hours with exercise, taking classes and keeping up with the world.

"When I look at the negatives of aging – diminished physical strength, chronic illnesses, decreasing income, and the probability of living alone, I realize, as the old saying goes, getting old isn't for the weak. My pet peeve in the matter is that people tend to not "see" older people, and often dismiss us as unimportant and not to be taken seriously, as our opinions don't count and have nothing to do with the reality of the present day world. AARP reports that older employees are now being recruited for the labor market and perhaps the time is approaching when we're appreciated for our past business history and what we know about the world and good work ethics.

"When I was younger and thought about retirement and what I would do with all my free time, I didn't realize, as I do now, that too much free time tends to diminish the years one has left. Life shouldn't be boring at any age. Keeping as active as one can, being involved in the community, treasuring your family and friends and constantly reminding oneself that age is only a number is my way of coping with the growing number of candles on my birthday cake." – G.S.

2.9 SUMMARY

This chapter discusses the notion of successful aging and the psychosocial factors that contribute to successful aging. Impacting successful aging are indications of resilience and the ability to cope well with life stressors. Considerable research suggests that more people are resilient in the midst of crises and at-risk life conditions than had previously been thought. The chapter ends with a personal story about successful aging.

2.10 QUESTIONS FROM THE CHAPTER

1. Don't you think the notion of successful aging is a bit presumptuous? Shouldn't we be able to define for ourselves whether we're aging well or not?
2. The idea that healthy communities extend life span more than income and social class seems patently incorrect. Doesn't money buy great health care, healthy food and healthy environments?
3. Aren't there a number of people whose health and emotional lives are a mess at 50 as they go through mid-life crises but they make changes as they age? Isn't it wrong then to say that your health in older age is necessarily influenced by the bad health practices you had at 50?
4. Resilience is one of those nebulous terms that probably applies to all of us at some time or other. Aren't we all resilient in our own ways?
5. Coping with stress isn't an internal dynamic of healthy people, it's a condition affected by social and economic factors. The greater the external factors (poverty, lack of work), the more likely you are to cope badly with stress. Don't you agree?

REFERENCES

Abrams, M. S. (2001). Resilience in ambiguous loss. *American Journal of Psychotherapy, 2*, 283–291.

Anderson, K. M. (1997). Uncovering survival abilities in children who have been sexually abused: Families in Society. *The Journal of Contemporary Human Services, 78*(6), 592–599.

Arend, R., Gove, F., & Sroufe, L. (1979). Continuity of individual adaptation from infancy to kindergarten: A predictive study of ego-resiliency and curiosity in preschoolers. *Child Development, 50*, 950–959.

Baldwin, A., Baldwin, C., Kasser, T., Zax, M., Sameroff, A., & Seifer, R. (1993). Contextual risk and resiliency during adolescence. *Development and Psychopathology, 5*, 741–761.

Barnas, M., & Valaik, P. L. (1991). Life-span attachment: Relations between attachment and socioemotional functioning in adult women. *Genetic, Social and General Psychology Monographs, 117*(2), 177–200.

Baron, L., Eisman, H., Scuello, M., Veyzer, A., & Lieberman, M. (1996). Stress resilience, locus of control, and religion in children of Holocaust victims. *Journal of Psychology, 130*(5), 513–525.

Beardslee, W. R., & Podorefsky, D. (1988). Resilient adolescents whose parents have serious affective and other psychiatric disorders: Importance of self understanding and relationships. *American Journal of Psychiatry, 145*, 63–69.

Billings, A. G., & Moos, R. H. (1981). The role of coping responses and social resources in attenuating the stress of life events. *Journal of Behavioral Medicine, 4*, 139–157.

Billings, A. G., & Moos, R. H. (1984). Coping, stress and social resources among adults with unipoloar depression. *Journal of Personality and Social Psychology, 46*, 877–891.

Butler, R., Lewis, M., & Sunderland. (1991). *Aging and Mental Health: Positive Psychological and Bio-medical Approaches* (4th ed.). New York: Macmillan.

Carver, C. S., Scheirer, M. F., & Weintraub, J. K. (1989). Assessing coping strategies: A theoretically based approach. *Journal of Personality and Social Psychology, 56*, 267–283.

Cohler, B. (1987). Adversity, resilience, and the study of lives. In E. J. Anthony & B. J. Cohler (Eds.), *The Invulnerable Child* (pp. 363–424). New York: Guilford.

Courbasson, C., Endler, M. A., Kocovski, N. S., & Kocovski, N. L. (2002). Coping and psychological distress for men with substance use disorders. *Current Psychology, 21*(1), 35–50.

Danner, D. D., Snowdon, D. A., & Friesen, W. V. (2001). Positive emotions in early life and longevity: Findings from the nun study. *Journal of Personality and Social Psychology, 80*(5), 804–813.

Egeland, E., Carlson, E., & Sroufe, L. (1993). Resilience as process. *Development and Psychopathology, 5*, 517–528.

Endler, N. S., & Parker, J. D. A. (1999). *Coping Inventory of Stressful Situations (CISS): Manual* (rev. ed.). Toronto: Multi-Health Systems.

Farber, E., & Egeland, B. (1987). Invulnerability among abused and neglected children. In E. J. Anthony & B. J. Cohler (Eds.), *The Invulnerable Child* (pp. 289–314). New York: Guilford.

Fisher, B. J. (1992). Successful aging and life satisfaction: A pilot study for conceptual clarification. *Journal of Aging Studies, 6*(2), 191–202.

Furstenberg, F. F. (1998). Paternal involvement with adolescence in intact families: The influence of fathers over the life course. *Demography, 35*(2), 201–216.

Garmezy, N., Masten, A., & Tellegen, A. (1964). The study of stress and competence in children: A building block for developmental psychopathology. *Child Development, 55*, 97–111.

Gibson, R. C. (1995). Promoting successful and productive aging in minority populations. In L. A. Bond, S. J. Cutler, & A. Grams (Eds.), *Promoting successful and productive aging* (pp. 279–288). Thousand Oaks, CA: Sage.

Gist, R., & Devilly, G. J. (2002). Post-trauma debriefing: The road too frequently traveled. *Lancet, 360*(9335), 741–743.

Gladwell, M. (2002, August 12). Political heat. *The New Yorker, 1*, 76–80.

Glick, H.A. (1994). *Resilience research: How can it help city schools? NCRAL Available from: <http://www.ncrel.org/sdrs/cityschl/city1_1b.html>* Accessed 1.08.2004.

Gordon, K.A. (1996). *Infant and toddler resilience: Knowledge, predictions, policy, and practice.* (3rd ed.), *Paper presented at the head start national research conference.* Washington, DC. 20–23.06.1996.

Havighurst, R. J. (1961). Successful aging. *The Gerontologist, 1*(1), 8–13.

Henry, D. L. (1999). Resilience in maltreated children: Implications for special needs adoptions. *Child Welfare, 78*(5), 519–540.

Jeste, D. (2005). Successful aging is simply 'Mind over Matter.' American College of Neuropsychopharmacology (ACNP) Annual Program Meeting. 11–15.12.2005. Waikoloa, Hawaii. Available from: <http://www.seniorjournal.com/NEWS/Aging/5-12-12-AgingMindOverMatter.htm/> . Accessed 23.12.2006.

Last, U. (1989). The transgenerational impact of hollocaust trauma: Current state of evidence. *International Journal of Mental Health, 17*(4), 72–89.

Lawton, M. P. (1977). The impact of the environment on aging and behavior. In J. E. Birren & K. W. Schaie(Eds.), *Handbook of the Psychology of Aging* (pp. 276–301). New York: Van Nostrand Reinhold.

Lawton, M. P., & Nahemow, L. (1973). Ecology and the aging process. In C. Eisdorfer & M. P. Lawton (Eds.), *The Psychology of Adult Development and Aging* (pp. 619–674). Washington, DC: American Psychological Association.

Lazarus, R. S. (1966). *Psychological Stress and the Coping Process.* New York : McGraw-Hill.

Liveneh, H., Livneh, C. L., Maron, S., & Kaplan, J. (1996). A multidimensional approach to the study of the structure of coping with stress. *Journal of Psychology, 130*(5), 501–513.

Luthar, S. (1993). Annotation: Methodology and conceptual issues in research on childhood resilience. *Journal of Child Psychology and Psychiatry, 34*, 441–453.

Luthar, S., & Zigler, E. (1991). Vulnerability and competence: A review of research on resilience in childhood. *American Journal of Orthopsychiatry, 6*, 6–22.

Mandleco, B. L., & Peery, J. C. (2000). An organizational framework for conceptualizing resilience in children. *Journal of Child and Adolescent Psychiatric Nursing, 13*(3), 99–112.

Masten, A. S. (2001). Ordinary Magic: Resilience processes in development. *American Psychologist, 56*, 227–238.

McCrae, R. R. (1984). Situational determinants of coping responses: Loss, threat and challenge. *Journal of Personality and Social Psychology, 46*, 919–928.

Miller, L.H., & Smith, A.D. (2005). *The different kinds of stress.* American Psychological Association Help Line. Available from: <http://www.apahelpcenter.org/articles/article.php?id = 21/>. Accessed 13.05.2005.

Neighbors, B., Forehand, R., & McVicar, D. (1993). Resilient adolescents and interparental conflict. *American Journal of Orthopsychiatry, 63*, 462–471.

Ozer, E. J., Best, S. R., Lipsey, T. L., & Weiss, D. S. (2003). Predictors of posttraumatic stress disorder and symptoms in adults: A meta-analysis. *Psychological Bulletin, 129*(1), 52–73.

Palmore, E. B. (1995). Successful aging. In G. L. Maddox (Ed.), *Encyclopedia of Aging: A Comprehensive Resource in Gerontology and Geriatrics* (pp. 914–915) (2nd ed.). New York: Springer.

Parkes, K. R. (1984). Locus of control, cognitive appraisal, and coping in stressful episodes. *Journal of Personality and Social Psychology, 46*(3), 655–668.

Parkes, K. R. (1986). Coping with stressful episodes: The role of individual differences, enviromneta; factors, and situational characteristics. *Journal of Personality and Social Psychology, 51*, 1277–1292.

Pearlin, L. I., & Skaff, M. (1996). Stress and the life course: A paradigmatic alliance. *Gerontiologist, 36*(2), 239–248.

Polk, L. V. (1997). Toward a middle range theory of resilience. *Advances in Nursing Science, 1*(3), 1–13.

Radke-Yarrow, M., & Brown, E. (1993). Resilience and vulnerability in children of multiple-risk families. *Development and Psychopathology, 5*, 581–592.

Robert, S. A., & Li, L. W. (2001). Age variation in the relationship between community socioeconomic status and adult health. *Research on Aging, 23*(2), 233–258.

Rowe, J. W., & Kahn, R. L. (1987). Human aging: Usual and successful. *Science, 237*, 143–149.

Rowe, J. W., & Kahn, R. L. (1998). *Successful Aging: The MacArthur Foundation Study*. New York: Random House.

Rutter, M. (1990). Psychosocial resilience and protective mechanisms. In J. Roll, A. S. Masten, D. Ciccetti, K. Nuechterlein, & S. Weintraub (Eds.), *Risk and Protective Factors in the Development of Psychpathology* (pp. 181–215). New York: Cambridge University Press.

Rutter, M. (2003). Genetic influences on risk and protection: Implications for understanding resilience. In S. S. Luthar (Ed.), *Resilience and Vulnerability* (pp. 489–509). Cambridge, UK: Cambridge University Press.

Ryff, C. D. (1989). Successful aging: A developmental approach. *The Gerontologist, 22*(2), 209–214.

Seligman, M. (1992). *Learned Optimism: How to Change your Mind and your Life.* New York: Pocket Books.

Solomon, R. (1996). Coping with stress: A physician's guide to mental health in aging. *Geriatrics, 15*(7), 46–51.

Stone, & Neale (1984)

Tech, N. (2003). *Resilience and Courage: Women, Men, and the Holocaust.* New Haven, CT: Yale University Press.

Tiet, Q. Q., Bird, H., & Davies, M. R. (1998). Adverse life events and resilience. *Journal of the American Academy of Child and Adolescent Psychiatry, 37*(11), 1191–1200.

Tyler, K. A., & Hoyt, D. R. (2000). The effects of an acute stressor on depressive symptoms among older adults. *Research on Aging, 22*(2), 143–164.

Vaillant, G. E. (2002). *Aging Well.* New York: Little, Brown and Company.

Vaillant, G. E., & Mukamal, K. (2001). Successful aging. *American Journal of Psychiatry, 158*(6), 839–847.

Walsh, F. (2003). Family resilience: A framework for clinical practice – Theory and Practice. *Family Processes, 42,* 1–18.

Werner, E. (1989). High-risk children in young adulthood: A longitudinal study from birth to 32 years. *American Orthopsychiatric Association, 59,* 71–72.

Werner, E. (1996). Vulnerable but not invincible: High risk children from birth to adulthood. *European Journal of Child and Adolescent Psychiatry, 5*(Suppl. 1), 47–51.

Werner, E., & Smith, R. (1982). *Vulnerable but Invincible.* New York: Adams, Bannister and Cox.

Werner, E., & Smith, R. S. (1992). *Overcoming the Odds: High-Risk Children from Birth to Adulthood.* Ithaca, NY: Cornell University Press.

Werner, E., & Smith, R. S. (2001). *Journey from Childhood to Midlife: Risk, Resilience and Recovery.* Ithaca, NY: Cornell University Press.

Wilkes, G. (2002). Abused children to nonabused parent: Resilience and conceptual change. Journal of Clinical Psychology, 58(3), 229–232.

Part two

Understanding Evidence-Based Practice

An Explanation of Evidence-Based Practice and its Application to Clinical Work with Older Adults

3.1 INTRODUCTION

Please note that some of the material in this chapter comes in modified form from Glicken (2005, pp. 3–18). The author thanks Sage Publications for permission to reprint that material.

This book on evidence-based practice (EBP) is about the use of research and critical thinking in assisting practitioners to determine the most beneficial ways of helping older adult clients with intrusive social and emotional problems. This chapter explains EBP and offers both positive and negative evaluations of the approach from the practice and research literature.

3.2 THE CURRENT STATE OF CLINICAL PRACTICE

The current practice of psychotherapy, counseling, and much of our work as human service professionals often relies on clinical wisdom with little evidence that what we do actually works. Clinical wisdom is often a justification for beliefs and values that bond us together as professionals but often fails to serve clients since many of those beliefs and values may be comforting, but they may also be inherently incorrect. O'Donnell (1997) likens this process to making the same mistakes, with growing confidence, over a long number of years. Issacs (1999) calls practice wisdom vehemence-based practice, where one substitutes volumes of clinical experience for evidence which is "an effective technique for brow beating your more timorous colleagues and for convincing relatives of your ability" (p. 1).

Flaherty (2001) believes that there is a "murky mythology" behind certain treatment approaches that causes them to persist and that "Unfounded beliefs of uncertain provenance may be passed down as a kind of clinical lore from professors to students. Clinical shibboleths can remain unexamined for decades because they stem from respected authorities, such as time-honored textbooks, renowned experts, or well-publicized but flawed studies in major journals" (p. 1). Flaherty goes on to note that even when sound countervailing information becomes available, clinicians still hold on to myths. And more onerous, Flaherty points out that we may perpetuate myths "by indulging the mistaken beliefs of patients or by making stereotypical assumptions about patients based on age, ethnicity, or gender" (p. 1), concerns in the mental health field that still plague us.

In a review of the effectiveness of psychotherapy over a 40-year period, Bergin (1971) calls for an evidence-based practice approach when he writes, "It now seems apparent that psychotherapy has had an average effect that is modestly positive. It is clear, however, that the averaged group data on which this conclusion is based obscure the existence of a multiplicity of processes occurring in therapy, some of which are now known to be unproductive or actually harmful" (p. 263).

In a more recent evaluation of the effectiveness of psychotherapy, Kopta et al. (1999) report that "The traditional view that the different psychotherapies – similar to medication treatments – contain unique active ingredients resulting in specific effects, has not been validated [and that] the aforementioned situations are evidence of a profession in turmoil" (p. 22). Kopta and colleagues go on to say that new research designs might help provide needed answers about the efficacy of one form of therapy over another with specific group of clients; however, "The field is currently experiencing apparent turmoil in three areas: (a) theory development for psychotherapeutic effectiveness, (b) research designs, and (c) treatment techniques" (Kopta et al., 1999, p. 1). Kopta and colleagues go on to note that "Researchers have repeatedly failed to find convincing evidence that different psychotherapies are differentially effective" (p. 3) and when differences are taken into consideration, the differences noted often have to do with "researcher allegiance [which is] influenced by the superiority of some treatment classes over others for depressed patients" (p. 3).

Frequently, the clinical wisdom view of practice has been based on what the American Medical Association Evidence-Based Practice Working Group (1992) refers to as unsystematic observations from clinical experience, a belief in common sense, a feeling that clinical training and experience are a way of maintaining a certain level of effective practice and an assumption that there are wise and more experienced clinicians who we can go to when we need help with clients. All of these assumptions are grounded in a paradigm that tends to be subjective and is often clinician focused rather than client focused. Aware of the subjective nature of social work practice, Rosen (1994) calls on the social work profession to use a more systematic way of providing practice and writes, "Numerous studies indicate that guidelines [for clinical practice] can increase empirically based practice and improve clients' outcomes" (found in Howard and Jensen, 1999, p. 283). The authors continue by suggesting that guidelines for social work practice would also produce better clinical training, cooperative client decision making and cost-effective practice; improve clinical training in schools of social work; and compile knowledge about difficult-to-treat conditions, "[because] few of the practice decisions social workers make are empirically rationalized" (Found in Howard and Jensen, 1999, p. 283).

Clinicians often make an argument that what we do in practice is intuitive, subjective, artful, and is based on our long years of experience. Psychotherapy, as this argument goes, is something one learns with practice. The responses made to clients and the approaches used during treatment may be so spontaneous and inherently empathic that research paradigms and knowledge-guided practice are not useful in the moment when a response is required. This argument is, of course, a sound one. The moment-to-moment work of the clinical practitioner *is* often guided by experience. However, as Gambrill (1999) points out, we often overstep our boundaries as professionals when we make claims about our professional abilities that we cannot prove. She points to the following statement made in a professional newsletter, and then responds to it:

> Professional social workers possess the specialized knowledge necessary for an effective social services delivery system. Social work education provides a unique combination of knowledge, values, skills, and professional ethics, which cannot be obtained through other degree programs or by on-the-job training. Further, social work education adequately equips its individuals with skills to help clients solve problems that bring them to social services departments and human services agencies. (NASW News, p. 14)

Gambrill's response:

> These claims all relate to knowledge. To my knowledge, there is no evidence for any of these claims. In fact, there is counterevidence. In Dawes' (1994) review of hundreds of studies, he concluded that there is no evidence that licenses, experience, and training are related to helping clients. If this applies to social work and, given the overlap in helping efforts among social workers, counselors, and psychologists, it is likely that it does, what are the implications? (Gambrill, 1999, p. 341)

The psychotherapy literature is replete with concepts and assumptions that seem unequivocally subjective and imprecise (Brent, 1998). Consider, for example, the following definition of psychotherapy provided by Brent: "a type of social influence exerted by a trained and socially sanctioned healer on a person or persons who suffer and are seeking relief, through a series of defined contacts." One might use the same definition for faith healers, psychics, and others who have both social sanction and exert social influence. Or consider this whimsical definition of psychotherapy as "two people playing together," or a final definition of psychotherapy as a "systematic use of a human relationship for therapeutic purposes." The vagueness of such definitions certainly cannot convey to clients what we do and makes it more than a little difficult for clinical researchers to evaluate the effectiveness of treatment.

As a response to overly subjective and sometimes incorrect approaches to practice, evidence-based practice believes that we should consult the research and involve clients in decisions about the best therapeutic approaches to be used, the issues in a client's life that need to be resolved, and the need to form a positive alliance with clients to facilitate change. This requires a cooperative and equal relationship with clients. Evidence-based practice also suggests that we act in a facilitative way to help clients gather information and rationally and critically process it. This differs from authoritarian approaches that assume the worker knows more about the client than the client does, and that the worker is the sole judge of what is to be done in the helping process.

3.3 DEFINING EVIDENCE-BASED PRACTICE

Sackett et al. (1997) define evidence-based practice as "the conscientious, explicit, and judicious use of current best evidence in making decisions about the care of individuals" (p. 2). Gambrill (2000, p. 1) defines EBP as a process involving self-directed learning which requires professionals to access information that permits us to:

1. take our collected knowledge and provide questions we can answer;
2. find the best evidence with which to answer questions;
3. analyze the best evidence for its research validity as well as its applicability to the practice questions we have asked;
4. determine if the best evidence we've found can be used with a particular client;
5. consider the client's social and emotional background;
6. make the client a participant in decision-making;
7. evaluate the quality of practice with that specific client.

The Council for Training in Evidence-Based Practice (2007) defines EBP as follows: "making decisions about behavioral health by integrating the best available research evidence with practitioner expertise and, the characteristics of those who will be affected, and doing so in a manner that is compatible with the environmental and organizational context" (p. 1).

Gambrill (1999) believes that EBP "requires an atmosphere in which critical appraisal of practice-related claims flourishes, and clients are involved as informed participants" (Gambrill, 1999, p. 345). In describing the importance of evidence-based practice, The American Medical Association (1992) writes:

A new paradigm for medical practice is emerging. Evidence-based medicine de-emphasizes intuition, unsystematic clinical experience, and pathophysiologic rationale as sufficient grounds for clinical decision-making, and stresses the examination of evidence from clinical research. Evidence-based medicine requires new skills of the physician, including efficient literature-searching, and the application of formal rules of evidence in evaluating the clinical literature. (AMA, 1992, p. 2420)

Timmermans and Angell (2001) indicate that evidence-based clinical judgment has five important features:

1. It is composed of both research evidence and clinical experience.
2. There is skill involved in reading the literature that requires an ability to synthesize the information and make judgments about the quality of the evidence available.
3. The way in which information is used is a function of the practitioner's level of authority in an organization and his or her level of confidence in the effectiveness of the applied information.
4. Part of the use of evidence-based practice is the ability to independently evaluate the information used and to test its validity in the context of one's own practice.
5. Evidence-based clinical judgments are grounded in the western notions of professional conduct and professional roles, and are ultimately guided by a common value system.

Gambrill (1999) points out that one of the most important aspects of EBP is the sharing of information with clients and the cooperative relationship that ensues. She notes that in EBP, clinicians search for relevant research to help in practice decisions and share that information with clients. If no evidence is found to justify a specific treatment regimen, the client is informed and a discussion takes place about how best to approach treatment. This includes the risks and benefits of any treatment approach used. Clients are involved in all treatment decisions and are encouraged to independently search the literature. As Sackett et al. (1997) note, new information is constantly being added to our knowledge base. Informed clinicians and clients may often find elegant treatment approaches that help provide direction where none may have existed before.

Gambrill (1999) believes that the use of EBP can help us "avoid fooling ourselves that we have knowledge when we do not" (p. 342). She indicates that a complete search for effectiveness research will provide the following information relevant for work with all clients including the elderly (Gambrill, 1999, p. 343) first suggested by Enkin et al. (1995):

1. Beneficial forms of care demonstrated by clear evidence from controlled trials.
2. Forms of care likely to be beneficial. The evidence in favor of these forms of care is not as clear as for those in category one.

3. Forms of care with a trade-off between beneficial and adverse effects. Effects must be weighed according to individual circumstances and priorities.
4. Forms of care of unknown effectiveness. There are insufficient or inadequate quality data upon which to base a recommendation for practice.
5. Forms of care unlikely to be beneficial. The evidence against these forms of care is not as clear as for those in category two.
6. Forms of care likely to be ineffective or harmful. Ineffectiveness or harm is demonstrated by clear evidence.

Hines (2000) suggests that some fundamental steps are required by EBP to obtain usable information in a literature search. They are: (1) developing a well formulated clinical question; (2) finding the best possible answers to your questions; (3) determining the validity and reliability of the data found; and (4) testing the information with your client. Hines suggests that a well-formulated clinical question must accurately describe the problem you wish to look for, limit the interventions you think are feasible and acceptable to the client, search for alternative approaches, and indicate the outcomes you wish to achieve with the client. The advantage of EBP, according to Hines, is that it allows the practitioner to develop quality practice guidelines that can be applied to the client, identify appropriate literature that can be shared with the client, communicate with other professionals from a knowledge-guided frame of reference, and continue a process of self-learning that results in the best possible treatment for clients.

Haynes (1998) writes that the goal of evidence-based practice "is to provide the means by which current best evidence from research can be judiciously and conscientiously applied in the prevention, detection, and care of health disorders" (p. 273). Haynes believes that this goal is very ambitious given "how resistant practitioners are to withdrawing established treatments from practice even once their utility has been disproved" (p. 273).

Denton et al. (2002) suggest that most of the therapies used to treat depression, among other conditions, have no empirical evidence to prove their effectiveness. The authors believe that before we select a treatment approach, we should consult empirically validated research studies that indicate the effectiveness of a particular therapeutic approach with a particular individual. The authors describe evidence-based practice as the use of treatments with some evidence of effectiveness. They note that evidence-based practice requires a complete literature search, the use of formal rules of proof in evaluating the relevant literature, and evidence that the selection of a practice approach is effective with a particular population.

In describing the ease with which evidence-based practice can be used, Bailes (2002) writes, "Evidence-based practice is not beyond your capability, even if you do not engage in research. You do not have to perform research; you can read the results of published studies [including] clinical research studies, meta-analyses, and systematic reviews" (p. 1). Bailes also indicates that the Internet permits access to various databases that allow searches to be done quickly and efficiently. Chapters 4 and 5 in this book are devoted to ways of obtaining and analyzing information for use in making informed treatment decisions.

In clarifying the types of data EBP looks for in its attempt to find best practices, Sackett et al. (1996) write, "Evidence based practice… involves tracking down the best external evidence with which to answer our clinical questions" (p. 72). The authors note that non-experimental approaches should be avoided because they often result in positive conclusions about treatment efficacy that are false. If randomized trials have not been done, "we must follow the trail to the next best external evidence and work from there" (Sackett et al., 1996, p. 72).

The Council for Training in Evidence-Based Behaviroal Practice (2007, pp. 3–4) notes that EBP requires the following competencies:

1. **Questions asked:** Practitioners using EBP must be able to ask answerable questions, prioritize their importance and know the type of evidence needed to answer the question accurately.
2. **Gathering evidence:** Practitioners using EBP must be able to develop a plan to search for best evidence, effectively and efficiently seek best evidence by knowing where to look for it, and be able to separate well done from poorly done studies.
3. **Critical appraisal**: Practitioners using EBP must be able to critically evaluate the validity and applicability of best evidence to client groups. To do this, practitioners need to know the strengths and weaknesses of the research mythologies.
4. **Using best evidence**: When treatment plans are developed in cooperation with client groups, the decision to use the available information should be weighted to determine its applicability to the problem and its relevance to the change strategies you and the client group want to utilize.

5. **Doing quality research**: Practitioners using EBP should feel a responsibility to do and share research information even if it is small subject research with limited controls for validity and reliability. In this way others continue the process of determining best evidence and our knowledge base grows as practitioners refine and expand the research effort.

3.4 CONCERNS ABOUT EVIDENCE-BASED PRACTICE FROM THE PRACTICE COMMUNITY

There are a number of concerns about evidence-based practice. One major concern is that EBP is a paradigm that was originally developed in medicine. Psychotherapy, so the argument goes, is less precise than medicine and cannot be open to the same scrutiny or the same standard as medicine because it is often subjective in nature. Another concern is that EBP seems to ignore the importance of practice wisdom and the countless years of experience by effective and dedicated practitioners. Many clinicians believe that researchers don't easily evaluate what we do in practice and attempts to determine effectiveness usually result in inconclusive findings. Psychotherapy effectiveness seems to relate to worker experience, according to Bergin (1971), and lumping inexperienced workers with experienced workers together in a research study often results in inconclusive and misleading findings.

Witkin and Harrison (2001) offer another concern about EBP and the problems encountered in reviewing clinical research: "Small alterations in the definitions of problems or 'interventions' can lead to changes in what is considered best practice. A review of readily accessible online reports of EBP or evidence-based medicine studies (see, for example, Research Triangle Institute, 2000) shows that various types of 'psychosocial' treatments are sometimes aggregated across studies" (p. 293). The authors suggest that finding the strongest evidence for a particular intervention may require a great deal of research sophistication at a level many clinicians do not posses and may never be interested in possessing. The authors are also concerned that "best evidence" may deny the fact that therapy is a joint effort and while the therapist may have a certain treatment in mind that shows research promise, it may not be acceptable to the client. They ask, "But what if practice is viewed as a mutual activity in which what is best (not necessarily effective) is co-generated by clients and practitioners? What is the relative value of different sources and types of evidence in this scenario?" (Witkin and Harrison, 2000, p. 295).

In one of the more large-scale evaluations of the effectiveness of psychotherapy, Seligman (1995) found that most clients are generally well satisfied with the help they were receiving. Although Seligman found no difference in client satisfaction between short and long term treatment, one cannot deny that clients remain in treatment because of a need for ongoing support and encouragement. These two factors are not easy to reconcile with scientific notions of treatment effectiveness. Psychotherapy, unlike medicine, doesn't often result in a cure. Clients may have prolonged periods of relief followed by a return of symptoms and the need for additional treatment. Using that description of psychotherapy, however, few could deny that medical care also results in relief of symptoms followed by the need for additional treatment. Finally, clinicians are trained in a subjective form of help we incorrectly call treatment. It really isn't treatment, which implies a medical process, but a more didactic exercise in which two people focus on the client's hurts and try and provide relief. It is, necessarily, a softhearted and empathic approach to healing that exists outside of an objective framework. Findings in empirical studies of effectiveness are, therefore, likely to indicate vague and undramatic results.

Among the suggested benefits of evidence-based practice are practice guidelines that describe best practice with certain types of emotional problems. Commenting on the use of evidence-based guidelines for practice, Parry and Richardson (2000) believe that clinicians are often uncertain because they believe the research underlying the practice recommendations often incorrectly generalizes findings from a specific population of clients to all clients. The authors also believe that clinicians reject "the medical metaphor, that psychotherapies can be 'prescribed' in any 'dosage' in response to a 'diagnosis'. There is also a strong belief amongst psychotherapy practitioners, that clinical judgments cannot be reduced to algorithmic procedures" (p. 280).

Barker (2001) wonders if practitioners use best evidence in the form of manuals or standardized protocols, and says that the answer is, "rarely, if ever. Rather, the successful therapist tailors therapy to suit the individual needs of the person, or the contextual factors" (p. 22). He defines tailoring therapy as meeting the needs of "often changing characteristics of clients" (p. 22), a description of therapy that makes effectiveness research improbable. Baker goes on to say, "The practice of psychotherapy is increasingly compromised by the pressures of economic rationalism and the demands for evidence-based practice. The diversity, which has characterized psychotherapy practice to date, risks being compromised by the narrow bandwidth of therapies which are deemed to fulfill the 'gold standard' validation criteria of the randomized controlled trials" (p. 11).

Chambless and Ollendick (2001) confirm that attempts to use EBP in manuals and in other disseminated ways often meet with rejection by practitioners for some of the following reasons:

1. Concerns about effectiveness studies suggest that non-empirically based research may be rejected as unscientific but, "No matter how large or consistent the body of evidence found for identified empirically supported treatments (ESTs), findings will be dismissed as irrelevant by those with fundamentally different views, and such views characterize a number of practitioners and theorists in the psychotherapy area" (Chambless and Ollendick, 2001, p. 699).

2. Presenting evidence-based information about treatment effectiveness can be problematic since it is difficult to design a manual or report that meets the specific needs of all therapists. Therapists are often unlikely to use such reports or manuals even when provided.

3. ESTs are effective in clinical settings and with a diverse group of clients; however, the studies found to support evidence-based treatment were high in external validity but low on internal validity. Consequently, while the authors found no compelling evidence of why ESTs could not be used in agencies by trained clinicians, more research on their use was suggested.

4. Economic problems facing many social agencies suggest that manuals prescribing treatments for specific social and emotional problems will be more of an issue as the economy softens and services for social and emotional problems are curtailed. The authors write: "Whatever the reluctance of some to embrace ESTs, we expect that the economic and societal pressures on practitioners for accountability will encourage continued attention to these treatments" (Chambless and Ollendick, 2001, p. 700).

In discussing the effectiveness of psychotherapy, Kopta et al. (1999) raise the issue of whether research evidence even exists to support the use of EBP in practice, and write, "researchers have repeatedly failed to find convincing evidence that different psychotherapies are differentially effective" (p. 445). They also worry that the belief system of the researcher, as Robinson et al. (1990) discovered, actually influences the outcomes of effectiveness studies.

Witkin and Harrison (2001) discuss social work and EBP and conclude that what social workers do may not be open to the same level or type of evaluation as medicine. Social workers act as cultural bridges between systems, individualize the client and his or her problem in ways that may defy classification, and work with oppressed people so that what we do may not fit neatly into organized theories of practice. In response to the use of EBP, the authors write:

> Sometimes this involves using the logic of EBP with clients when there is credible evidence of some relevant knowledge available. Other times, however, the most important work is in educating decision makers or those who have control of resources about how irrelevant the best scientific evidence is to the world of people whose experiences brought them into contact with the professionals. (Witkin and Harrison, 2001, p. 295)

Witkin and Harrison (2001) raise the issue of whether the helping professions should be placed in the same precarious position as medicine when it relates to issues of managed care. The authors write, "Is it a coincidence that EBP is favored by managed care providers pushing practice toward an emphasis on specificity in problem identification and rapid responses to the identified conditions?" (p. 246). The AMA (EBP Working Group, 1992) reinforces this concern when it states that "Economic constraints and counter-productive incentives may compete with the dictates of evidence as determinants of clinical decisions. The relevant literature may not be readily accessible. Time may be insufficient to carefully review the evidence (which may be voluminous) relevant to a pressing clinical problem" (p. 2423).

3.5 RESPONSES TO CRITICISMS OF EVIDENCE-BASED PRACTICE

In response to concerns that managed care may use EBP to lower costs, Sackett et al. (1996) write, "Some fear that evidence based medicine will be hijacked by purchasers and managers to cut the costs of health care. Doctors practicing evidence based medicine will identify and apply the most efficacious interventions to maximize the quality and quantity of life for individual patients; this may raise rather than lower the cost of their care" (p. 71). An editorial in *Mental Health Weekly* (2001) challenges the idea that EBP is being pushed by the health care crisis. The editorial argues that

> Tight budgets make adoption of best practices difficult. Their implementation often requires a restructuring of existing services. And once a best practice is implemented, fidelity to its key elements is

critical to success. However, methods of ensuring fidelity in real practice settings remain unproven. (2001, Internet).

The AMA Working Group (1992) identifies three misinterpretations about EBP that create barriers to its use, and then responds to those misinterpretations in the following statements:

1. Evidence-based practice ignores clinical experience and clinical intuition.
   - On the contrary, it is important to expose learners to exceptional clinicians who have a gift for intuitive diagnosis, a talent for precise observation, and excellent judgment in making difficult management decisions. Untested signs and symptoms should not be rejected out of hand. They may prove extremely useful, and ultimately be proved valid through rigorous testing. The more experienced clinicians can dissect the process they use in diagnosis, and clearly present it to learners, the greater the benefit (p. 2423).

2. Understanding of basic investigation and pathology plays no part in evidence-based medicine.
   - The dearth of adequate evidence demands that clinical problem-solving must rely on an understanding of underlying pathology. Moreover, a good understanding of pathology is necessary for interpreting clinical observations and for appropriate interpretation of evidence (especially in deciding on its generalizability) (p. 2423).

3. Evidence-based practice ignores standard aspects of clinical training such history taking.
   - A careful history and physical examination provides much, and often the best, evidence for diagnosis and directs treatment decisions. The clinical teacher of evidence-based medicine must give considerable attention to teaching the methods of history and diagnosis, with particular attention to which items have demonstrated validity and to strategies to enhance observer agreement (p. 2423).

In a review of the most effective practices in psychotherapy, Chambless (2001) notes that one argument used against EBP is that there is no difference in the effectiveness of various forms of psychotherapy and that identifying best practices is therefore unnecessary. However, Chambless found considerable evidence that in the treatment of anxiety disorders and childhood depression, cognitive and behavioral methods were fairly clearly defined and that positive results often ensued from the treatment.

The British Medical Association raises other issues with EBP in an editorial appearing in the July 1998 *British Medical Journal*. The editorial calls into question the implied ease with which good evidence is available in medicine and by implication, whether it is readily available to the helping professional. The editorial notes that most published research in medical journals is too poorly done or not relevant enough to useful to physicians. In surveys, more than 95% of the published articles in medical journals did not achieve minimum standards of quality or relevance. Clinical practice guidelines are slow to produce, costly, have poor quality, and are difficult to update. (p. 6)

By way of response, Straus and Sackett (1998) report that evidence-based practice has been quite successful in general medical and psychiatric settings and that practitioners read the research accurately and make correct decisions. They write, "a general medicine service at a district general hospital affiliated with a university found that 53% of patients admitted to the service received primary treatments that had been validated in randomized controlled trials" (p. 341). The authors also note that three quarters of the evidence used in the treatment of clients was immediately available through empirically evaluated topic summaries, and the remaining quarter was "identified and applied by asking answerable questions at the time of admission, rapidly finding good evidence, quickly determining its validity and usefulness, swiftly integrating it with clinical expertise and each patient's unique features, and offering it to the patients" (p. 341). Similar results, according to Strauss and Sackett (1998), have been found in studies of a psychiatric hospital (p. 341).

3.6 WHY PRACTITIONERS SOMETIMES RESIST THE USE OF EBP

In a personal correspondence, Bushfield (2007) gives the following reasons for the resistance to EBP:

> Recent developments in Evidence Based Practice (EBP) suggest the need to combine the best "clinical practice" skills used in engaging and assessing the person in his/her situation, and then apply the best evidence-based interventions. In the absence of evidence regarding the specific aspects of the individual client in his/her situation, what should the practitioner do? Too often, we do what we like or what we are used to doing. We use "clinical wisdom" or "trial and error."

> The discussion on EBP digs at our roots. Flexner raised the question, "are we really professionals?" Despite nearly a century of development

of the social work profession, the core arguments remain: do we have empirical evidence as the basis of our work? Other questions include: is practice wisdom evidence? Whose knowledge do we value? Are there other ways of knowing? Has evidence caught up with the reality of our encounters within a rapidly changing environment?

Even when one embraces the need for evidence, it seems that empiricism, attempting to clean up the messiness of subjectivity, has it own messiness. How was data obtained, and from whom? Under what circumstances? What about missing data, and do techniques to handle this merely reinforce the status quo, including stereotypes?

Some argue that evidence, even when it has its merits, is missing the nuances discovered in a single subject study. While we can easily agree that the snapshot does not capture reality, it is less obvious that videos, attempting to more accurately capture reality, still carry the influence of the videographer's eye. Even more problematic, when we are aware that the camera is running, we may show a different side of ourselves.

So how should practitioners greet EBP? With healthy skepticism, and with a willingness to participate in the building of evidence from the ground up. In social work, we are compelled to know both the general and the unique. Since little evidence addresses the multiple aspects of person and environment, the multiple dimensions of time – both life course and life events – and little evidence makes sufficient accounting for both the researcher and the setting, as well as the meaning of the research to its participants, I for one, will offer a different kind of skepticism: not the rejection of evidence, but rather the closer scrutiny of the latest and best evidence for its broader and relevant application to the most vulnerable.

There is still strong evidence that clients prefer the caring relationship, time spent, and provision of hope: engagement and caring presence. To the extent that the latest evidence reflects the influence of these variables on client outcomes, I stand ready to embrace it. Even the best evidence based interventions may depend on the ability to engage the client in the intervention. However, engagement and caring may be insufficient, without effective approaches beyond engagement. So, perhaps we need to think of a "both/and" approach. I would like to communicate both that I want to help, that I believe that help is helpful, and that there is evidence that my ways of helping have a great likelihood of working. Are interventions effective in the absence of relationship? Does the evidence suggest that workers are interchangeable widgets which, when performing the appropriate function, can create effective outcomes? I think not. What is needed is more focus on engaging the client in evaluating the evidence for its application to the client's situation. Strengths and empowerment, sometimes missing in the rush toward evidence, are powerful tools. Further, as an ethical practitioner, I want to have sufficient evidence that what I am doing will work, and therefore am compelled to be a critical consumer of new evidence – and refuse to be "left out" of the discussion. This requires me to understand research and statistical analysis, and to search out the best that evidence has to offer.

3.7 IS EVIDENCE-BASED PRACTICE APPLICABLE TO THE HUMAN SERVICES?

Reynolds and Richardson (2000) argue that despite concerns among clinicians that EBP may impede their freedom, new opportunities in practice research suggest that clinician freedom will be enhanced because more options will be available as creative research methodologies suggest new forms of treatment. As new research opportunities develop, the profile of psychotherapy will rise. And while evidence-based practice has been called "cookbook practice" and a "new type of authority" that threatens the autonomy of professionals, the possibility exists that research in psychotherapy effectiveness will have the same positive effect that medical research has had on the practice of medicine. In discussing the benefits of practice guidelines, Parry and Richardson (2000) believe that well-done practice guidelines will help clinicians crystallize their thinking about treatment. Published guidelines will also give clients more information and consequently give them additional power to decide on their own treatment. High quality guidelines help in training new professionals and influence the writing of textbooks that must increasingly contain evidence of best practices. Parry and Richardson (2000, p. 279) provide the following examples of well-done guidelines for professional practice:

1. The American Psychiatric Association has published practice guidelines for eating disorders (APA, 1993a) and for major depressive disorder in adults (APA, 1993b).
2. The Australian and New Zealand College of Psychiatrists ran a quality assurance project which has produced several treatment outlines; for agoraphobia (Quality Assurance Project, 1982a), depressive disorders (1982b), for borderline, narcissistic and histrionic personality disorders (1991b) and for antisocial personality disorders (1991a).

3. The US Agency for Health Care Policy and Research has been influential. For example, their depression in primary care guideline (Agency for Health Care Policy and Research, 1993a,b) was widely discussed (Persons et al., 1996; Munoz et al., 1994). More recently, Schulberg et al. (1998)reviewed research published between 1992 and 1998 to update this guideline.

4. Other guidelines worth exploring include those on the treatment of bipolar disorder (Frances et al., 1996), choice of antidepressants in primary care (North of England Evidence-Based Guideline Development Project, 1997) and treatment of obsessive-compulsive disorder (March et al., 1997).

We are in the midst of a health care crisis in America that directly affects the human services. As Witkin and Harrison (2000) and others have repeatedly noted, the human service professions have not embraced the concept of best practices or the need to function from a knowledge-guided frame of reference. The result is a growing suspicion among health care analysts and providers that what we do is expendable. In providing a warning to mental health professionals to begin close cooperative relationships with self-help groups, Humphreys and Ribisl (1999) give a prophetic view of what the current thinking is regarding the health of the helping professions by asking, "Why should public health and medical professionals be interested in collaborating with a grassroots movement of untrained citizens?" (p. 326). The reasons the authors provide are that money for health care is contracting and is likely to continue doing so, and that self-help groups often provide "benefits that the best health care often does not: identification with other sufferers, long-term support and companionship, and a sense of competence and empowerment" (p. 326).

Professions have a body of knowledge that should be based, not on practice wisdom or practice experience, but on the evidence that we are collecting empirical data that supports our interventions. Without such a body of knowledge, we begin to lose our status as professions and the future of psychotherapy in the USA seems clear: less therapy provided, irrespective of client need; therapy provided by the least highly trained workers with heavy reliance on self-help groups; psycho-educational materials in the form of reading for clients in lieu of therapy; and the hope that clients will be resilient and wise enough to get better, essentially, by themselves.

3.8 A PERSONAL STORY: LIFE IS GOOD AT 86

Jack is an 86-year old tennis player and raconteur. He graciously let me interview him, and while these aren't always his exact words, I've tried to be faithful to what he said.

"Until I remarried and began a successful business in my mid-fifties, I guess you could say that I had no point of view and did what I thought other people wanted me to do. The change took place while I was look-ing at a property to buy in east Los Angels and I was shot and seriously wounded in a random shooting. The bullet took out part of my liver. It took me six months to get over the shock and the physical pain.

"During the time I was recuperating my wife and I decided to move to Hawaii and start a new business. I had very little money and we knew we were taking a chance, but in the 10 years we worked at building our business we were able to plan for our eventual retirement, sell our business at a nice profit, and find this community in paradise. (He points to the pines and the mountains nearby. We're sitting outside watching a tennis match and talking, and it's a perfect day, sunny and warm with the smells of springs in the Arizona high country.)

"I surround myself with people who are optimistic and make me laugh. I think laughter is the healthiest emotion, and even though I have some serious health problems, I take care of myself and I don't dwell on them. I know my tennis is limited and that there are many things I can't do any-more, but getting out with a bunch of guys, hitting the ball, and then going out for coffee and laughing together – it's the best thing about my life.

"My wife is someone who takes care of me when I need it and who helped me develop our business that ultimately allowed us to retire and enjoy life. My first wife was someone who always had us in debt, and who I think never loved me or felt anything about me except that that I was a provider. My current wife and I met while we were developing a new syna-gogue in Los Angeles. We had time to get to know each other and to appre-ciate how many things we had in common and how well we got along.

"One of our sons was gay and died of AIDS. He had a doctor-assisted suicide in Oregon and it was a very powerful experience. He had close friends over and the minister of his church said some words about his life that still make me cry when I think about (pauses and wipes tears from his eyes). I know that death isn't beautiful, but in its own way it was. Since then, I've never feared dying. It took a while to get over his death but I think about the joy he gave me when he was alive and well. I have another son we help out financially who's a graphic designer and talented but not very good with money. When

I die we'll be worth a lot of money and I guess the family will get it. I think about spending it all now but my needs are few and the traveling I wanted to do when I was younger we've already done. My wife had a hip replacement and she'd rather stay at home anyway. It's fine with me.

"I don't think of myself as being religious. The guys joke about my being Jewish, but I'm just like them in most ways. While I'm proud of being a Jew, the religion never mattered much to me just as their religions don't matter much to them. I was raised in a religious home but it didn't stick.

"I have many friends and I know that I could count on them if I needed their help. That's the best thing about life now, being able to be with people I like and who I think genuinely like me. I stay away from people who seem unhappy, and I know I flirt a lot with young women and say things to ladies at the tennis club most guys couldn't get away with. What the hell, I can't do anything about it anyway and they know it, so why not? It's one of the privileges of being old. You can say things that would be offensive if you were younger and everyone thinks it's charming now.

"I began mentoring a young boy in the first grade who was having some behavioral problems after his parents divorced. One of my friend's wives suggested that I'd be a good mentor for a young child so I volunteered at the public school and he was assigned to me. We hung out together and I gave him a little support and encouragement. He's a senor in high school now and a colonel in the Civilian Air Patrol. I'm really proud of him. I think I did a better job with him than with my own sons, but then you get wiser as you age. Maybe I was good all along, but I felt more confident and comfortable with myself as I got older so that I could be a good friend instead of a parent.

"I started to become a real human being in my fifties and it's just gotten better and better. I would say to anyone reading your book that you should make the most of your time and enjoy yourself. There's so little time to live that you should do it to the fullest. More than half my life was spent being unhappy, in debt, and feeling unloved. This opportunity I've had since I met my present wife has been a blessing, and we should all be open to change and to the possibilities of life. Good friends, laughter, enough money to be comfortable, and good health. That's all anyone can ask for when they're 86 – J.S.

3.9 SUMMARY

This chapter discusses the definitions of evidence-based practice and some of the criticisms of the approach found in the literature. Among the strongest criticism of EBP is that we fail to have a well-defined literature at present and what we do have is difficult to read and comprehend, and too time-consuming for most practitioners. There is evidence that clinicians do not use manuals that contain best evidence. On the positive side, there is a need to organize best practices and to assure clients and third party providers that what we do actually works. EBP is an approach that tries to organize a way of providing the best possible service to clients using a knowledge-guided approach to practice and substantial involvement of clients in decision-making to assure that the client–worker relationship is cooperative. The chapter ends with a personal story about aging.

3.10 QUESTIONS FROM THE CHAPTER

1. Do you think it's possible to organize best practice in ways that capture the individual nature of the client? Isn't this the problem with EBP, that it cannot individualize what's actually best for a specific client and his or her needs?
2. Why do you think training manuals are so unpopular with clinicians?
3. There is evidence in this chapter that we don't have enough conclusive data accumulated to indicate best evidence with most client problems. Doesn't this suggest that EBP cannot function adequately until we have considerably more research evidence?
4. EBP originated in medicine. Do you think that medicine and therapy are similar enough to utilize an approach developed for medical practice?
5. Because therapy requires a more highly involved participation by the client than medicine, do you accept Gambrill's criticism that we make statements in the helping professions about what we do and its effectiveness that are unsupported by the data that create false impressions?

REFERENCES

Agency for Health Care Policy and Research (1993a). *Depression in primary care: Detection and diagnosis.* Washington, DC: US Department of Health and Human Services.

Agency for Health Care Policy and Research (1993b). *Depression in primary care: Treatment of major depression.* Washington, DC: US Department of Health and Human Services.

American Psychiatric Association (1993a). Practice guideline for eating disorders. *American Journal of Psychiatry, 150,* 207–228.

American Psychiatric Association (1993b). Practice guideline for major depressive disorder in adults. *American Journal of Psychiatry Supplement, 150* (Suppl. 4).

Bailes, B. K. (2002, June). Evidence-based practice guidelines – one way to enhance clinical practice. *AORN Journal.*

Barker, P. (2001). The ripples of knowledge and the boundaries of practice: The problem of evidence in psychotherapy research. *International Journal of Psychotherapy, 6*(1), 11–24.

Bergin, A. E. (1971). The evaluation of therapeutic outcomes. In A. E. Bergin & S. Garfield (Eds.), *Handbook of psychotherapy and behavior change* (pp. 170–217). New York: John Wiley and Sons.

Brent, D. A. (1998, February). Psychotherapy: Definitions, mechanisms of action, and relationship to etiological models. *Journal of Abnormal Child Psychology.*

Chambless, D. L. (2001). Empirically supported psychological interventions: Controversies and evidence. Chamblesshttp://www.findarticles.com/cf_0/m0961/2001_Annual/73232726/print.jhtml. *Annual Review of Psychology.*

Council for Training in Evidence-Based Behavioral Practice. (2007). Definition and competencies for evidence-based behavioral practice. *Supported in part by contract N01-LM-6-3512 from the National Institutes of Health Office of Behavioral and Social Sciences Research to Northwestern University.*

Dawes, R. M. (1994). *House of cards: Psychology and psychotherapy built on myth.* New York: Free Press.

Denton, W. H., Walsh, S. R., & Daniel, S. S. (2002). Evidence-based practice in family therapy: Adolescent depression as an example. *Journal of Marital and Family Therapy, 28*(1), 39–45.

Department of Health and Human Services (US) (1990). Bureau of Maternal and Child Health and Resource Development. In: *Surgeon General's Workshop on Self-Help and Public Health.* Washington: Government Printing Office.

Editorial. (1998, July 4). Getting evidence into practice. *British Medical Journal, 317,* 6.

Editorial. (2001, August 20). Project to bring evidence-based treatment into real world. *Mental Health Weekly.* <http://www.findarticles.com/cf_0/m0BSC/32_11/77610655/print.jhtml/>.

Enkin, M., Keirse, M. J. N., Renfrew, M., & Neilson, J. (1995). *A guide to effective care in pregnancy and childbirth* (2nd ed). New York: Oxford University Press.

Evidence-Based Medicine Working Group. (1992). Evidence-based medicine: A new approach to teaching the practice of medicine. *Journal of the American Medical Association, 268,* 2420–2425.

Flaherty, R. J. (2001, September 15). Medical myths: Today's perspectives. *PatientCare.* <http://www.findarticles.com/cf_0/m3233/17_35/78547389/print.jhtml/>

Frances, A., Docherty, J. P., & Kahn, D. A. (1996). Treatment of bipolar disorder. *The Journal of Clinical Psychiatry, 57* (Suppl. 12a).

Gambrill, E. (2000, October). Evidence-based practice. *A handout to the dean and directors of schools of social work.* Huntington, Beach, CA.

Gambrill, E. (1999). Evidence-based practice: An alternative to authority-based practice. *Journal of Contemporary Human Services, 80*(4), 341–350.

Haynes, B. (1998, July 25). Barriers and bridges to evidence based clinical practice (Getting Research Findings into Practice, part 4.). *British Medical Journal, 317,* 273–276.

Hines, S. E. (2000, February 29). Enhance your practice with evidence-based medicine. *Patient Care.*

Howard, M. O., & Jenson, J. M. (1999). Clinical practice guidelines: Should social work develop them? *Research on Social Work Practice, 9*(3), 283–301.

Humphreys, K., & Ribisl, K. M. (1999). The case for partnership with self-help groups. *Public Health Reports, 114*(4), 322–329.

Issacs, D. (1999, December 18). Seven alternatives to evidence based medicine. *British Medical Journal.*

Kopta, M. S., Lueger, R. J., Saunders, S. M., & Howard, K. I. (Annual 1999). Individual psychotherapy outcome and process research: Challenges leading to greater turmoil or a positive transition? http://www.findarticles.com/cf_0/m0961/1999_Annual/54442307/print.jhtml. *Annual Review of Psychology.*

Luborsky, L. (1994). Therapeutic alliances as predictors of psychotherapy outcomes: Factors explaining the predictive success. In A. O. Horvath & L. S. Greenberg (Eds.), *The working alliance: Theory, research, and practice* (pp. 38–50). New York: Wiley & Sons.

Luborsky, L., Singer, B., & Luborsky, L. (1975). Comparative studies of psychotherapy. *Archives of General Psychiatry, 32,* 995–1008.

March, J. S., Frances, A., Carpenter, D., & Kahn, D. A. (Eds.), (1997). *Treatment of obsessive-compulsive disorder.* The Expert Consensus Guideline Series.

Munoz, R., Hollon, S., McGrath, E., Rehm, L., & VandenBos, G. (1994). On the AHCPR guidelines: Further considerations for practitioners. *American Psychologist, 49,* 42–61.

National Association of Social Work Board of Directors. (1999, January). Proposed public policies of NASW. *NASW News, 44*(3), 12–17.

North of England Evidence Based Guideline Development Project (1997). *Evidence based clinical practice guideline: The choice of antidepressants for depression in primary care.* Newcastle upon Tyne: Centre for Health Services Research.

O'Donnell, M. (1997). *A skeptic's medical dictionary.* London: BMJ Books.

Parry, G., & Richardson, P. (2000). Developing treatment choice guidelines in psychotherapy. *Journal of Mental Health, 9*(3), 273–282.

Persons, J. B., Thase, M. E., & Crits-Christoph, P. (1996). The role of psychotherapy in the treatment of depression: Review of two practice guidelines. *Archives of General Psychiatry, 53,* 283–290.

Quality Assurance Project. (1982a). A treatment outline for agoraphobia. *Australian and New Zealand Journal of Psychiatry, 16*, 25–33.

Quality Assurance Project. (1982b). A treatment outline for depressive disorders. *Australian and New Zealand Journal of Psychiatry, 17*, 129–148.

Quality Assurance Project. (1991a). Treatment outlines for antisocial personality disorders. *Australian and New Zealand Journal of Psychiatry, 25*, 541–547.

Quality Assurance Project. (1991b). Treatment outlines for borderline, narcissistic and histrionic personality disorders. *Australian and New Zealand Journal of Psychiatry, 25*, 392–403.

Research Triangle Institute. (2000). Assessing "best evidence": *Grading the quality of articles and rating the strength of evidence.* <www.rti.org/epc/grading-article. html/> Available.

Reynolds, R., & Richardson, P. (2000). Evidence based practice and psychotherapy research. *Journal of Mental Health, 9*(3), 257–267.

Robinson, L. A., Berman, J. S., & Neimeyer, R. A. (1990). Psychotherapy for the treatment of depression: A comprehensive review of controlled outcome research. *Psychological Bulletin, 108*, 30–49.

Rosen, A. (1994). Knowledge use in direct practice. *Social Service Review, 68*, 561–577.

Sackett, D. L., Rosenberg, W. M. C., Muir Gray, J. A., Haynes, R. B., & Richardson, W. S. (1996, January 13). Evidence based medicine: What it is and what it isn't http://bmj. com/cgi/content/full/312/7023/71?ijkey = JflK2VHyVI2F6. *British Medical Journal, 312*, 71–72.

Sackett, D. L., Richardson, W. S., Rosenberg, W., & Haynes, R. B. (1997). *Evidence-based medicine: How to practice and teach EMB.* New York: Churchill Livingstone.

Schulberg, H. C., Katon, W., Simon, G. E., & Rush, A. J. (1998). Treating major depression in primary care practice: An update of the agency for health care policy and research practice guidelines. *Archives of General Psychiatry, 55*, 1121–1127.

Seligman, M. E. P. (1995). The effectiveness of psychotherapy: The consumers report study. *American Psychologist, 50*(12), 965–974.

Strauss, S. E., & Sackett, D. L. (1998, August 1). Using research findings in clinical practice. http://bmj.com/cgi/content/full/317/7154/339. *British Medical Journal, 317*, 339–342.

Timmermans, S., & Angell, A. (2001). Evidence-based medicine, clinical uncertainty, and learning to doctor. *Journal of Health & Social Behavior, 42*(4), 342.

Users' Guides to Evidence-based Medicine. (1992). Evidence-based medicine: A new approach to teaching the practice of medicine. *Journal of the American Medical Association, 268*(17), 2420–2425.

Witkin, S. L., & Harrison, W. D. (2001, October). Editorial: Whose evidence and for what purpose? *Social Work, 46*(4), 293–296.

Chapter four

Using Evidence-Based Practice to Diagnosis and Assess Psychosocial Difficulties in Older Adults

4.1 INTRODUCTION

This chapter discusses the important distinctions made when diagnosing older adults with emotional problems, distinctions that are often influenced by physical problems unique to older adults. The chapter also provides an example of a strengths perspective psychosocial assessment of an older adult experiencing a variety of serious health and emotional problems.

In describing the unique aspects of diagnosing emotional problems of older adults, the Guidelines for Psychological Practice with Older Adults of the American Psychological Association (APA, 2003) indicates that assessment tools should be appropriately validated and normed for use with older adults. When that isn't possible, the report worries that clinicians might use instruments that are not well suited to determine the social, emotional, and cognitive functioning of older adults. Even when assessment procedures are modified to take into consideration special frailties and impairments, the results of assessments may be too flawed to accept. The report encourages clinicians to make certain that assessment is done with sensitivity to hearing and reading problems and medications that may alter behavior and cognitive functioning before assigning a diagnosis, and encourages clinicians to conduct "repeated-measures assessments at more than a single time point. Such longitudinal assessment is useful particularly with respect to such matters as the older adult's affective state or functional capacities, and can help in examining the degree to which these are stable or vary according to situational factors, time of day, or the like" (p. 23).

The report goes on to say that "Other special challenges in assessing older adults include interpreting the significance of somatic complaints; appraising the nature and extent of familial and other social support; evaluating potential elder abuse or neglect; and identification of strengths and potential compensatory skills" (pp. 23–25). Assessments may also affect the efficacy of treatment and knowing when referrals to nursing home and day care programs are most appropriate. Recognizing emotional problems in older adults poses additional challenges. Aging brings with it a higher prevalence of certain medical conditions, realistic concerns about physical problems, and a higher use of prescription medications. As a result, separating a medical condition from physical symptoms may be more complicated with older adults.

Because of the complex relationship between emotional problems, drug interactions, and serious physical illness in the elderly, an accurate diagnosis is not always straightforward. Additionally, some older adults may be aware of their emotional difficulties but believe that nothing can be done about it, or they may only report physical symptoms such as aches and pains. Often their symptoms are ignored or confused with other ailments common in the elderly, including Parkinson's or Alzheimer's disease, dementia, thyroid disorders, arthritis, strokes, cancer, heart disease, medication, and other chronic conditions. Depression may even be a predictor of Alzheimer's disease or an impending physical illness before the symptoms of the disease itself become evident.

To make more accurate diagnostic decisions, Cloud (2003) suggests the use of four categories of disorders: "Those arising from brain disease, those arising from problems controlling one's drive, those arising from problematic personal dispositions, and those arising from life circumstances" (p. 106).

The Guidelines for Psychological Practice with Older Adults of the American Psychological Association (APA, 2003, p. 7) list the following inaccurate stereotypes of older adults that can contribute to negative biases and may affect the way an older adult is viewed diagnostically:

> (1) With age inevitably comes senility; (2) older adults have increased rates of mental illness, particularly depression; (3) older adults are inefficient in the workplace; (4) most older adults are frail and ill; (5) older adults are socially isolated; (6) older adults have no interest in sex or intimacy; and (7) older adults are inflexible and stubborn (Edelstein and Kalish, 1999). Such views, the report cautions can lead to "misdiagnosis of disorders and inappropriately decreased expectations for improvement, so-called "therapeutic nihilism" (Goodstein, 1985), and to the lack of preventive actions and treatment (Dupree and Paterson, 1985).

The report also cautions that badly informed therapists may assume that older adults are too old to change or less likely than younger adults to benefit from counseling and psychotherapy. Some health and mental health professionals may avoid working with older adults because it creates discomfort about their own aging or their relationships with parents or other older family members, a phenomenon sometimes termed "gerophobia" (Verwoerdt, 1976).

Smyer (1984) suggests that in assessing older adults we use a transition approach that believes development occurs throughout the life span and "contradicts the previous therapeutic pessimism which equated old age with rigid defenses, lack of therapeutic motivation, and generally poor prospects for change or growth and a time of life not worthy of therapeutic investment" (p. 17). Smyer has developed a typology of potential transitions, containing four types of life stresses: (1) biological, (2) personal/psychological, (3) physical/environmental, and (4) social/cultural. Smyer has also identified 14 different contexts in which life events occur, including family, love and marriage, parenting, health, self, friendships, social relations, finances, and work (1984, pp. 18 and 19).

To understand an older adult, Schlossberg (1990) writes, "Clinicians need to know the transitions, life events, stresses. Is the transition a personal one at work, a personal one with neighbors, or a family conflict? By taking a life-events approach, rather than an age approach, we begin to identify what prompts the need for help" (p. 9). The author continues,

> Beyond identifying the transition or change in the client's life, counselors benefit from knowing the degree to which the events (like retirement or promotion) or "nonevents" (like being passed over for a promotion or failing to have a wanted child or grandchild) alter the client's life. We need to ask whether the change (whether biological,

personal, physical, or social) alters the client's roles, relationships, routines, and assumptions about self. The more the event or nonevent alters an adult's roles, routines, assumptions, and relationships, the more the person will be affected by the transition and have to cope with it. (Schlossberg, 1990, p. 9)

Groopman (2007) reports three primary errors made in diagnoses:

1. anchoring, which means that clinicians grab onto the first symptom or abnormality and use it to make snap judgments about a client's condition;
2. availability, which means that an easily remembered prior experience with a client – a memory that is most available to the clinician – is used to explain a new situation the clinician is trying to diagnose;
3. attribution, which means that the clinician is diagnosing from stereotypes. Groopman believes this later error is the one most likely to harm older adults because many of us harbor untrue preconceived notions about aging that becomes stereotypic in time.

Another serious error in diagnosis relates to views on race. Whaley (2001) is concerned that Causcasian clinicians often see African American clients as having paranoid symptoms that are more fundamentally a cultural distrust of Caucasians because of historical experiences with racism. He believes that the diagnostic process with African American clients tends to discount the negative impact of racism and leads to diagnostic judgments about Black clients implying that they are more dysfunctional than they really are. This tendency to misdiagnose, or to diagnose a more serious condition than may be warranted, is what Whaley calls "pseudo-transference" and has its origins in cultural stereotyping by clinicians who fail to understand the impact of racism. Whaley believes that cultural stereotyping ultimately leads to, "more severe diagnoses and restrictive interventions" (p. 558) with African American clients. Whaley's work suggests that clinicians may incorrectly use diagnostic labels with clients they either feel uncomfortable with or whose cultural differences create some degree of hostility, casting doubt on the accuracy of diagnostic labels with an entire range of older clients who may differ educationally, racially and culturally from clinicians. These concerns reinforce the subjective nature of the diagnostic process in general and the DSM in particular.

In an anchoring, or the use of an incorrect diagnosis that is based on first impressions, Robertson and Fitzgerald (1990) randomly assigned 47 counselors to watch videos of a depressed male portrayed by an actor.

The only changes made in the videos were the client's type of employment (professional vs. blue collar) and the client's family or origin (traditional or nontraditional). The researcher found that counselors made more negative diagnostic judgments when the actor portrayed a blue-collar worker and came from a non-traditional family. The signs and symptoms of any specific emotional disorders were secondary to the worker's bias.

In an example of another type of bias, self-confirmatory bias, or diagnosis based only on the information collected by the clinician that confirms his or her original diagnosis, Haverkamp (1993) had counseling and counseling psychology students watch a video of an initial counseling session and then write down the questions they wanted to ask in a follow up session with the client. The results were that the majority of students (64%) wanted to ask questions that confirmed their original diagnostic impression of the client. A follow up study by Pfeiffer et al. (2000) came to a similar conclusion.

Gladwell (2007) discusses the reasons crime profilers often make serious errors in their profiles (diagnosis) of unknown criminals who have committed heinous criminal acts. He says that profilers often use three general statements about criminals they are profiling that one often sees in clinical assessments of clients:

1. the Rainbow Ruse, a statement that suggests a personality trait and then its opposite ("The client is quiet and unassuming but in the right circumstance he may be vindictive and hostile");
2. the Jacques Statement that tailors a diagnosis to the age of the client ("By 65, most of a man's hostility toward women will likely be gone");
3. the Barnum Statement, or what we used to call an *Aunt Fanny Diagnosis* because it was so vague that it could fit everyone in the world, including our Aunt Fanny.

These techniques are frequently used in diagnostic statements when clinicians either haven't a clue about what's really wrong or they fail to collect reliable and valid information on which diagnostic category is evident by applying the behaviors noted in the DSM IV. Here's an example of an actual profile of the Wichita Kansas serial killer known as BTK (Gladwell, 2007, p. 44):

> Look for an American male with a possibility of a connection to the military. He will drive a decent car. He won't be comfortable with women. He will be a lone wolf. But he may have women friends. He will be either never married, divorced, or married. He may or may not live in a rental, and might be lower class, lower middle class or middle class.

[Gladwell then notes that the profile had nothing in common with the real BTK Killer who was] a pillar of his community, the president of his church, and the married father of two].

Croskerry (2002) believes that most diagnostic errors occur because clinicians make decisions far too soon and without enough evidence to support a diagnosis. He calls these "representative errors" since they are based on what clinicians have been trained to observe and believe, and therefore tend to overwhelm an observation with preconceived beliefs about a person and what may be wrong.

Yet another type of bias that often provides incorrect diagnosis in older adults is "confirmation bias" where clinicians confirm what they believe by ignoring or selectively accepting certain information about the client. As Groopman (2007) notes, "When people are confronted with uncertainty, they are susceptible to unconscious emotions and personal biases, and are more likely to make cognitive errors" (p. 41).

McLaughlin (2000) suggests the following ways of reducing errors in diagnosing:

1. Don't make too much or too little of the evidence at hand.
2. Try and note the biasing effect of your workplace that may routinely diagnose everyone in the same way.
3. Try and disprove a diagnosis.
4. Consistently use all of the DSM diagnostic criteria and keep current about revisions.
5. Be aware of other disorders or a dual diagnosis, and delay making a diagnosis until you have more data.
6. Use symptom checklists to make certain your diagnosis adheres to DSM categories, and follow a logical protocol to collect and evaluate data about the client before finalizing a diagnosis.
7. If you use psychological instruments in diagnosis, make certain they're valid and reliable with the type of client you're diagnosing (by age, gender, ethnicity, etc.).
8. Make absolutely certain your expectations of clients don't reflect racial, ethnic, gender, religious bias, or self-fulfilling prophesies about certain categories of diagnosis.
9. Remember the importance of social factors in diagnosis and that the DSM may have a built in bias against certain groups.
10. Consider other diagnostic possibilities and understand that the more time you take getting to know the client, the more likely you are to arrive at a correct diagnosis.

11. Consider the pros and the cons of a diagnosis before formally using it with a client.
12. Use multiple diagnostic instruments to determine a diagnosis, and accept a diagnosis only if those instruments are in agreement with one another.
13. Focus on what may be atypical about a client and follow those leads to help determine a diagnosis.
14. Follow ethical standards.
15. Use training to improve your diagnostic work particularly with diverse ethnic and cultural groups.

Grounded theory (Glaser, 1992) may be another way to help clinicians make accurate assessments of clients. In grounded theory we are not testing a predetermined belief (an hypothesis) as we normally would in most research. Instead, we are trying to come up with a theory about the client and the current problem the client is experiencing. Diagnosis develops through the following series of steps:

1. Collect sufficient information about the client including current functioning, past functioning, and the client's theory of why he or she is experiencing difficulty now.
2. Take notes that clarify the information we have collected and refer back to the notes to see patterns or themes in the information collected. To help see patterns and themes in the information collected create categories of issues, problems, and patterns.
3. Summarize the patterns and themes until an emerging theory about the client develops.
4. Test that theory against accumulating information to see if patterns and themes persist.
5. Begin to consider a diagnosis that, while theoretically accurate now, may change as more data is collected.
6. Test the diagnosis by determining if it fits the situation and whether it helps clients make sense of their experience and manage their lives more effectively.
7. Have a way to double check a diagnosis (i.e., audio taping an interview and letting a colleague go through the data collection to theory process, or continually checking your notes and comparing them to emerging information).
8. Frequently ask the client to provide feedback on the information accumulated to see if your data is accurate.

4.2 DIAGNOSTIC CHECKLISTS

Gawande (2007) reports the significant benefits of short checklists in hospital settings. Simply asking physicians to abide by several important questions posed about their practice with patients in emergency room and ICU facilities significantly reduced infections, length of stay in the facility, long-term improvement in conditions, and a number of other important areas of concern to medical practice. Gawande (2007) notes that by following simple procedures contained in a checklist "within the first 3 months of using the checklist, the infection rate in Michigan's ICU's dropped by 66% saving hospitals seventy-five million dollars in costs and more than 1500 lives, a figured sustained for over four years because of a stupid little checklist" (p. 94). While the following checklist may not have such dramatic results, it includes the four large areas of information needed to accurately access older adults proposed by Smyer (1984).

4.2.1 A checklist to determine the psychosocial functioning of older adults

1. Check for past and current illnesses, accidents, disabilities, surgeries, emotional problems, past counseling, hospitalizations and medications.
2. Have the client bring all medications they are taking for the initial interview including over-the-counter medications and vitamins.
3. If possible, have the client's physician write a brief history of the client's current medical condition.
4. Check on sleeping problems and length of time the client sleeps.
5. Check for language problems, hearing problems, and memory loss.
6. Check to find out how the client spends his/her day.
7. Find out the type of housing the client owns or rents, who if anyone lives with him or her, its cost, and the client's satisfaction with his/her lodging and ability to pay for it.
8. Ask the client to bring financial records to determine the client's current financial state.
9. Ask the client to bring a spouse, mate or friend to provide additional information about the client's life.
10. Get a complete psychosocial history including the current problem, its duration, and what the client has done to resolve the problem.

11. Get a complete past and current family history including relationships with parents, siblings, and children.
12. Check for past work experience, satisfaction with work and whether the client works at present.
13. Get a general life satisfaction indication from the client.
14. Check on the client's religious beliefs and practices.
15. Check for suicidal tendencies.
16. Check for alcohol and drug use.
17. Check to find out about friends and how if the client feels isolated or friendless.
18. Check for sexual problems, unprotected sex, STDS, and HIV/AIDS.

4.3 AN EVIDENCE-BASED PRACTICE PSYCHOSOCIAL ASSESSMENT USING THE STRENGTHS PERSPECTIVE WITH OLDER ADULT CLIENTS

4.3.1 Introduction

Rather than using a diagnostic label with older adult clients that may fail to accurately describe the client's unique qualities, a psychosocial assessment summarizes the relevant information we know about a client and places it into concise statements that allows other helping professionals to understand the client and his or her problem(s) as well as we do. Psychosocial assessments differ from DSM diagnostic categories in that they provide brief historical information about the possible cause of the problem. Included in the assessment are the client's strengths as well as the problems that might interfere with the client's life at present.

For those readers unfamiliar with the strengths perspective (also called positive psychology and the wellness model), Van Wormer (1999) describes the elements of the strength approach as follows:

> The first step in promoting the client's well-being is through assessing the client's strengths. A belief in human potential is tied to the notion that people have untapped resources – physically, emotionally, socially, and spiritually – that they can mobilize in times of need. This is where professional helping comes into play – in tapping into the possibilities, into what can be, not what is. (p. 51)

A key idea of the strengths perspective is that skills in one area of life can be transferred to other less functional areas of life. Contrary to the adage that people learn from their mistakes, they generally repeat their mistakes. Success is far more instructive and motivating than failure. Anderson (1997) suggests the benefits of focusing on the positive qualities of children who have been sexually abused. She believes that the focus of work should not be on the damage done to the child but on the child's survival abilities to cope with the abuse. This means that practitioners must look for themes of resilience in the "survival stories" of older clients and help them recognize the active role they played in their ability to survive serious life problems.

In Table 4.1, Orsulik-Jerus et al. (2003, p. 237) suggest a way of differentiating pathology models and the way they view important elements of treatment from wellness models such as the strengths perspective.

Table 4.1 Traditional versus Strength-Based Models

Traditional	vs.	Strength-based
Diagnostic assessment involves identifying symptoms and pathology		Assessment includes identifying strengths, uses a biopsychosocial model
Focus is on illness		Focus is on strengths
Counseling directed at suppressing negative symptoms		Counseling directed at supporting coping behavior, change, and growth
Emphasis on insight of emotional problems through understanding of past events		Emphasizes new possibilities, options, and amplifying successes
Client receives treatment		Client is active in treatment
Therapist is the expert		Therapist is a partner
Client is categorized and labeled		Each client is unique
Focus on what is wrong and why		Focus on what is right and how

A CASE STUDY: EVIDENCE-BASED PRACTICE AND THE ASSESSMENT PROCESS

This case study is used to show an evidence-based practice approach to assessing an older client experiencing life-long depression and social isolation. The outline used in the case is for illustrative purposes only. Under each heading there is a description of the information one might include. The important thing to remember is that the assessment provides information to other professionals. It necessarily includes all of the information relevant to the case. Some of that information might pertain to ongoing difficulties or prior life problems experienced by the client. Most important, however, is that it tries to be as objective as possible to support observations, impressions, initial diagnosis, and ultimately, treatment.

THE PSYCHOSOCIAL ASSESSMENT OUTLINE AND THE RELEVANT INFORMATION PERTAINING TO THE CASE

Section I: Brief description of the client and the problem

In this section of the psychosocial assessment, we should include relevant socio-demographic information about the client including the client's age, marital status, the composition of the client's family of origin and their current level of interaction, what the client is wearing, the client's verbal and non-verbal communications, his or her affect, and anything of significance that took place during the interview(s), including the defined problem(s). Interpretations are normally not made in this section. The following is an example of how this section might be written from an evidence-based practice perspective:

Since the death of her husband three years ago, Mrs. Joann Snyder, 75, has been in a state of extreme bereavement. She never leaves the house, won't answer calls from her children, often fails to take the dog out so that her apartment has a terrible smell, and is unwilling to talk to anyone about her depression.

Mrs. Snyder was referred to adult services by her daughter, Susan, after her daughter was called to her mother's home by the police because she wouldn't respond to neighbors who had not seen her in days and who knocked on her door to find out if she was all right. Before entering her mother's home she asked that an adult services worker accompany her and work with her mother because the mother–daughter relationship was troubled.

At the time the worker first met Mrs. Snyder, she was in bed and unable to move without great pain because of a hip injury she sustained in a fall two weeks earlier. With extraordinary effort she was able to get herself food or have it delivered, although the pain from her hip was extreme. Partially eaten food was strewn about the apartment and dog excrement was everywhere. Mrs. Snyder was taken from the home by ambulance to the hospital where she had her hip surgically repaired and remained on bed rest. The first sustained contact with the client took place in the hospital two days post-surgery.

Mrs. Snyder told the worker that she resented the intrusion into her life and at first would not talk to her. The worker noted that she was morbidly obese, her hair was unkempt, and she exuded considerable body odor. She wouldn't let the nurses bathe her. She ignored the worker for the first 30 minutes, occasionally looking at her and pursing her lips. Gradually, and in a fleeting way, she began to explain her life after her husband died. She told the worker she was extremely depressed and had hoped that she would die after her hip injury. She said the worker hadn't done her any favor by coming to the home and that Susan, her daughter, was not welcome to see her in the hospital.

QUESTIONS ABOUT THIS INITIAL INFORMATION

Question: How depressed is Mrs. Snyder?

Answer: Mrs. Snyder's behavior suggests serious depression. An aspect of the DSM-IV to consider in rating Mrs. Snyder's overall functioning is the Global Assessment Functioning Scale of the DSM-IV, also known as the GAF Score (APA, 1994, p. 32). The GAF Score ranges from 100 ("Superior functioning in a wide range of activities. Life problems never seem to get out of hand. Is sought after by others because of his or her many qualities. No symptoms") (APA, 1994, p. 32) to 10 and below ("Danger to self and to others. Inability to maintain hygiene and the possibility of suicidal acts") (APA, 1994, p. 32). In reviewing the GAF, an appropriate score for Mrs. Snyder might be in the 50–41 range: "Serious symptoms (e.g., suicidal ideation) or any impairment in social, occupational or school functioning (e.g., no friends)" (APA, 1994, p. 32). How serious is this score? It's serious enough to warrant treatment, and serious enough to worry about a more extreme depression and the possibility of suicide. Living for two weeks in severe pain and not asking for help suggests serious symptoms of social isolation, But we don't know for certain without more information. Let's see if we change our minds as we learn more about Mrs. Snyder.

Section II: Historical Issues

This section includes any past issues of importance in understanding the client's current problems. The following might be relevant points to include in the historical section of our report:

Her daughter Susan said that Mrs. Snyder has always been a difficult woman who is prone to depressions and can be very uncommunicative. After her father died, Susan was called to the mother's apartment on numerous occasions by the apartment manager or the police because of smells from the apartment and fear that she had become disabled or had died. For three years after her husband died Mrs. Snyder wouldn't let her two daughters or son inside the house, wouldn't answer calls, and refused to respond to the concerns of her children about her welfare.

In the second meeting in the hospital, Mrs. Snyder began to talk about the fears she'd had all of her life that something terrible would happen to her. Her parents were Holocaust survivors and she grew up in a home with two older brothers (now deceased) where everyone was fearful. Even the smallest deviation from planned schedules threw her parents into a panic. She described her parents as serious, fearful, pessimistic, and emotionally aloof. Stories of the Holocaust were regularly told to the children to keep them in line and to keep them hyper-vigilant so they could prevent any unforeseen problem that could arise and threaten their safety. Mrs. Snyder said that she could never remember a time when she fully trusted anyone or thought her life was safe. She admitted that her marriage had been rocky and that her relationships with her children were problematic. She knew things weren't good while they were growing up but felt unable to do anything about it. Perhaps, she admitted, she had been very depressed throughout their childhood. She had no friends and told the worker that she felt lonely and isolated. She wished she could have friends but didn't think she had the skills to make and keep them and, anyway, she said, "People always let you down. You can be sure of that."

Mrs. Snyder is an avid reader. Although she didn't go to college, she is highly educated in the classics and learned three languages on her own so that she could read books she admired in their original language. At the worker's suggestion, Mrs. Snyder was lent a laptop and shown how to access the Internet. After working on the computer for several days she remarked to the worker that she had found a few articles online about people just like her and would the worker like to hear about them. They chatted for a while about the articles. Mrs. Snyder said she could see that there was lots of "gold" online and maybe she could use the Internet to learn about herself. And she did. Each time the worker came back to see her Mrs. Snyder would point out similarities between herself and material in the articles she had read. She was particularly interested in the dynamics of children of survivors and how other people had the same upbringing that she did, but ended up differently. She wondered why, which led to long discussions of Mrs. Snyder's approach to coping with life.

Out of the blue Mrs. Snyder asked to see her two daughters, and the three of them talked an entire afternoon. Susan told the worker that it was thrilling to see how perceptive and intuitive her mother was. Her mother could see that she hadn't done much of a job of parenting and apologized to her daughters. She explained to them how frightened and depressed she'd been since her husband died, and how she thought the children hated her. Susan had never seen her mother so animated and thought it was the beginning of a much better relationship for both daughters.

After several months in a rehabilitation facility, the worker helped Mrs. Snyder prepare to go home. She had the apartment cleaned and the daughters stocked it with food. Mrs. Snyder had lost a great deal of weight during rehabilitation and felt certain that this would continue when she went home. The daughters agreed to see their mother every weekend. In the meantime, they hired someone to be with her part of the day to help her bathe, dress, and make certain she has sufficient food. The daughters also bought her a computer and she regularly goes on line to have long chats with other people who are having later-life medical problems. She says it's a godsend.

The worker and the public health nurse see Mrs. Snyder in her home every week to make certain she is in good physical and emotional condition. Before returning home from the rehab facility where Mrs. Snyder had been sent after a short hospital stay, Mrs. Snyder asked if the worker could help her "sort out" some things about herself that concerned her. Wondering if she could be more specific, Mrs. Snyder told the worker, "Sex always made me physically ill. Being touched, even by my children, made me feel dirty. I'd push them away instead of holding them like most mothers do. Loving someone seemed theoretical, but I could never feel the emotion that goes with love. I don't like or trust most people. I feel a lot of self-hatred. I've felt that way all of my life. I feel cynical about the world. I don't think I understand what it feels like to be happy. I've had thoughts about suicide almost all of my life. If I wasn't so concerned about going to hell, something I don't even believe in, I'd have done it a long time ago. I binge eat to the point of vomiting, and then I eat more. I can't stop myself. The thought of going outside alone frightens me. Sometimes I'm so scared I hide in the bathroom. I'm a miserable person and I hoped I'd die when I fell, but I didn't, and I can't go on this way."

Mrs. Snyder described a life in which her only connection to the world has been though books. "I feel as if I was laid down on the planet by aliens," she told her worker. "I've never felt part of anything. My husband put up with more from me than I can imagine. He was a good man in his own way. He left me alone to read and live in my little fantasy world. I didn't have to work and I could pursue my interest in languages and fiction. My children somehow made it into adulthood without me. Luckily for them, my husband Larry was good with the kids and gave of himself. Personally, I found them an inconvenience and resented my pregnancies. My parents were, as always, so negative that by the time I had the kids they'd gone through every imaginable illness and disease the kids could ever get and were convinced the babies would all be terribly deformed and retarded. My parents lived their life as if everything that could go wrong would. I was sick and tired of listening to them make me even more worried than I was. I really hated them.

"Something happened at some point in our family and we all went our own way. When Larry proposed to me, I accepted even though I felt nothing for him and worried that we would have sex, and that it would be despicable. And it was. We stopped after the 3 kids. I'd vomit when we'd have sex. It was pretty hard on Larry. Maybe he saw someone else. I didn't care. It didn't matter at all to me. I felt nothing. I still don't. I have curiosity about my life. I must have blocked out some things and I'd like to know what they are and why. I feel relieved that my girls are back in life. I was a lousy mother. They stuck with me when they shouldn't have. My mother was a terrible woman. Just thinking about her brings up many hurtful memories. I think she thought my father loved me more than her. Maybe he did. He was a fine man and he deserved better than that mean old bag.

"I never wanted to do anything with my life. I had no ambition, and I wasn't excited about anything except literature. The lives I could read about in books were much more exciting than mine. I guess I lived in a perpetual fantasy world. When I broke my hip, I didn't care if I lived or died. All I cared about was whether I had enough books to read. I know this makes me sound awful but what I'm telling you is the truth. I've read about how people feel emotions and I envy them. I feel nothing, I just exist. Maybe you're not doing me any favor by listening to my problems. I'm an old woman who hasn't done anything with her life, and I regret nothing.

"My brothers became big shots in business, but we stopped talking a long time ago. I never saw their kids or went to a wedding, or anything. Why should I? What they did to me as a kid was despicable. I can't talk about that now, but take it from me, it wasn't pretty. I hated my parents for letting it happen. The old bag probably put them up to it."

Questions

1. Question: Is there a relationship between parents who survive genocide and emotional problems in their children?

Answer: Sometimes. Baron et al. (1996) report that many clinicians who first saw survivors of the Holocaust believed that they would be very poor parents and that their children would suffer from a range of emotional difficulties. Children of survivors, however, have shown no pattern of mal-adjustment or psychopathology in most research. Last (1989) reviewed the research on Holocaust survivors and hypothesized that the effect of the Holocaust on parents, "will be manifest in the offspring of those who suffered, more often in the form of specific character formations than in any psychopathological symptoms" (p. 87). Does this negate the possibil-ity of a relationship between parental survival of genocide and depres-sion in a child? No, but neither is it necessarily a strong indicator.

2. Question: Has the lack of intimacy Mrs. Snyder experienced with her parents, her siblings, her husband and children led to depression?

Answer: People who grow up in an environment with limited intimacy sometimes develop what Weiss (1961) calls an "existential crisis." An exis-tential crisis usually develops after some important life event such as the death of loved ones or health problems. It may also develop without any apparent reason and usually does not move into a clinical depression. Clients with an existential depression lose their sense of newness in life and often feel isolated and withdrawn. They may think of the world as a place of suffering and obsess about the unhappiness they see around them. If Mrs. Snyder had an existential crisis it may also be seen as a pro-longed bereavement related to the death of the client's parents and the end of her marriage. As Weiss (1961) writes in paraphrasing Karen Horney, "[I]t [an existential crisis] is a remoteness of the client in crisis from his own feelings, wishes, beliefs and energies. It is a loss of feeling of being an active, determining force in his own life [and results in] an alienation from the real self" (p. 464).

3. Question: She doesn't tell us what her brothers did, but we suspect physical and/or sexual abuse. She also doesn't tell us what happened in the family that caused them all to disperse, but again, we wonder about abuse or something so traumatic that it split the family apart. Of course we only have Mrs. Snyder's version to rely on and it could be inaccurate. Assuming abuse *did* take place, could it have such a long-term impact?

Answer: If one can assume that any severe trauma will result in a degree of behavioral change in most people, and if the trauma is severe and continues for a prolonged period (as in the case of physical and sex-ual abuse), Ozer et al. (2003) suggest that PTSD will develop and sustain itself as a behavior when several primary reasons for developing PTSD exist, including the following:

1. a history of prior traumas;
2. existence of emotional problems prior to the traumatic event;
3. emotional problems in the victim's family of origin;
4. the extent a person believes the traumatic event will endanger his or her life;

5. the lack of a support system to help the client cope;
6. the level of emotional responsiveness of a person during and after the trauma; and,
7. the existence of a dissociative state during and following the trauma.

According to the authors, no single variable predicts PTSD but a cluster of variables strengthens the probability of developing. Would the symptoms last so long? Reports of lifetime rates of PTSD of between 30% and 50% have been noted in women who were sexually assaulted or raped (Foa et al., 1995; Meadows and Foa, 1998). The Harvard Health Letter (2002) reports that PTSD is most likely to occur in those people who have experienced some form of assault. Seventy percent of the patients in the Harvard Health Letter report who had current or lifetime PTSD said that the assault was their very worst traumatic experience. So, yes, it's possible that long-term sexual abuse by the brothers, if it happened, could be related to Mrs. Snyder's symptoms.

Section III: Diagnostic Statement

The diagnostic statement is a summary of the reasons the client is experiencing problems now. The diagnostic statement combines material from the prior two sections and summarizes the most important information into a brief statement. The following diagnostic statement was written after Mrs. Snyder's last day in a rehab facility and before returning to her own apartment:

Joann Snyder is a 75 year-old widowed mother of two adult daughters and a son who was seen initially because of her emotional and physical state after a fall in which her hip was broken leaving her unable to freely move about the house. Mrs. Snyder has a long history of isolation from her children and severe depression since the death of her husband three years ago. She says that she has always felt depressed and has been openly suicidal for many years, especially since her husband's death. She describes herself as emotionally distant, aloof, without friends, and unable to provide affection to others, particularly her children and husband. Her parents were Holocaust survivors whom she describes as cold and distant, and who focused on issues of safety using the terrible things that occurred to them during the Holocaust to reinforce their parenting of Mrs. Snyder and her two deceased older brothers. She indicates serious problems with her brothers, but doesn't describe what they were, and suggests a very poor relationship with her mother, even indicating that whatever the brothers did to her may have been initiated and approved of by her mother. She says her father was a fine man and deserved a much better wife than her mother.

Mrs. Snyder doesn't believe her two daughters care much for her. Both daughter's note the difficult time they've had with their mother throughout their lives, but especially since their father died. They describe her as cold, uninterested in having contact with them, and self-absorbed. The recent attempts on the part of the daughters and their mother to reconcile seem to be working. This is certainly a positive sign, as is the fact that an otherwise uncommunicative person has confided so much information to the worker, interacts with others via e-mail, and is now asking for help.

In summarizing the client's history and its impact on her, but remembering that we have no confirming evidence for much of what she says about her early life, it would appear that the cold, aloof family life she experienced, coupled with the possibility of physical or sexual abuse by her older brothers and a very poor relationship with her mother have led to serious intimacy issues, poor relationships with others, particularly her daughters and husband, severe depression with suicidal thoughts throughout her life, distrust of the motives of others, and social isolation.

Her husband's role in keeping Mrs. Snyder from an even more severe depression needs to be evaluated, but the evidence provided by the client and her daughters suggests that he was a stabilizing factor in the family and a potentially co-dependent relationship with his wife allowed Mrs. Snyder to continue her long-term behavior without any pressure to change. Once he died, her caretaker was lost and Mrs. Snyder fell into an even deeper depression.

There is almost no indication of happiness in her life other than the joy she gets from reading and a formidable intelligence that allows her to learn languages so that she can read books in their original language. She has no formal education yet she has read widely and, in conversations with the worker, spoke with considerable understanding about a number of writers who have written about psychology and psychiatry. She has begun to use the Internet to find reading material on subjects that seem related to her behavior and finds satisfaction in e-mailing people she has met online.

Given her desire to find out more about herself, her improved relationship with her daughters, and new friends made on the Internet, the prognosis seems good at this point, although lifelong depressions with thoughts of suicide and social isolation are always serious and could return. The worker will focus on helping her develop awareness of her behavior, on maintaining a positive relationship with her children, and on assessing changes in her behavior, which might indicate a return of depression and social withdrawal.

QUESTIONS

1. Question: Is it possible for grief to endure during the entirety of the three years since the death of her husband, and still play such a significant role in her current functioning?

Answer: Balk (1999) notes that bereavement (the loss of a significant person in one's life) can result in physical and emotional problems, the most significant of which may include:

> [I]ntense and long-lasting reactions such as fear, anger, and sorrow. Bereavement affects cognitive functioning (e.g., memory distortions, attention deficits, and ongoing vigilance for danger) and behavior (e.g., sleep disturbances, excessive drinking, increased cigarette smoking, and reckless risk taking). It impacts social relationships as outsiders to the grief become noticeably uncomfortable when around the bereaved. And bereavement affects spirituality by challenging the griever's very assumptions about the meaning of human existence. (Balk, 1999, p. 486)

Jacobs and Prigerson (2000) warn that bereavement sometimes develops into a complicated or prolonged grief lasting more than a year. The symptoms of complicated grief include intrusive thoughts about the deceased, numbness, disbelief that a loved one has passed away, feeling confused, and a diminished sense of security. Prolonged grief may be unresponsive to interpersonal therapy or to the use of antidepressants. So yes, prolonged bereavement can last three years and in Mrs. Snyder's case, longer without an intervention.

2. Question: This diagnosis is nothing more that a recap of what we already know. Wouldn't it be helpful to give Mrs. Snyder a diagnosis at the end so that we know what we're dealing with?

Answer: A diagnosis is a cluster of symptoms with indications of duration and severity. The medical model would insist that before we can treat, we need a solid diagnosis, much as we would if the client had a physical problem or an illness. Mrs. Snyder has a cluster of problems but we have seen changes in her behavior that make it difficult to know whether a diagnosis would be useful or accurate now. There are symptoms of PTSD (emotional numbing, hypervigilance, anxiety), of depression (suicidal thoughts and a form of slow suicide in which she allows her physical condition to deteriorate), and of schizoid personality disorder in which people are aloof from others, unable to enjoy close relationships, do not enjoy life, lack friends, and are cold, aloof and detached (DSM-IV, p. 641). It's hard to know which of these many likely diagnoses fits, and even if they all do, of what value they are in treatment while the client is currently showing indications of change.

Section IV: The Treatment Plan

The treatment plan describes the goals of treatment during a specific period of time and comes from the agreement made between the worker and the client in the contractual phase of treatment. In this example, 12 sessions are used over a three-month period, although in reality Mrs. Snyder has the right to continue or discontinue the contact with her worker at any time. Mrs. Snyder agreed to the following treatment plan:

1. To enlist Mrs. Snyder in a cooperative effort to find the best treatment approaches for her current problems by reading the existing literature and discussing it with the worker.
2. To help her understand and possibly resolve a prolonged absence of emotion and intimacy that seems related to a troubled relationship with her parents and brothers and has resulted in a persistent depression and social isolation.
3. To discuss issues of intimacy that might help in promoting new and more satisfying relationships.
4. To evaluate the extent of her depression and to possibly ask for a psychiatric consultation to consider medication to relieve persistent symptoms of depression.
5. To help her develop satisfying relationships with her children.
6. To encourage involvement in group activities, including self-help groups on bereavement and depression that might also help her develop better relationship skills.

QUESTIONS

1. Question: Doesn't the lack of a diagnosis limit our ability to treat Mrs. Snyder?

Answer: We don't know with certainty what Mrs. Snyder's condition really is, other than that she experiences depression and has feelings of aloofness and self-loathing. One way to objectify the process would be to determine her level of depression by using an instrument such as The Beck Depression Inventory (BDI) (Beck et al., 1961). The BDI would help determine the seriousness of the problem and evaluate any risk of suicide. The BDI has good reliability (0.80 to 0.90) and good validity for measuring depression, according to Wilcox et al. (1998). Another depression inventory, the CES-D (Radloff, 1977), is also a good instrument and has a high comparative correlation (0.70) with the BDI when the two instruments test the same people and the test results are compared (Wilcox et al., 1998). A second professional opinion might also help.

For the time being, let's consider the GAF Score of 50-41 as an indication of her current social functioning and let's assume that Weiss's description of an existential crisis is applicable. How might this affect our treatment? In describing treatment for an existential crisis, Weiss (1961) writes that, "To defrost, to open up, to experience and to accept himself becomes possible for the patient only in a warm, mutually trusting relationship in which, often for the first time in his life, he feels truly accepted as he is, accepted with those aspects of himself which early in life he had felt compelled to reject or repress" (p. 474). Weiss goes on to say that as treatment progresses, the client who may appear so devoid of self-awareness and who seems emotionally lacking in feeling and introspection will "begin to reveal surprising aliveness and depth, passionate longings, and strong feelings of loss" (p. 475).

2. Question: Isn't there a good chance that use of the right antidepressant might bring about behavioral changes without the need for therapy?

Answer: Mrs. Snyder wants to find out about herself. We hope that process leads to an improvement in functioning, but it may not and the depression may have a physical basis. The reason for a psychiatric consultation in the treatment plan is to make certain that Mrs. Snyder's behavior isn't bio-chemical in nature. If it is, then certainly the correct psychotropic medication is in order. The issues she has identified might do well with a combination of medication and psychotherapy. The research evidence seems to suggest that antidepressants alone are no more effective than therapy. However, we have no control over whether the client actually takes an antidepressant and no way to judge his or her functioning unless the client sees us often. That's why therapy can be highly beneficial since it keeps close tabs on the client and can help identify depression that seems to be non-responsive to medication or to therapy.

To help answer the question of the best efficacy of medication for depression versus the efficacy of therapy alone, several studies are provided that show the relationship between improvement in depression and the use of antidepressants and/or therapy.

STUDY 1

It is clear that antidepressant medications produce a 60% recovery rate when prescribed within proper dosages and for adequate duration. Depression-specific time-limited psychotherapies achieve similar outcomes, even with patients experiencing moderate to severe symptomatology. Two principles emerge from this body of work: (1) major depression should not be treated with anxiolytic medications alone or with long-term psychotherapy; and (2) patient preference for a particular guideline-based treatment should be considered when it is clinically and practically feasible. (Kopta, 1998, p. 2)

STUDY 2

The most frequently cited results were reported by the National Institute of Mental Health Treatment of Depression Collaborative Research Program. Two hundred-fifty unipolar depressed patients at three sites were randomly assigned to one of four conditions: cognitive-behavior therapy (CBT), interpersonal therapy (IPT), imipramine (a tricyclic antidepressant) plus clinical management (IMI-CM), and pill placebo with clinical management (PLA-CM). Results were generally as follows: (a) all four conditions resulted in significant improvement; (b) neither form of psychotherapy was superior to the other; (c) the only significant treatment difference for all patients occurred between IMI-CM and PLA-CM; (d) for the more severe cases, IMI-CM and IPT produced more improvement than PLA-CM whereas CBT did not; and (e) IMI-CM generally produced more rapid effects than the other conditions. (Kopta, 1999, Internet, p. 14)

SOME THOUGHTS ABOUT WHY CLIENTS CHANGE

Before we leave the treatment plan, perhaps a brief discussion of why clients change their behavior as a result of treatment might be helpful. McConnaughy et al. (1983) believe that client change requires both the worker and the client to be at the same state of readiness in understanding the client's problems and the emotional commitment to change them. Howard et al. (1993) suggest that clients start therapy in a state of demoralization. Through the development of trust, the therapist helps them identify their primary problems, instills hope, and helps them develop a sense of well-being. As their sense of well-being increases, problems that seemed unsolvable to the client can be discussed and remedied. Remediation suggests that clients practice new behaviors that reinforce change through stages of treatment. Howard et al. (1993) add,

> From a psychotherapy practice point of view, the phase model suggests that different change processes will be appropriate for different phases of therapy and that certain tasks may have to be accomplished before others are undertaken. It also suggests that different therapeutic processes may characterize each phase. Therapeutic interventions are likely to be most effective when they focus on changing phase-specific problems when those problems are most accessible to change. (p. 684)

Howard et al. (1996) caution that while these phases are distinct, they suggest different treatment goals and, "thus the selection and assessment of different outcome variables to measure progress in each phase" (p. 1061). These are, of course, untested ideas from the literature, but they may help in better understanding the change process with a client like Mrs. Snyder.

Section V: Contract

The contract is an agreement between the worker and the client that specifies the problems to be worked on in treatment, the number of sessions agreed on, and rules related to being on time, the length of each session, payment, and the cancellation policy. Many workers write up the contract and have both the client and worker sign it. Since the worker is visiting Mrs. Snyder once a week to evaluate her social and emotional functioning, the contract would be part of that arrangement. A contract with Mrs. Snyder might read as follows:

> Mrs. Snyder has agreed to meet with the worker in her home for 12 consecutive one-hour weekly sessions. She agrees that more meetings might be required. The effectiveness of treatment and the progress made will be evaluated after each session and at the end of the 12 sessions using client feedback and a depression instrument. Mrs. Snyder agrees to consult the research, share the research she's read with her worker, and to write summaries of what took place during each session with questions to be discussed in future sessions, and to send them to the worker by e-mail. The summaries will be provided to the therapist two days after a prior session, or sooner. After 12 sessions, the client and worker will jointly determine whether additional sessions are needed. Mrs. Snyder has agreed to other conditions in the contract- including the non-cancellation of session clause without 24 hours notice with a reason given in writing to the worker.

QUESTIONS

1. Question: Can significant change take place in 12 sessions?

Answer: Very often it can. Seligman (1995) found no difference in client satisfaction with treatment among clients who had been seen for an average of six months and those who had been seen for an average of two years. Kopta (1999) reports a study in which clients with severe substance abuse problems were provided 12 sessions using three different types of treatment (twelve-step-based counseling, psychodynamic therapy, and cognitive-behavioral therapy). The author writes, "Significant and sustained improvements in drinking outcomes were observed for all three groups" (p. 21). Fleming and Manwell (1998) report that people with alcohol-related problems including persistent depressions often receive counseling from primary care physicians or nursing staff in five or fewer standard office visits with very good results.

2. Question: Will Mrs. Snyder continue seeing the worker for 12 sessions? She seems to have a contrarian's approach to life and might discontinue treatment at any point.

Answer: No doubt she might, but in the meantime she may have gained a great deal. Her introduction to the Internet may also help if she discontinues treatment. Clients stop treatment when they believe it isn't doing them any good or when the subject matter becomes too troubling. Mrs. Snyder intellectualizes at a very high level and uses the information gained in treatment to satisfy her curiosity. Will the emotions she begins to feel affect the continuation of treatment? It's hard to know whether treatment will improve her emotional life. The general idea behind treatment is to develop introspection and improve social and emotional functioning. Whether this can happen without some change in the aloof, unemotional way she approaches life is hard to say. The strengths approach would say that clients change in their own way, at their own pace, and for reasons that make sense to them. If Mrs. Snyder just wants closure on some troubling issues in her past, that's as good a reason to initiate treatment as any. If it helps with closure but doesn't change her behavior, that's unfortunate but still, the client has the right to determine how they will use treatment, understanding the consequences if treatment isn't properly used to change troubling behaviors. That's as much as we can expect. It is likely Mrs. Snyder will continue seeing the therapist as long as the contact is interesting. When it stops being interesting, she may look elsewhere for information including people she meets online, books, and articles on the Internet. Who's to say this isn't as effective a form of treatment as direct therapy?

One additional type of treatment that may work with Mrs. Snyder is Bibliotherapy. Bibliotherapy is the use of literature to facilitate the therapeutic process. Myers (1998) defines Bibliotherapy as "a dynamic process of interaction between the individual and literature, which emphasizes the reader's emotional response to what has been read" (p. 243). Pardeck (1995) gives six goals of Bibliotherapy: (1) to provide information; (2) to gain insight; (3) to find solutions; (4) to stimulate discussion of problems; (5) to suggest new values and attitudes; and (6) to show clients how others have coped with problems similar to their own. "Bibliotherapy provides metaphors for life experiences that help clients verbalize their thoughts and feelings and learn new ways to cope with problems" (Myers, 1998, p. 246). Suggesting books with themes that resonate with Mrs. Snyder might certainly have an impact and could be used for discussion of their relevance to her life.

Discussion of the Case

Mrs. Snyder presents a confusing assortment of symptoms. She describes herself as aloof, unemotional, detached from people (most of whom she doesn't like), and incapable of intimacy. These are not positive indications of someone who would benefit from treatment. And yet, she has asked for help and has begun showing an improved relationship with her daughters. On the assumption that we can all benefit from self-awareness the worker is helping her develop insight into her behavior. She has a variety of options available that might help her achieve her goal.

While much of the current literature seems to suggest that a form of cognitive-behavioral therapy works best with depression, it's not entirely certain that it would work well with Mrs. Snyder. The active and directive nature of cognitive therapy could remind the client of similar communication patterns used by her domineering parents. One approach that might be worth considering is the strengths perspective. Glicken (2004) defines the strengths perspective as, "a way of viewing the positive behaviors of all clients by helping them see that problem areas are secondary to areas of strength and that out of what they do well can come helping solutions based upon the successful strategies they use daily in their lives to cope with a variety of issues and problems" (p. 3).

Understanding her parents and their behavior could help Mrs. Snyder better understand herself. The strengths approach tries to frame behavior as positively as possible and, "[w]hile clients need to understand any harm done to them by parental conduct and to understand its impact, they benefit from a more complete and potentially positive view of their parents" (Glicken, 2004, p. 5). The ability to understand her parents as they might have explained and defended their own behavior is an important aspect of treatment with Mrs. Snyder and could help satisfy her "curiosity" about her life.

By involving Mrs. Snyder in a cooperative relationship where she works closely with the worker in trying to understand herself, She may come to learn how one develops and maintains relationships. Her treatment also calls for a very empathic approach, one which Saleebey (2000) believes, "obligates us to understand . . . to believe that everyone (no exceptions here) has external and internal assets, competencies and resources" (p.128), and that these resources, regardless of how dormant or untested they might be, are able to provide the wise helper with the ability to facilitate the relationship in a way that permits the client to work through relationship concerns and discomforts.

4.4 SUMMARY

This chapter discusses the difficulty of making correct and accurate diagnoses for emotional problems with older adults and the many clinician biases that may result in incorrect diagnosis. An example of a psychosocial assessment that focuses on client strength is provided. Used correctly, a psychosocial assessment can provide the practitioner with an understanding of the connecting elements that have created the current crisis in a client's life. It can also help clinicians develop strategies that may move the older client in positive ways. A key to the use of the psychosocial assessment is to recognize positive client behaviors and to support assumptions about the cause of a problem and the most efficacious treatment with a recognition of the best evidence available from the research literature.

4.5 QUESTIONS FROM THE CHAPTER

1. We're assuming Mrs. Snyder is depressed because of the serious problems she had with her family. Are there alternative reasons for her depression?
2. We tend to assume that children of parents who have been traumatized will suffer negative consequences because parental traumas create problems in parenting. Do you believe that's necessarily true?
3. Many survivors of the Holocaust went on to live healthy, normal, and productive lives. Don't we make the mistake of assuming that most people aren't resilient enough to cope with severe traumas when, in fact, they are?
4. We often think of depression as biochemical when it continues on for long periods of time. Given the complexities of her problem, do you think medication will help Mrs. Snyder reduce her symptoms of depression?
5. The GAF score of 50–41 seems high for someone who spent two weeks alone with a broken hip and didn't call anyone for help. What might a more accurate GAF score be, in your opinion?

REFERENCES

Anderson, K. M. (1997, November). Uncovering survival abilities in children who have been sexually molested. *Families in Society: The Journal of Contemporary Human Services, 78,* 592–599.

Balk, D. E. (1999). Bereavement and spiritual change. *Death Studies, 23*(6), 485–493.

Baron, L., Eisman, H., Scuello, M., Veyzer, A., & Lieberman, M. (1996, September). Stress resilience, locus of control, and religion in children of Holocaust victims. *Journal of Psychology, 130*(5).

Beck, A. T., Ward, C. H., Mendelson, M., Mock, J., & Erbaugh, J. (1961). An inventory for measuring depression. *Archives of General Psychiatry, 4,* 561–571.

Cloud, J. (2003, January 30). How we get labeled. *Time, 16*(13), 102–106.

Croskerry, P. (2002). Achieving quality clinical decision-making: Cognitive strategies and detection of bias. *Academic Emergency Medicine, 9(11), 1108–1115.*

Edelstein, B., & Kalish, K. (1999). Clinical assessment of older adults. In J. C. Cavanaugh & S. Whitbourne (Eds.), *Gerontology: An interdisciplinary perspective* (pp. 269–304). New York: Oxford University Press.

Fleming, M., & Manwell, L. B. (1998). Brief intervention in primary care settings: A primary treatment method for at-risk, problem, and dependent drinkers. *Alcohol Research and Health, 23*(2), 128–137.

Foa, E. B., Hearst-Ikeda, D., & Perry, K. J. (1995). Evaluation of a brief cognitive-behavioral program for the prevention of chronic PTSD in recent assault victims. *Journal of Consulting and Clinical Psychology, 63,* 948–955.

Gentilello, L. M., Donovan, D. M., Dunn, C. W., & Rivara, F. P. (1995). Alcohol interventions in trauma centers: Current practice and future directions. *JAMA, 274*(13), 1043–1048.

Gladwell, M. (2007, November 12). Dangerous minds: Criminal profiling made easy. *The New Yorker, LXXXIII*(35), 36–45.

Glaser, B. G. (1992). *Basics of grounded theory analysis: Emergence vs forcing.* Mill Valley, CA: Sociology Press.

Glicken, M. D. (2004). *Using the strengths perspective in social work practice.* Boston, MA: Pearson Education, Inc.

Goodstein, R. K. (1985). Common clinical problems in the elderly: Camouflaged by ageism and atypical presentation. *Psychiatric Annals, 15,* 299–312.

Groopman, J. (2007, January 29). What's the trouble: How doctors think. *The New Yorker, LXXXII*(47), 36–41.

Guidelines for Psychological Practice with Older Adults. American Psychological Association Approved as APA Policy by the APA Council of Representatives, August, 2003 American Psychological Association, 750 First Street, NE, Washington, DC 20002–4242.

Harvard Mental Health Letter (2002). . What causes post-traumatic stress disorder: Two views. *Harvard Mental Health Letter, 19*(4), 8.

Haverkamp, B. (1993). Confirmatory bias in hypothesis testing for client-identified and counselor self-generated hypotheses. *Journal of Consulting Psychology, 40,* 305–315.

Henry, D. L. (1999, September). Resilience in maltreated children: Implications for special needs adoptions. *Child Welfare, 78*(5), 519–540.

Howard, K. I., Lueger, R. J., Mailing, M. S., & Martinovich, Z. (1993). A phase model of psychotherapy outcome: Causal mediation of change. *Journal of Consulting and Clinical Psychology, 61,* 678–685.

Howard, K. I., Moras, K., Brill, P. B., Martinovich, Z., & Lutz, W. (1996). Evaluation of psychotherapy: Efficacy, effectiveness, and client change. *American Psychologist, 51,* 1059–1064.

Jacobs, S., & Prigerson, H. (2000). Psychotherapy of traumatic grief: A review of evidence for psychotherapeutic treatments. *Death Studies, 24*(6), 479–496.

Kopta, S. M. (Annual 1999). Individual psychotherapy outcome and process research: Challenges leading to greater turmoil or a positive transition? <http://www.find-articles.com/cf_0/m0961/1999_Annual/54442307/print.jhtm>. *Annual review of psychology.*

Last, U. (1989). The transgenerational impact of holocaust trauma: Current state of the evidence. *International Journal of Mental Health, 17*(4), 72–89.

McConnaughy, E. A., Prochaska, J. O., & Velcer, W. F. (1983). Stages of change in psychotherapy: Measurement and sample profile. *Psychotherapy: Theory, Research and Practice, 20*, 375–388.

McLaughlin, J. E. (2002). Reducing diagnostic bias. *Journal of Mental Health Counseling, 24*(3), 256–270.

Meadows, E. A., & Foa, E. B. (1998). Intrusion, arousal, and avoidance: Sexual trauma survivors. In V. Follette, I. Ruzek, & F. Abueg (Eds.), *Cognitive-behavioral therapies for trauma* (pp. 100–123). New York: Guilford.

Monti, P. M., Colby, S. M., Barnett, N. P., et al. (1999). Brief intervention for harm reduction with alcohol-positive older adolescents in a hospital emergency department. *Journal of Consulting and Clinical Psychology, 67*(6), 989–994.

Myers, J. E. (1998). Bibliotherapy and the DCT: Co-constructing the therapeutic metaphor. *Journal of Counseling and Development, 76*, 225–234.

Orsulik-Jerus, S., Shepard, J. B., & Britton, P. J. (2003). Counseling older adults with HIV/AIDS: A strengths-based model of treatment. *Journal of Mental health Counseling, 25*(3), 233–244.

Ozer, E. J., Best, S. R., Lipsey, T. L., & Weiss, D. S. (2003). Predictors of posttraumatic stress disorder and symptoms in adults: A meta-analysis. *Psychological Bulletin, 129*(1), 52–73.

Pardeck, J. T. (1995). Bibliotherapy's innovative approach for helping children. *Early Childhood Development and Care, 110*, 83–88.

Radloff, L. S. (1977). The CES-D Scale: A self-report depression scale for research in the general population. *Journal of Applied Psychological Measures, 1*(3), 385–401.

Riley, B. B., Perna, R., & Tate, DG. (1998). Spiritual patients have a better quality of life than those who aren't. *Modern Medicine, 66*(5), 45–48.

Robertson, J., & Fitzgerald, L. F. (1990). The (mis) treatment of men: Effects of client gender role and life-style on diagnosis and attribution of pathology. *Journal of Counseling Psychology, 37*, 3–9.

Saleebey, D. (2000). Power to the people; strength and hope. *Advancements in Social Work, 1*(2), 127–136.

Schulberg, C. (2001, June 10). Treating depression in primary care practice: Applications of research findings <http://www.findarticles.com/cf_0/m0689/6_50/75995854/print.jhtml>. *Journal of family practice.*

Schlossberg, N. K. (1990). Training counselors to work with older adults. *Generations, 14*(1), 7–11.

Seligman, M. E. P. (1995). The effectiveness of psychotherapy: The consumers report study. *American Psychologist, 50*(12), 965–974.

Sigal, J. J., & Weinfeld, M. (2001). Do children cope better than adults with potentially traumatic stress? A 40-year follow-up of Holocaust survivors. *Psychiatry, 64*(1), 69–80.

Smyer, M. A. (1984). Life transitions and aging: Implications for counseling older adults. *The Counseling Psychologist, 12*(2), 1728.

Van Wormer, K. (1999, June). The strengths perspective: A paradigm for correctional counseling. *Federal Probation, 63*(1).

Verwoerdt, A. (1976). *Clinical geropsychiatry.* Baltimore, MD: Williams and Wilkins Co.

Weiss F.M. In Josephson E., & Josephson M. (Eds.), (1961). *Man alone.* New York: Laurel (pp. 463–479).

Weiss, J. R., Weiss, B., Hanns, S. S., Granger, D. A., & Morton, T. (1995). Effects of psychotherapy with children and adolescents revisited: A metaanalysis of treatment outcomes. *Psychological Bulletin, 117,* 450–468.

Whaley, A. L. (2001). Cultural mistrust: An important psychological construct for diagnosis and treatment of African Americans. *Psychology: Research and Practice, 32*(6), 555–562.

Wilcox, H., Prodromidis, M., & Scafidi, F. (1998). Correlations between BDI and CES-D in a sample of adolescent mothers. (Beck Depression Inventory; Center for Epidemiologic Studies Depression Scale) <http://www.findarticles.com/cf_0/m2248/131_33/53368535/p1/article.jhtml?term=beck+depression+inventory>. Fall: Series *Adolescence.*

Chapter five

Evidence-Based Practice and the Client-Worker Relationship with Older Adults

5.1 INTRODUCTION

This chapter considers the significance of the therapeutic relationship in effective counseling and psychotherapy with older adults and offers evidence that the relationship is a key factor in helping older adults, who tend to personalize the relationship with workers to an even greater degree than do younger clients.

Evidence-based practice (EBP) believes in the need to form a positive alliance with clients to facilitate change. This requires a cooperative and equal relationship with clients, particularly older clients who have a wealth of knowledge about life and may have achieved at very high levels of success. EBP also suggests that we act in a facilitative way to help clients gather information and rationally and critically process it. This differs from authoritarian approaches that assume the worker knows more about the client than the client does, and that the worker is the sole judge of what is to be done in the helping process. Gambrill (1999) points out that one of the most important aspects of EBP is the sharing of information with clients and the cooperative relationship that ensues.

In recognizing the importance of the relationship, Warren (2001) reports that "The relationship between the quality of the patient-therapist relationship and the outcome of treatment has been one of the most consistently cited findings in the empirical search for the basis of psychotherapeutic efficacy" (p. 357). Writing about the power of the therapeutic relationship, Saleebey (2000) argues that "If healers are seen as non-judgmental, trustworthy, caring and expert, they have some influential tools at hand, whether they are addressing depression or the disappointments and pains of unemployment" (p. 131). In a review of EBP for psychotherapy, Kopta et al. (1999) conclude that the relationship is of key importance in the helping process, while Greenfield et al. (1985) note the beneficial effects of increasing a patient's involvement with their own care as a result of a positive client–worker relationship.

5.2 DEFINING THE THERAPEUTIC RELATIONSHIP

Brent (1998) defines psychotherapy as a "modality of treatment in which therapists and patients work together to ameliorate psychopathological conditions and functional impairment by focusing on (1) the therapeutic relationship; (2) the patient's attitudes, thoughts, affect, and behavior; and (3) social context and development" (p. 1). Entwistle et al. (1998) believe that clients are actively involved in decisions regarding their treatment in four ways: (1) through the care a patient will or will not receive; (2) through the research information indicating the effectiveness of certain interventions, including their risks and benefits; (3) through the use of recommended approaches showing good research validity, or doing nothing; and (4) through involvement in all decisions regarding treatment. The Evidence-Based Practice Working Group of the American Medical Association (1992) writes that all EBP practitioners must be sensitive to the emotional needs of clients and that "[u]nderstanding patients' suffering and how that suffering can be ameliorated by the caring and compassionate practitioner are fundamental requirements for practice" (p. 2422). The Working Group also calls for more research to better understand how the interaction between clients and practitioners affects the outcome of treatment.

In an assessment of a study done using *Consumers Report* data on the effectiveness of psychotherapy, Seligman (1995) found that clients have the wisdom to "shop around" for therapists who meet their own particular needs, and that the type of therapy they receive is less important than the intangible aspects of whether they like the therapist and think that he or she will be able to help them. Seligman writes, "Patients in psychotherapy in the field often get there by active shopping, entering a kind of treatment they actively sought with a therapist they screened and chose" (p. 970).

Commenting on the importance of the therapeutic relationship in the change process and the hope that research will find evidence of the best fit between clients and the type of alliances that work best, Warren (2001) suggests that research on therapeutic relationships, "make[s] possible the development of treatment protocols that can then increase [treatment] efficacy, influence the training of psychotherapists, and provide standard treatment protocols for the purposes of further treatment process research" (p. 357).

Orlinsky et al. (1994) report that there are five variables that have consistently been demonstrated to positively affect the quality of both the therapeutic alliance and treatment effectiveness: (a) the overall quality of the therapeutic relationship; (b) the skill of the therapist; (c) patient cooperation versus resistance; (d) patient openness versus defensiveness; and (e) the duration of treatment.

Keith-Lucas (1972) defines the relationship as "the medium, which is offered to people in trouble and through which they are given an opportunity to make choices, both about taking help and the use they will make of it" (p. 47). Keith-Lucas says that the key elements of the helping relationship are "mutuality, reality, feeling, knowledge, concern for the other person, purpose, the fact that it takes place in the here and now, its ability to offer something new and its nonjudgmental nature" (p. 48).

In describing the significant elements of the relationship, Bisman (1994) says that therapeutic relationships are a form of "belief bonding" between the worker and the client, and that both parties need to believe that "the worker has something applicable for the client, the worker is competent, and that the client is worthwhile and has the capacities to change" (p. 77). Hamilton (1940) suggests that bonding takes place when the clinician and client work together and that "[t]reatment starts only when mutual confidence is established, only when the client accepts your interest in him and conversely feels an interest in you" (pp. 189–190).

Weiss et al. (1995) report that clients are highly motivated to resolve their problems and that they actively work throughout their treatment to recall experiences and obtain knowledge that will help them so that they can coach their therapist about what needs to been done and the best way to do it. The effective therapist recognizes the significance of client coaching and rather than seeing it as controlling or divisive, accepts it as an important part of the client's need for significant involvement in the process. Writing about the importance of the relationship, Glicken (2004) says that

> The relationship is a bond between two strangers. It is formed by an essential trust in the process and a belief that it will lead to change. The worker's expertise is to facilitate communications, enter into a dialogue with the client about its meaning, and help the client decide the best ways of using the information found in searches for best evidence. (p. 50)

Not all older clients like a cooperative relationship. Older adult clients who view the therapist as an authority figure may want advice and expect the clinician to be an expert in the issues that are troubling them, while other clients may want a prolonged analysis of the reasons for their current problems. What the client wants and needs is primary, and the worker should be responsive to the needs and desires of the client while helping him or her develop skills in working cooperatively. As Saleebey (1996) suggests:

> [H]ow social workers encounter their fellow human beings is critical. They must engage individuals as equals. They must be willing to meet them eye-to-eye and to engage in dialogue and a mutual sharing of knowledge, tools, concerns, aspirations, and respect. The process of coming to know is a mutual and collaborative one. (p. 303)

In describing the client-centered approach with older adults, Dacey and Newcomer (2005) write that forming a relationship with the older client requires that we establish rapport, set an agenda for discussion, respect the client's freedom of choice, and by carefully listening to the client, seek to understand and encourage the client to make his or her own decisions. "While practitioners can give 'advice' as part of the counseling intervention, this should be provided in a nonjudgmental manner, and only when the client has stated a willingness to hear it" (Dacey and Newcomer, 2005, p. 199).

5.3 EVIDENCE OF THE IMPORTANCE OF THE THERAPEUTIC RELATIONSHIP TO TREATMENT OUTCOMES

Noting the importance of the therapeutic alliance in the professional literature, Gelso and Hayes (1998) wonder if we have a clear understanding of what is meant by the worker–client relationship, and write, "Because the therapy relationship has been given such a central place in our field for such a long period of time, one might expect that many definitions of the relationship have been put forth. In fact, there has been little definitional work" (p. 5). But in a review of EBP for psychotherapy, Kopta et al. (1999) say that the relationship is of key importance in the helping process. Horvath and Greenberg (1994) found research evidence of the central role of the relationship in successful therapies. Major advances, according to Horvath and Greenberg (1994), have been made in (1) understanding the important role of relationships in the helping process; (2) having a better concept of how one operationalizes the relationship for research purposes; (3) having an increased awareness of variables prior to treatment that suggest potential for a successful therapeutic relationship; and (4) understanding the ways in which the relationship may change as treatment progresses, including "ruptures" in the relationship.

Krupnick et al. (1996) evaluated data from the large-scale National Institute of Mental Health Treatment of Depression Collaborative Research Program, which compared treatments for depression. The authors found that a positive therapeutic relationship was predictive of treatment success for all conditions. In another large study of diverse forms of therapy for alcoholism, the therapeutic relationship was also significantly predictive of success (Connors et al. 1997). Horvath and Symonds (1991) note that a positive relationship between scores on the quality of the initial (early) relationship and positive outcomes have been repeatedly found regardless of how the relationship is described by the practitioner. Kopta et al. (1999) write that

> Bordin (1994) argued that – regardless of the modality – the alliance always involves agreement on tasks and goals as well as a sense of compatibility or bonding. This latter viewpoint has been confirmed in the Working Alliance Inventory (Horvath, 1994). Both Luborsky's and Bordin's programs have consistently found a predictive association between alliance [relationship] and outcome. (p. 8)

Commenting further on the importance of the relationship in outcome studies of therapy, Brent (1998) reports that "[t]he contribution of therapeutic empathy and a good working alliance to positive clinical outcome has been demonstrated in several clinical trials of adult patients (Burns and Nolen-Hoeksema, 1992; Cooley and Lajoy, 1980; Luborsky et al., 1985; Murphy et al., 1984)" (p. 2). Brent goes on to say that

"From the patients' points of view, provision of support, understanding, and advice have been reported as most critical to good outcome (Cooley and Lajoy, 1980; Murphy et al., 1984)" (p. 2). In further comments about the relationship and effective therapeutic outcomes, Brent (1998) reports that, "The adult psychotherapy literature strongly supports the central role of the therapeutic relationship and therapeutic empathy in mediating the efficacy of treatment across many treatment models and psychopathological conditions" (p. 8). Finally, Brent writes that

> There appears to be a reciprocal relationship between therapist and patient behavior in both good and poor outcome psychotherapy. According to Henry et al., (1986) in "good outcome" therapy, the therapist is described as "helping and protecting, affirming and understanding," whereas the patient is seen as "disclosing and expressing." In "poor outcome" psychotherapy, the therapist tends to be "blaming and belittling," whereas the patient is depicted as "walling off and avoiding." Not surprisingly, therapists tend to attribute success to technique, whereas patients attribute a good outcome to the therapist's support and understanding (Feifel and Eells, 1963; Mathews, Johnson, Shaw, and Geller, 1974). (Brent, 1998, p. 2)

5.4 SPECIAL CONCERNS ABOUT THE THERAPEUTIC RELATIONSHIP WITH OLDER ADULTS

Myers and Harper (2004) suggest that "common life experiences and transitions in later life often create specific needs for counseling" (p. 208). The authors note that each of the life transitions and problems experienced by older adults require problem-solving skills that may or may not work, particularly when there are multiple transitions requiring, in many cases, the need for counseling interventions. Counselors are usually younger than their clients and need to consider the "impact of differences in age and life experience on the counseling relationship" (p. 208). The authors caution that it may take longer to build rapport, particularly in clients who are reluctant to seek help (see Chapter 9 on elder abuse clients as an example). Older clients may not be familiar with counseling, or they may have problems discussing and dealing with feelings, as is sometimes the case with older adults from more traditional cultures and for male clients. The authors point out that physical limitations may require changes in the length of sessions, the assessment process, and when there are cognitive or sight impairments, the use of standardized assessment measures that require reading.

It may also be wise to focus discussion on a single topic and not let the session flow into other issues, since memory may be impaired and too many subjects may cause confusion.

Myers and Harper (2004) believe that older persons often view human services workers in the same way they view medical personnel, anticipating that the relationship will be hierarchical and directive and that they will experience some degree of difficulty coping with relationships that ask their opinion or give the client a great deal of personal authority. This can be dealt with by explaining how the clinician works and why it is so important for the client to have maximum input. Often, however, older clients are very therapy-savvy, having seen therapy on television and in various films and dramas. The authors also note that young-old adults, those aged 50 to 75, tend to "share more common concerns with younger persons, although the dynamics of the aging process complicate treatment planning even for those older adults, regardless of age, who remain physically healthy."

Woolfe and Biggs (1997) confirm that therapists frequently avoid working with older adults and suggest that age bias among therapists can be understood by looking at the following issues of counter transference, first described by Knight (1986, 1996a, 1996b):

1. **Parental counter transference:** "The therapist may find clients who remind them of their own mother or father, which may lead to over-commitment to seeing a client change; irrational anger with a client; and feeling wounded if the client questions their expertise" (p. 190).

2. **Grandparent counter transference:** This involves a somewhat "fuzzily" perceived older adult whom the therapist must protect from others, especially the therapist's parents. Grandparent counter transference can be problematic when it clouds the therapist's judgment and stops them from seeing the seriousness of an older adult's problems. "Grandparent fantasies can also be negative, leading the counselor into being overly ready to see the older person as senile, complaining and making irrational demands of a good, kind, younger family that must be protected" (p. 190).

Woolfe and Biggs (1997) suggest that the way therapists view older clients and the general lack of research on therapy with the elderly indicate a "tendency to perceive old age in stereotyped and negative ways with the result that later-life potential is often severely underestimated" (p. 193).

Morgan (2003) believes that age differences between the client and therapist may lead the client to relate to the therapist as a son or a daughter. Morgan (p. 1593) writes

> Less obvious may be more subtle transference manifestations occurring around issues of dependency. For instance, a healthier elderly patient who sees the therapist as a parent or an educator may sell short his or her own abilities. Some frail elderly persons may see the therapist as a rescuer, whereas other frail elderly persons may feel as though the therapist represents an envied competitor with whom they can no longer compete, thereby leading them to view therapy as a demeaning circumstance. Romantic transferences, with their unrequited nature, can also be a source of humiliation for the patient. Awareness of these and other transference possibilities among older patients is important in order to allow therapy to progress.

Morgan (2003) goes on to suggest that a therapist's fears of aging may prompt memories of parents or grandparents that affect the work done with older adults, particularly if those memories are painful. Another relationship problem occurs when an older adult's feelings of hopelessness stimulate feelings of hopelessness in the therapist, often negating a better understanding of the client's feelings of vulnerability and leading the therapist to become punitive or withdrawing needed help from the client.

According to the Guidelines for Psychological Practice with Older Adults (APA, 2003), clinicians have a number of inaccurate stereotypes of older adults that may contribute to negative bias and affect the delivery of services, including: (1) with age inevitably comes senility; (2) older adults are likely to have higher rates of mental illness and depression; (3) older adults do badly in the workplace; (4) most older adults are frail and ill; (5) older adults are socially isolated and lonely; (6) older adults have no sexual desires or need for intimacy; and (7) older adults are inflexible, rigid, and stubborn. The report believes that these views "become self-fulfilling prophecies, leading to misdiagnosis of disorders, inappropriately decreased expectations for improvement, and to the lack of preventive actions and treatment" (p. 5). Some clinicians may avoid serving older adults because doing so evokes discomfort with their own aging or their relationships with parents or other older family members, a phenomenon sometimes termed "gerophobia." The report suggests that

> [P]aternalistic attitudes and behavior can potentially compromise the therapeutic relationship and reinforce dependency. Positive

stereotypes (e.g., the viewpoint that older adults are "cute," "child-like," or "grandparentlike"), which are often overlooked in discussions of age-related biases, can also adversely affect the assessment and therapeutic process and outcomes. (p. 6)

Culture and ethnicity also play an important role in developing relationships with older clients. For example, Latino clients with traditional or immigrant backgrounds usually take time to get to know the worker and talk around the problem. This is partly done as a way of gauging the worker's competence, but it also serves as a way of processing the problem in a manner that is familiar to the client. The client may also be very suspicious of the worker's motives. Indirectness helps the client maintain control over the interview until the worker can be better evaluated for his or her competence and level of kindness.

Feelings are highly valued in many cultures. With Latino clients, one approach to making feelings part of the therapeutic relationship is to tell the client that you will communicate with them, "de corazon a corazon", or, heart to heart. In Mexico, this concept of a close personal relationship in which true feelings can be communicated has various levels of meaning. It is sometimes associated with the process called "el desague de las penas," (unburdening oneself) or what North American therapists might call venting. It may also be a part of the process of opening one's soul to a *compadre* or a close personal friend so that the friend can see inside a person's heart and therefore feel his or her sorrow and despair. Allowing Latino clients to unburden themselves may significantly improve the quality of work with older Latino clients.

Stickle and Onedera (2006) write that, as part of the therapeutic relationship, "[o]lder clients may need to be educated on the therapeutic process including expectations, the expression of feelings, length of therapy, work toward goals, and confidentiality" (p. 43). In discussing depressed older clients the authors believe that older clients may need physical contact to reinforce verbal interaction, and suggest actions such as "stroking the individual's arm or shoulder, holding a hand for a while or touching a forehead, or simply leaning toward the client" (p. 43). According to the authors, use of physical contact suggests that you value them and that it may indicate to older clients the nature of the work we do and its importance in resolving the client's problems. This approach should be used with caution because it can also be interpreted as condescension.

Bergin and Walsh (2005) believe that one of the most important aspects of the client–worker relationship with older clients is to impart hope in older clients who often experience despair because of failing health, the death of loved ones, and diminished abilities to do what came so easily when they were younger. Dufault and Martocchio (1985) define hope as being "characterized by a confident yet uncertain expectation of achieving a future good, which, to the hoping person, is realistically possible and personally significant" (p. 380). In attempting to define hope in a therapeutic context, Farran et al. (1995) summarize hope as an essential way of feeling, thinking, behaving and relating to oneself and one's world that is "fluid in its expectations and in the event that the desired object or outcome does not occur, hope can still be present" (p. 6).

Bergin and Walsh (2005) view the worker as an "ambassador of hope" whose knowledge and skill will make the client's life better. Snyder (1994) suggests that clients' hopes for a successful outcome are fuelled by the therapist's explicit positive messages about treatment prognosis. Buechler (1995), on the other hand, sees hope as an ongoing process throughout therapy, which is engendered by the client's experience of a therapist who struggles with problems without giving up, and who maintains "humor and courage in situations that seem to inspire neither" (p. 72). Bergin and Walsh (2005) believe that most older adult clients have experienced positive relationships in the past that can be mirrored "[I]n the therapeutic dyad where a therapeutic rapport is easily established. The client will be able to recount times in their life when their hopes have been fulfilled which can be used by the clinician to 'challenging unrealistic hopes' and the reinstallation of realistic hope" (p. 11). Attaining realistic hope can be achieved by

> helping the client to adjust to his/her limitations, while "reinstalling" the hope that life may still be satisfying. The reinstallation of hope can also be seen to play an essential part in bereavement therapy, which involves the older adult client adjusting [to such issues as] the loss of the loved one, i.e., that their life may be different but it is still worth having (Knight, 1996). (Bergin and Walsh, 2005, p. 11)

In the development of relationships with older clients, Berg and Miller (1992) have identified seven characteristics of well-formed goals that might enhance the working relationship with older adults:

1. Goals for the work done together should be well formed and expressed in the client's language. They should include the client's thinking about ways of changing. Worker goals should be thoroughly processed by the client, and if the client believes the goal

is unrealistic or is disconnected from the client's notion of how best to proceed with change, the worker and client should negotiate the goal until both feel they are ready to proceed. Setting goals is a type of negotiation in which the process is cooperative.

2. The goals for treatment are small because, as Berg and Miller point out, small goals are easier to achieve than large ones.
3. The goals should focus on social functioning and should be very concrete. Rather than suggesting a goal of more involvement with others, the goal may be to have coffee with a friend several times a week. Such a goal is measurable and gives the client something concrete to do.
4. The goals should be positive and include doing something rather than not doing something.
5. Goals are small steps necessary to achieve desired change.
6. Goals are realistic given the client's motivation, cognitive abilities, and willingness to stick with the incremental nature of the change process.
7. Goals may be perceived by the client as sometimes difficult, but necessary to achieve a desired level of improvement.

5.5 GENDER AND THE THERAPEUTIC RELATIONSHIPS

Clinical wisdom usually suggests that gender is a neutral variable in clinical outcomes and that the quality of the help is more significant than issues related to the genders of the worker and the client. However, studies by Gehart-Brooks and Lyle (1999), and Sells et al. (1994) suggest that a therapist's gender *is* an important factor affecting the client's therapy experience. While clients specifically state that gender is important, parallel interviews with therapists suggest that it isn't important. Gerhart (2001) believes that this "potential oversight has significant implications for the practice of ethical, gender-sensitive therapy and training" (p. 444), and she goes on to say that, "Jones and Zoppel (1982) found that clients, regardless of gender, agreed that female therapists formed more effective therapeutic alliances than male therapists; however, both male and female clients of male therapists also reported significant improvements as a result of therapy" (p. 444).

Gerhart (2001) also reports that further inquiry into the relationship between gender and therapeutic outcomes indicates that "male and female therapists interrupted females three times more often than male clients (Werner-Wilson et al., 1997)" (p. 444). Shields and McDaniel (1992) found that families made more directive statements to male therapists, but disagreed more openly with each other in front of females. Shields and McDaniel (1992) found that male therapists explained issues more fully than female therapists and that male therapists provided more advice and direction than female therapists. Werner-Wilson et al. (1999) report that men were more successful at suggesting issues for discussion in family treatment, while women did better in marital therapy. Gerhart (2001) believes that these "studies provide further evidence that gender may significantly affect the therapeutic process in ways in which therapists are currently unaware" (p. 444).

Gerhart (2001) describes three possible types of gender-related connections made by clients: (1) The connection is stronger with a therapist of the same gender because it offers a common language and knowledge base; (2) the connection is stronger with a therapist of the opposite gender because gender differences may provide motivation to work harder in treatment; (3) the client develops a good relationship with a therapist of the same gender but often reports that therapists of the opposite gender are also effective. (p. 451). In summarizing her work on gender, Gerhart writes

> Perhaps the most striking pattern is that what one viewed as a therapist's strength, another viewed as a detriment. For example, clients described women as more feeling-focused, but only half found this helpful. Conversely, almost all clients described male therapists as more direct and problem-focused, yet only half found this approach helpful. What is consistent is that clients reported that they experienced a distinct and consistent difference between male and female therapists. (p. 452)

5.6   RACIAL AND ETHNIC VARIABLES IN THERAPEUTIC EFFECTIVENESS

A number of studies have examined the relationship between racial bias and psychiatric diagnoses. Adebimpe (1981) found that a high number of African-American patients were misdiagnosed as schizophrenic, a finding, according to Laszloffy and Hardy (2000), supported in subsequent studies that examined white, black and Latino patients. Even though the symptoms were the same, African-American and Latino patients were often diagnosed as schizophrenic, while white patients were almost always correctly diagnosed with emotional or affective disorders (Garretson, 1993; Lopez and Nunez, 1987; Loring and Powell, 1988; Malgady et al., 1987; Pakov et al., 1989; Solomon, 1992). Laszloffy and Hardy (2000) believe that underlying the misdiagnosis is a "subtle, unintentional racism" (p. 35). In defining racism, the authors write that "all expressions of racism are rooted in an ideology of racial superiority/inferiority that assumes some racial groups are superior to others, and therefore deserve preferential treatment" (p. 35), a definition that makes unintentional or subtle racism difficult to accept.

Flaherty and Meagher (1980) found that among African-American and Caucasian male schizophrenic inpatients who had similar global pathology ratings,

> African-American patients spent less time in the hospital, obtained lower privilege levels, were given more p.r.n. medications, and were less likely to receive recreation therapy and occupational therapy. Seclusion and restraints were more likely to be used with black patients. (p. 679)

While the authors avoid suggesting a direct relationship between racial bias and the treatment of minority patients, they conclude that it is an important intervening variable.

In a report on race and mental health, the US Surgeon General (Satcher, 2001) notes that the cultures of clinicians and the way services are provided influence the therapeutic alliance and by extension, diagnosis and treatment. Service providers, according to the report, need to be able to build upon the cultural strengths of the people they serve. The Surgeon General suggests that "while not the sole determinants, cultural and social influences do play important roles in mental health, mental illness and service use, when added to biological, psychological and environmental factors" (p. 1). In trying to understand barriers to treatment that affect ethnic and racial minorities, the Surgeon General says that the mental health system often creates impediments that lead to distrust and fear of treatment, which ultimately deter racial and ethnic minorities from seeking and receiving needed services. Importantly, the Surgeon General adds, "Mental health care disparities may also stem from minorities' historical and present day struggles with racism and discrimination, which affect their mental health and contribute to their lower economic, social, and political status" (Satcher, 2001, p. 1). In an earlier report on mental health, the Surgeon General (Satcher, 1999) wrote that while mental illness is at least as prevalent among racial and ethnic minorities as in the majority white population, "many racial and ethnic minority group members find the organized mental health system to be uninformed about cultural context and, thus, unresponsive and/or irrelevant" (p. 1), and may prefer clinicians who share their racial, ethnic, and socio-economic backgrounds (Satcher, 1999, Chapter 8, p. 4, Internet version of the report).

Laszloffy and Hardy (2000) believe that as long as racism occupies such a significant role in our everyday lives, it cannot be completely eliminated without carefully examining what we say to clients, what we do with clients, and, as a strong reminder of the importance of EBP, what we really believe. In validating the need for cultural and racial sensitivity, Peña et al. (2000) write that, "In work with African-American patients, the therapist's skill in recognizing when problems do or do not revolve around the condition of being black could have serious implications for the acceptability of treatment, the development of the treatment alliance, and in psychotherapy, the accuracy of interpretations" (p. 14). The authors report that each of these variables has a significant impact on treatment outcomes and that therapists with limited awareness of the significance of race may experience problems in "listening empathically" and in actually understanding the client's conflicts.

CASE STUDY: AN EVIDENCE-BASED PRACTICE APPROACH TO THE THERAPEUTIC RELATIONSHIP

Natasha Putkin is a 67-year-old Russian immigrant who came to the USA with her family when she was 28 years-old. She considers herself thoroughly assimilated and is married to an American man. Her family has had a difficult time in America and has been unable to resume the professional careers they had in Russia. Much of their interaction with Natasha contains negative messages about all things American, including her husband. Natasha considers herself to be a strong and competent woman, but her relationship with her family has become strained because her husband is beginning to disengage from Natasha's family. Natasha worries that the disengagement will ultimately include her. Like many clients new to therapy, Natasha is looking for someone to give her advice. She expects that therapy will last just a few sessions and told the therapist she chose, "I just want some help with my family and my marriage. Just be honest with me and give me good information."

The therapist was very business-like with Natasha, and helped her tell her story in a way that satisfied Natasha's need for advice. He then suggested several articles she could find on the Internet that related to the issues she needed help with and recommended that she carefully write down some concrete questions to ask in their next session. Natasha left the interview feeling very satisfied with the therapist. He was a no-nonsense person who was giving her exactly what she was looking for, and he wasn't condescending in the way some people are who work with older adults. Natasha read the articles, found them very useful, but had some questions she needed to ask the therapist about several parts of each article she found unclear. She e-mailed the therapist her questions and within a short time received clear answers. Once again, he urged her to carefully construct the questions she would like to discuss in their next session. Natasha spent over two hours writing her questions down but began to realize that she had more questions than the therapist could possibly answer in one session. She decided that perhaps the treatment might take several more sessions than she'd originally planned for. The questions she wrote covered three pages, single-spaced.

Natasha shared the questions with her therapist who took a few minutes to read them. He noted that there were some similarities in several of them and asked if they could meld the questions together. Natasha thought this was a good idea. He then said that there were three fundamental areas covered by the questions and asked if they could focus on each area and the questions included to save time. Natasha was delighted with the efficient way the therapist was responding. In one session, they covered two areas and all of the questions included. Once again, the therapist suggested that she read some additional articles, specifically articles on the immigrant experience, assimilation, family issues with older adults, and marriages where cultural differences existed. Natasha found the articles very helpful and, having learned to use the Internet, was able to find other articles of a similar nature.

In the third session, the therapist answered all of the remaining questions, and wondered if there were some other things Natasha would like to discuss. Natasha felt that, for the time being, she was very satisfied with the results of their work together and terminated treatment after three informative and useful sessions. Her evaluation of the treatment was highly positive and she referred several of her older friends to the therapist. Each friend was surprised at how differently the therapist responded to them. When the three women compared the therapist's style, Natasha said it was business-like, one of her friends described it as very warm and supportive, and a second friend described the style as relaxed, slow and intimate. Each client was looking for something different from the therapist and each received it. They agreed that it took a very competent person to relate to their stated needs and to the style of interaction they found most comfortable. All three women felt that the therapist had involved them at a very high level and that he had done exactly what each client had asked of him. He didn't argue that they needed more help or criticize their agenda. They all believed that they had benefited significantly from the experience and that their presenting problems had been resolved. None felt the need for more treatment, and all felt that termination occurred at just the right moment in time.

In describing his work with the three clients, the therapist said that he believed that clients should set the therapeutic agenda and that unless he felt the agenda was harmful, he usually believed that clients selected the correct issues to discuss. He believed this was the essence of a cooperative relationship. He also felt that it was important to enter the client's world and to try and relate to it in ways that clients felt would be most helpful. He always asked for client input in decisions about treatment, suggested additional reading, asked them to come in with questions and, when asked a question, answered it. If he didn't know the answer, he said he would do some research and suggested that the client do the same. He encouraged e-mails and tried to answer them quickly. He always asked clients to e-mail him a summary of what they had learned in their prior session and to read as much as they could about the questions they were going to ask him in the next session. He believed that being an informed client made for much faster and more effective therapy.

5.7 SUMMARY

This chapter covers some important issues related to the therapeutic relationship and its significance to treatment effectiveness. While some of the authors cited in this chapter believe that the relationship is a key element in treatment effectiveness, many also believe that much more research is needed to establish the specific aspects of the relationship that help or hinder client change. Issues of the significance of client-worker gender and race\ethnicity were also raised, with many authors believing that both issues have an impact on treatment efficacy and that much more time must be spent in training new workers for effective work with diverse client populations. A case study is included in the chapter which describes a cooperative worker-client relationship.

5.8 QUESTIONS FROM THE CHAPTER

1. In thinking about older adult clients seeking professional help, what might be the worker characteristics (style of relating, race, gender, religious background, etc.) that you believe would make the initial relationship easiest? Why?
2. Can you think of some instances with older adults when the therapeutic relationship might hinder client change or actually cause harm?

3. The case study makes the therapist sound like a chameleon. Do you think it's possible for therapists to dramatically change their style of relating to meet the very different needs of clients?
4. In what ways might differences in the expectations of a relationship between the worker and the older adult client result in conflict?
5. One of the authors cited in this chapter suggests using physical touch and other forms of contact with older clients. Might this not be felt to be condescending by the client and a breach of the formality that should exist between client and helper? Explain your answer.

REFERENCES

Adebimpe, V. R. (1981). Overview: White norms and psychiatric diagnosis of black patients. *American Journal of Psychiatry, 138*, 279–285.

Berg, I. K., & Miller, S. D. (1992). *Working with the problem drinker: A solution-focused approach.* New York: W. W. Norton.

Bergin, L., & Walsh, S. (2003). The role of hope in psychotherapy with older adults: Guidelines for psychological practice with older adults. *American Psychological Association, 1*(August).

Bisman, C. (1994). *Social work practice: Cases and principles.* Belmont, CA: Brooks/Cole.

Bordin, E. S. (1994). Theory and research on the therapeutic working alliance: New directions. In Horvath and Greenberg (pp. 13–37).

Brent, D. A. (1998). Psychotherapy: Definitions, mechanisms of action, and relationship to etiological models <http://www.findarticles.com/cf_0/m0902/n1_v26/20565425/print.jhtml>. *Journal of abnormal child psychology* (February).

Buechler, S. (1995). Hope as inspiration in psychoanalysis. *Psychoanalytic Dialogues, 5*(1), 63–74.

Burns, D. D., & Nolen-Hoeksema, S. (1992). Therapeutic empathy and recovery from depression in cognitive-behavioral therapy: A structural equation model. *Journal of Consulting and Clinical Psychology, 60*, 441–449.

Connors, G. J., Carroll, K. M., DiClemente, C. C., Longabaugh, R., & Donovan, D. M. (1997). The therapeutic alliance and its relationship to alcoholism treatment participation and outcome. *Journal of Consulting Clinical Psychology, 65*, 588–598.

Consumer Reports. (1995). Mental health: Does therapy help? November, 734–739.

Cooley, E. J., & Lajoy, R. (1980). Therapeutic relationship and improvement as perceived by clients and therapists. *Journal of Clinical Psychology, 36*, 562–570.

Dacey, M. L., & Newcomer, R. A. (2005). A client-centered counseling approach for motivating older adults toward physical activity. *Topics in Geriatric Rehabilitation, 21*(3), 194–205.

Dufault, K., & Martocchio, B. C. (1985). Hope: Its spheres and dimensions. *Nursing Clinics of North America, 20*(2), 379–391.

Entwistle, V. A., Sheldon, T. A., Sowden, A., & Watt, I. S. (1998). Evidence-informed patient choice. Practical issues of involving patients in decisions about health care technologies. *International Journal of Technology Assessment in Health Care, 14*, 212–225.

Evidence-Based Medicine Working Group. (1992). Evidence-based medicine: A new approach to teaching the practice of medicine. *Journal of the American Medical Association, 268*, 2420–2425.

Farran, C. J., Herth, K. A., & Popovich, J. M. (1995). *Hope and hopelessness: Critical clinical constructs*. California: Sage Publications.

Feifel, H., & Eells, J. (1963). Patients and therapists assess the same psychotherapy. *Journal of Consulting Psychology, 27*, 310–318.

Flaherty, J. A., & Meagher, R. (1980). Measuring racial bias in inpatient treatment. *American Journal of Psychiatry, 137*, 679–682.

Gambrill, E. (1999). Evidence-based practice: An alternative to authority-based practice. *Journal of Contemporary Human Services, 80*(4), 341–350.

Garretson, D. J. (1993). Psychological misdiagnosis of African Americans. *Journal of Multicultural Counseling and Development, 21*, 119–126.

Gelso, J., & Hayes, J. A. (1998). *The psychotherapy relationship: Theory, research and practice*. New York: Wiley.

Gerhart, D. R., & Lyle, R. D. (2001). Client experience of gender in therapeutic relationships: an interpretive ethnography (December 22). *Family Process, 40*, 443–458.

Gerhart-Brooks, D. R., & Lyle, R. R. (1999). Client and therapist perspectives of change in collaborative language systems: An interpretive ethnography. *Journal of Systemic Therapies, 18*(4), 78–97.

Glicken, M. D. (2004). *Using the strengths perspective in social work practice*. Boston, MA: Allynand Bacon/Longman.

Greenfield, S., Kaplan, S., & Ware, J. E., Jr. (1985). Expanding patient involvement in care. Effects on patient outcomes. *Annals of Internal Medicine, 102*(4), 520–528.

Hamilton, G. (1940). *Social casework*. New York: Columbia University Press.

Henry, W. P., Schacht, T. E., & Strupp, H. H. (1986). Structural analysis of social behavior: Application to a study of interpersonal process in differential psychotherapeutic outcome. *Journal of Consulting and Clinical Psychology, 54*, 27–31.

Horvath, A. O., & Greenberg, L. S. (Eds.), (1994). *The working alliance: Theory, research and practice*. New York: Wiley.

Horvath, A. O., & Symonds, B. D. (1991). Relation between working alliance and outcome in psychotherapy: A meta-analysis. *Journal of Consulting Clinical Psychology, 38*, 139–149.

Jones, E. E., & Zoppel, C. L. (1982). Impact of client and therapist gender on psychotherapy process and outcome. *Journal of Consulting and Clinical Psychology, 50*, 259–272.

Keith-Lucas, A. (1972). *Giving and taking help*. Chapel Hill: University of North Carolina Press.

Knight, B. G. (1986). *Psychotherapy with older adults*. London: Sage.

Knight, B. G. (1996a). *Psychotherapy with older adults* (2nd ed.). California: Sage.

Knight, B. G. (1996b). Psychodynamic therapy with older adults: Lessons from scientific gerontology. In R. T. Wood (Ed.), *Handbook of the clinical psychology of ageing*. Chichester: Wiley.

Kopta, M. S., Lueger, R. J., Saunders, S. M., & Howard, K. I. (1999). Individual psychotherapy outcome and process research: Challenges leading to greater turmoil or a positive transition? <http://www.findarticles.com/cf_0/m0961/1999_Annual/54442307/print.jhtml>. *Annual Review of Psychology*.

Krupnick, J. L., Sotsky, S. M., Simmens, S., Moyer, J., Elkin, I., et al. (1996). The role of the therapeutic alliance in psychotherapy and pharmacotherapy outcome: Findings in the National Institute of Mental Health Treatment of Depression Collaborative Research Program. *Journal of Consulting Clinical Psychology, 6*, 532–539.

Laszloffy, T. A., & Hardy, K. V. (2000). Uncommon strategies for a common problem: Addressing racism in family therapy. *Family Process, 39*, 35–50.

Lopez, S., & Nunez, J. A. (1987). The consideration of cultural factors in selected diagnostic criteria and interview schedules. *Journal of Abnormal Psychology, 96*, 270–272.

Loring, M., & Powell, B. (1988). Gender, race, and DSM-III: A study of the objectivity of psychiatric diagnostic behavior. *Journal of Health and Social Behavior, 29*, 1–22.

Luborsky, L., McLellan, A. T., Woody, G. E., O'Brien, C. P., & Auerbach, A. (1985). Therapist success and its determinants. *Archives of General Psychiatry, 42*, 602–611.

Malgady, R. G., Rogler, L. H., & Constantino, G. (1987). Ethnocultural and linguistic bias in mental health evaluation of Hispanics. *American Psychologist, 42*, 228–234.

Mathews, A. M., Johnson, D. W., Shaw, P. M., & Geller, M. G. (1974). Process variables and the prediction of outcome in behavior therapy. *British Journal of Psychiatry, 125*, 256–264.

Morgan, A. C. (2005, Jan.). Practical geriatrics; psychodynamic psychotherapy with older adults. *Aging and Mental Health, 9*(1), 71–75.

Murphy, G. E., Simons, A. D., Wetzel, R. D., & Lustman, P. J. (1984). Cognitive therapy and pharmacotherapy: Singly and together in the treatment of depression. *Archives of General Psychiatry, 41*, 33–41.

Myers, J. E., & Harper, M. C. (2004, Spring). Evidence-based effective practices with older adults. *Journal of Counseling and Development, 82*, 207–218.

Orlinsky, D. E., Grawe, K., & Parks, B. K. (1994). Process and outcome in psychotherapy – noch einmal. In A. E. Bergin & S. L. Garfield (Eds.), *Handbook of psychotherapy and behavior change* (pp. 270–378) (4th ed.). New York: Wiley.

Pakov, T. W., Lewis, D. A., & Lyons, J. S. (1989). Psychiatric diagnosis and racial bias: An empirical investigation. Professional Psychology. *Research and Practice, 20*, 364–368.

Peña, J. M., Bland, I. J., Shervinton, D., Rice, J. C., & Foulks, E. F. (2000). Racial identity and its assessment in a sample of African-American men in treatment for cocaine dependence <http://www.findarticles.com/cf_0/PI/search.jhtml?magR = all + magazinesandkey = psychotherapy + %2B + race>. *American Journal of Drug and Alcohol Abuse.* (1February), 13.

Saleebey, D. (1996). The strengths perspective in social work practice: Extensions and cautions. *Social Work, 41*(3), 296–305.

Saleebey, D. (2000, Fall). Power to the people; strength and hope. *Advancements in Social Work, 1*(2), 127–136.

Satcher, D. (1999) Mental health, a report of the surgeon general. <http://www.mental-health.org/features/surgeongeneralreport/chapter8/sec1.asp#ensure>

Satcher, D. (2001). Mental health: Culture, race, and ethnicity. A supplement to mental health: A report of the surgeon general. <http://www.surgeongeneral.gov/library/mentalhealth/cre/release.asp>

Seligman, M. E. P. (1995). The effectiveness of psychotherapy: the consumers report study. *American Psychologist, 50*(12), 965–974.

Sells, S. P., Smith, T. E., Coe, M. J., Yoshioka, M., & Robbins, J. (1994). An ethnography of couple and therapist experiences in reflecting team practice. *Journal of Marital and Family Therapy, 20*, 247–266.

Shields, C. G., & McDaniel, S. H. (1992). Process differences between male and female therapists in a first family interview. *Journal of Marital and Family Therapy, 18*, 143–151.

Snyder, C. R. (1994). *The psychology of hope: You can get there from here*. New York: Free Press.

Solomon, A. (1992). Clinical diagnosis among diverse populations: A multicultural perspective. *Families in Society, 73*, 371–377.

Stickle, F., & Onedera, J. D. (2006, Spring). Depression in older adults. *AQUITSPAN, 5*(1), 36–46.

Warren, C.S. (2001). Book review of *Negotiating the Therapeutic Alliance: A Relational Treatment Guide*, J.D. Safran & J.C. Muran. (2000). New York: Guilford Press, in *Psychotherapy Research, 11* (3), 2001, 357–359.

Weiss, W. D., Sampson, H., & O'Connor, L. (1995, Spring). How psychotherapy works: the findings of the San Francisco Psychotherapy Research Group. *Bulleting of the Psychoanalytic Research Society, IV*(1).

Werner-Wilson, R. J., Price, S. J., Zimmerman, T. S., & Murphy, M. J. (1997). Client gender as a process variable in marriage and family therapy: Are women clients interrupted more than men clients? *Journal of Family Psychotherapy, 11*, 373–377.

Werner-Wilson, R. J., Zimmerman, T. S., & Price, S. J. (1999). Are goals and topics influenced by gender modality in the initial marriage and family therapy session? *Journal of Marital and Family Therapy, 25*, 253–262.

Woolfe, Ray, & Biggs, Simon (1997). Counselling older adults: Issues and awareness. *Counselling Psychology Quarterly, 10*(20), 189–195.

Part three

Evidence-Based Practice and Psychosocial Problems of Older Adults

Chapter six

Love and Intimacy in Older Adulthood

6.1 INTRODUCTION

This chapter explores two important issues in aging: love and intimacy, and the practice issues that pertain to both. While older adults often experience a remarkable adaptation to love and value a mature notion of love that is more accepting and emotionally healthy, there are many older adults who maintain dysfunctional approaches to love, and "who are just as jealous, just as infantile, just as filled with irrationality when they fall in love in their 70s and 80s as [they were at earlier ages]. And it still is possible to have a broken heart in old age. A broken heart looks different in somebody old. You don't yell and scream like you might when you were 20" (Zernike, 2007, p.1).

Older love is often more patient. Older adults recognize that the bad times pass and the good times pass. "As you experience the good and bad times, they're more precious, they're richer" (Zernike, 2007, p. 1). It's also that older people may simply be better able to deal with the emotional aspects of love. As it ages, the brain becomes more programmed to be happy in relationships, according to brain researchers. Zernike adds,

As people get older, they seem to naturally look at the world through positivity and be willing to accept things that when we're young we would find disturbing and vexing. It is not rationalization: the reaction is instantaneous. Instead of what would be most disturbing for somebody, feeling betrayed or discomfort, the other thoughts – about how from his perspective it's not betrayal – can be accommodated much more easily, it paves the way for you to be sympathetic to the situation from his perspective, to be less disturbed from her perspective. (p. 1)

Walsh (1988) sees married older people as having unique concerns that center around the fact that older couples usually experience increased marital satisfaction and intimacy and yet realize that they have only a limited time left to be a couple. With the positives of wisdom and integrity (Erikson, 1963) that often come as couples age is the psychological paradox that these benefits of life are limited in a way possibly unknown in earlier years.

6.2 SEX AND INTIMACY

Stein (2007) reports the results of a study of 3,000 US adults aged 57–85 which found that half to three quarters of the respondents remained sexually active, with a "significant population engaging in frequent and varied sex" (p. A1). The study indicates, not surprisingly, that healthier people reported the highest rates of sexual activity and that a healthy sex life may itself help keep people vibrant. According to Stein the study noted that 28% of the men and 14% of the women said sex was very important and those with partners reported being as sexually active as adults in their forties and fifties. "But even among the oldest age group (80–85), 54% of those who were sexually active reported having sex at least two to three times per month, and 23% reported having sex once a week or more" (p. A1).

The study also found that among those who remained sexually active, nearly half reported at least one sexual problem. Forty-three percent of the women in the survey reported a lack of sexual desire, 39% reported vaginal dryness, while 37% of men reported problems achieving an erection. The study suggests that older sexually active adults with sexual problems might benefit from "more frank and open discussions about sex with their doctors" (p. A1) and that human service professionals should be developing skills in working with older adults in the areas of love and sexuality. Funding in this important area of life for older adults is very limited, according to the study, and more studies to determine the extent of sexual problems in older adults are needed.

In a National Council on the Aging study (1998), the following data were found:

- 48% of men and women over 60 are sexually active (some form of sexual activity once a month).
- 39% of men and women over 60 would like to be more active than they are.

- About 75% of sexually active older Americans say their sex life today is as emotionally satisfying or even more satisfying than it was when they were in their forties.

Data for women over 60:

- 37% are sexually active.
- 62% say sex is better or at least equally as physically satisfying as it was at 40.
- Women who are not sexually active often give lack of a partner as the reason.
- 69% say sex is equally as emotionally satisfying as it was at 40.
- 47% say sex is important to a relationship.

Data for men over 60:

- 61% are sexually active.
- 61% say sex is better or at least equally as physically satisfying as it was at 40.
- 76% say sex is equally as emotionally satisfying as it was at 40.
- 72% say sex is important to a relationship.

Reasons given for less sexual activity and less satisfaction:

- Medical condition prevents one from having sex (51% men, 12% women).
- Partner has a medical condition that prevents having sex.
- Person has less physical desire to have sex (55% of both men and women).
- Taking some medications seem to reduce sexual desire (44% men, 16 % women).

Bancroft (2007) reports that despite the high prevalence of sexual problems among the participants in the study cited by Stein (above), only 38% of the men and 22% of women

> reported having discussed sex with a doctor since the age of 50 years. Until recently, older adults tended to keep quiet about their sexuality because younger people assumed that they were not and should not be sexually active. (Bancroft, 2007, p. 820)

Bancroft believes that the helping professions, including the medical profession, "should encourage older patients to feel comfortable in discussing sexual problems" (p. 822). In determining the options for resolving sexual problems in older adults, Bancroft argues that

For some older couples, sex can continue to play an important part in their relationship and well-being, and some may benefit from counseling or medication for that purpose. Other couples choose to leave sex behind as they settle into their later life. Often there may be the need for negotiation between partners. (p. 822)

Genevay (1999, p.2) indicates that the following may define sexual problems as people age: "*Women*: Arousal time increases; less lubrication may result in pain; vaginal thinning may result in pain. *Men:* Increased time to achieve erection; more control over ejaculation, but flow is reduced; increased refractory period before second erection is possible."

A University of Missouri at Kansas City report (2007) indicates that the following psychosocial factors may result in sexual problems for older adults:

1. sexual activity in middle age is a strong predictor of sexual activity in old age;
2. negative attitudes toward sexual activities other than intercourse, such as kissing and masturbation, interfere with the openness to try new ways of expressing intimacy;
3. reactions and beliefs about physiological changes or illness-induced changes have a negative impact on sexual functioning;
4. reactions to attitudes of others, society or adult children have a powerful impact on self-concept; and
5. living arrangements that do not allow for privacy, such as long-term care facilities, create a barrier to sexual activity.

According to Huffstetler (2006), older adults may internalize society's prejudice against sexuality in older adults. The Geriatric Sexuality Breakdown Syndrome identified by Kaas (1981) categorizes breakdowns in sexual functioning that result from an older person internalizing ageist attitudes. Huffstetler (2006) notes that while not all older adults experience this syndrome, "those who do typically go through seven stages: precondition susceptibility, dependence on available cues, societal labeling, sick role, learning of behaviors, atrophy of social skills, and internalization of labels" (p. 7).

6.3 NATURAL CHANGES MAY AFFECT INTIMACY

The following is summarized from a Mayo Clinic (2007) online discussion of sexuality and older adults.

6.3.1 Physical changes in women

Testosterone regulates sex drive for both men and women. Most aging men and women produce enough testosterone to maintain their interest in sex. Although physical changes may affect some aspects of sex, these changes give people reasons to try new positions and techniques and, in general, to experiment with new aspects of sexuality which both partners find acceptable. Changes women experience are most often linked to menopause and reduced estrogen levels. As women age, it may take longer for the vagina to swell and lubricate when sexually aroused. A woman's vagina may also lose elasticity. Together these two conditions can make intercourse less comfortable or even painful. Women might also feel a burning sensation during vaginal penetration or discover vaginal bleeding afterward. Longer foreplay sometimes helps stimulate natural lubrication or women can try water-based lubricants such as K-Y jelly, or talk to a physician about estrogen cream or estrogen replacement therapy. Vaginal penetration helps maintain lubrication and elasticity if done regularly. If a woman hasn't been sexually active for a while because of illness or absence from a mate, it's a good idea to talk to the partner about slowly moving back to having intercourse to minimize pain, or to opt for other ways to be intimate.

6.3.2 Physical changes in men

As men age, it might take longer to achieve an erection. Erections may be less firm and may not last as long. Aging also increases the time between possible ejaculations. Trying different positions may make intercourse easier for both partners. If a man is having problems maintaining an erection or reaching orgasm a doctor can discuss medications that can help men achieve and maintain an erection. Partners can help distinguish physical from other aspects of erectile problems by noting that healthy men have an erection while they sleep every 90 minutes or so. When an erection fails to take place during sleep, as it does for about 10% of all men, it may suggest a physical problem such as diabetes, high blood pressure, cardio-vascular problems, spinal injuries, or medications that inhibit sexual functioning including medications for depression, high blood pressure, antihistamines, acid-blocking drugs, and drugs used to treat sleep problems.

6.3.3 Psychological changes in men and women as they age

Often the same sexual problems that affect men and women earlier in life affect them as they age. Feeling embarrassed or ashamed about sexual needs and performance anxiety may affect a person's ability to become aroused. Changes in appearance might also affect the ability to emotionally and physically connect with a partner. A poor body image often reduces sex drive because one of the partners no longer feels worthy of sexual attention from the other partner. The stress of worrying too much about how one will perform can trigger impotence in men or a lack of arousal in women. Urging clients experiencing sexual difficulties to take things slowly can help reduce performance anxiety – the main cause of sexual difficulties in the young and the old.

6.4 SUGGESTIONS FOR HELPING OLDER ADULTS IMPROVE THEIR SEX LIVES

1. **Help clients expand their definition of sex** to include touch, sensual massage, masturbation, and oral sex.
2. **Help clients improve communications with partners.** When sexual problems exist it can be helpful to have partners discuss any physical or emotional changes they may be going through, and what partners can do to accommodate those changes during intimacy. Communication itself can be arousing.
3. **Make changes in sexual routines.** Simple changes can improve one's sex life, including changing the time of day when a couple usually has sex to a time when both partners have the most energy (for example, mornings, when a couple has just had a refreshing night of sleep). Because it might take longer to become aroused, couples might take more time to set the stage for romance, such as a romantic dinner or an evening of dancing.
4. **Managing expectations.** If a couple hasn't had sex very often as younger adults, they shouldn't expect to have a great deal of sex as older adults. Partners who enjoyed frequent sex when they were younger are more likely to continue to do so as they age.
5. **Caring for one's health.** Older couples should be urged to have a healthy diet and regular exercise to keep their bodies fit, since this keeps a person ready for sex at any age. Couples should also be urged to avoid alcohol, since it often decreases sexual functioning in men and women. Illegal drugs such as marijuana and cocaine impair sexual functioning, as do a number of prescription drugs. Couples on medication should be urged to determine sexual side effects from doctors, pharmacists and websites where side effects are discussed. If a medication has a sexual side effect, perhaps other medications with less adverse effects might be used.

6. **Sex and single older adults.** Almost half of the people 65 and older in the USA are single. New romances can be exciting and may lead to sexual intimacy, but couples should be urged to practice safe sex. Contrary to popular belief, AIDS is not a younger person's disease. According to a Mayo Clinic report, people over 50 make up about 19% of the AIDS cases in the USA. All sexually active people – no matter their age – can contract STDs. Couples should be urged to stay monogamous with a new partner, practice safe sex by using condoms, and both partners should be tested for HIV. Older adults are less likely than are younger adults to have ever been tested.

According to Perman (2006), many older adults simply date without necessarily wanting to remarry. Living Apart Together (LAT) is a form of relationship in which partners define themselves as a couple, see each other often but maintain separate residences. Creating this form of relationship may stem from job demands, responsibilities to family members, etc., but for others it provides sufficient intimacy but also time to see friends, have secure finances, and be involved in activities they enjoy, but which their partners may not. For women, maintaining their own homes constitutes a resource base that provides financial security and avoids co-mingling finances and the problems that may arise from misunderstandings about money, unequal responsibilities, or broken relationships.

Some states have wisely given older adults the opportunity to have domestic partnerships in which one of the partners might receive the medical benefits of the other. Many people who enter into domestic partnerships have a form of pre-nuptial agreement that serves to protect them financially should the relationship end. Entering a domestic partnership has many of the legal constraints of marriage but fewer of the benefits. Income tax, for example, must be paid as a single tax payer and joint returns are disallowed under federal and state guidelines.

6.5 DETERMINING THE CAUSE OF SEXUAL DIFFICULTIES IN OLDER ADULTS

Huffstetler (2006) suggests that the theory of deconstruction helps older adult clients with sexual problems understand the historical reasons they may be experiencing sexual problems and to rewrite their personal narratives about their sexual lives and their experiences with love and intimacy by developing alternative meanings in order to "examine the meaning of sexuality in their own lives and to determine ways to overcome any taboos related to sexual expression" (p. 10). Sexual assessment tools might also be helpful in firming up a diagnosis. The Clinical Effectiveness Group (2005) using best evidence suggests that the following information is necessary to establish a firm diagnosis of sexual problems:

1. **Presenting complaint:** Start the sexual history with less intrusive questions regarding presenting concerns and symptoms before asking more sensitive questions regarding sexual behavior. The reason for attendance should be ascertained. After this has been determined, the clinician should then ask direct questions regarding the duration and nature of any reported symptoms (Clinical Effectiveness Group, 2005, p. 3).

2. **Attitudes toward love:** It's important to obtain a history of the client's experiences with love. Often those experiences and the attitudes and beliefs that underlie them may have a great deal to do with current problems in sexuality and intimacy. In obtaining the history, the following should be ascertained:
   - Their description of romantic love.
   - Have any of their partners met that description and if so indicate why and who they were.
   - Did marriage or long-term relationships develop from a love experience?
   - Any unrequited loves?
   - Any love experiences that were heart-breaking?
   - Any divorces? Find out why a marriage ended in divorce.
   - Children? How many and what is the quality of the relationship?
   - Relationships with ex-spouses or long-time relationships.

3. **Sexual history:** The following are important pieces of information that might explain why the client is having a sexual problem now:
   - Attitudes of parents toward love and sexuality.
   - Religious or other barriers to the enjoyment of sex which associate sex with guilt and denial.
   - Physical limitations, which have made sexual relations problematic.
   - First sexual experience and how it affected the client.
   - Early experiences and whether any resulted in a sexual problem.

- Any sexual problems preceding the problem the client is currently having.
- Sexual histories with spouses or sexual partners.
- Whether having children affected sexuality.
- Period of not having sex and why.
- If the client is male, has he ever had sexual contact with another man?
- Has the client been sexually molested? If so, at what age and what was the impact?
- Sexually transmitted infections or brief sexual encounters.
- Has the client been tested for HIV/AIDS, Hepatitis B, or any other STD? When and what was the diagnosis?
- Past medical problems, surgeries and medications.
- Past use of counseling for sexual and non-sexual problems. Reasons for counseling and changes made, if any.

4. **Current sexual issues:** In this part of the sexual history it's vital that accurate information be obtained. Having the client's partner come to the interview may be helpful, particularly if the partner is experiencing unhappiness because of the sexual problem. The following topics should be covered:
   - What is the current sexual problem? Be sure to have the client be very specific.
   - How long has it been since the client last had intercourse or other sexual activities?
   - How long has the problem lasted?
   - What has the client done to resolve the problem and how effective have those attempts been?
   - Are they currently in a relationship?
   - Define the relationship (marriage, steady committed, partner, occasional sexual partner).
   - The client's assessment of the relationship.
   - What has the client's sexual partner done to help or harm the problem (if the client has a sexual partner)?
   - Has the client sought professional help? If so from whom and with what impact?
   - Current medications, surgeries or medical problems that might create problems in sexual functioning.
   - Are there positions or sexual acts the client finds unacceptable and would not be willing to try? Ask the same question about the client's sexual partner.

A CASE STUDY: LOSING SEXUAL INTEREST IN A PARTNER

The following case involves a 67-year-old male and a 64-year-old female who have been married for 35 years and are the parents of three grown and successful children. The wife tells the first part of the case, followed by the husband.

Her Story

"We've been married over 35 years and have what I think is an exceptional life by any measure. We have good friends, loving children, and we're financially in very good shape. Jack started losing interest in having sex with me two years ago. When I asked why our sex life wasn't as good as it used to be (we'd previously had sex at least three times a week), he said that he'd just didn't have much of a sex drive, yet I caught him masturbating at the computer on one of those porn sites. I didn't say anything, but I know he goes into those sites once or twice a day. It's hurtful to me that he masturbates instead of having sex with me, but I can't get up the courage to discuss it. He seems happy with me otherwise, but I miss sex and I'm feeling pretty rejected a lot of time."

His Story

"I love my wife but the truth is that I don't find her attractive any more. She's put on a lot of weight and she looks old to me. She's losing her hair and when I see her naked it repulses me. After 35 years the passion wanes but this is much more serious, I think. The thought of having sex with her makes me physically ill and a couple of times, during oral sex, I've gotten so ill I've vomited. I masturbate while looking at porno sites. It seems a harmless way to deal with my sexual needs, but my guess is that Jackie knows and resents it. I can't get myself to talk to her about it since I think it would break her heart, and anyway, it makes me feel like a complete ass."

Intervention

The clinician who ultimately saw this couple did so for the purpose of divorce mediation since Jackie, much against her true wishes but because of deeply hurt feelings, initiated divorce proceedings against Jack. The clinician, a licensed and highly experienced clinical social worker, quickly realized that neither partner wanted a divorce, but that the sexual problem was daunting. Jack had no desire to have sex with other women and felt fine masturbating to porn sites. Jackie finds that an unacceptable solution. The worker asked the couple to discuss their sexual problem. Jack said, "You've put on at least 100 pounds since we married. You don't dress up or put on makeup the way you used to. You wear old lady clothes, and you never try and look nice for me. Your sleep apnea, which the doctor said was due to your weight, requires that you wear a breathing mask at night. How appealing do you think that is for me?"

Jackie responded by saying, "If I lost weight and started to look better would that even make a difference? Much of the weight I've put on happened in the past couple of years when you clearly didn't want to have sex with me. And when this all started, I was dressing up and I looked good but you stopped having interest in me anyway, so stop putting the blame for your problem on me. You just find those bimbos on the Internet a lot sexier than a 64-year-old woman, any 64-year-old woman. Admit it."

Jack told Jackie, "Maybe that's true. Maybe young women turn me on but we have a relationship I treasure. I've never been unfaithful, I still love you. You want to break up a marriage because after 35 years we don't have a sex life? That seems pretty extreme to me. Do you think you'll go out there in the world and a prince charming who wants to have sex with you all the time will come along?"

"No," Jackie replied, "no I don't, but I won't have to live with the humiliation of sleeping with a man who doesn't want to touch me, will I?"

In further discussions Jackie agreed to lose weight and begin taking better care of her self. She joined a tennis club, began working out and went to people who would help her choose more attractive clothing and better makeup. Jack agreed to stop using porn sites and to stop masturbating. As Jack's sexual needs increased and Jackie began looking better, the sex life they enjoyed earlier slowly began to return. The clinician who worked with them said:

"You see a lot of older adults like Jack and Jackie who still love one another but the passion has left and it's hurtful. Many of them describe their partners as roommates or business partners. I went to the literature and read what little I could find on older sexuality and discovered that sexual distance often develops when partners begin to find one another unattractive. I also felt that with Jack not masturbating he would pay more attention to Jackie to have his sexual needs met if Jackie did something to improve her attractiveness to Jack. She readily agreed to lose weight since she felt uncomfortable and unattractive at her current weight. Joining a weight loss program and the tennis club helped her lose weight and improve her self-esteem. She also began to discover that as she lost weight and dressed more attractively that men in her age group began to look at her in ways they hadn't in awhile. Jack also noticed, which helped improve the frequency of sexual contact. Feeling a bit worried that someone might take Jackie away from him increased his desire to please her. It's not an ideal solution, since you would hope that love, mutual concern, and the desire to please one another would resolve this problem naturally without the need for a professional. In my experience sex is a difficult thing for people to talk about to one another. Sometimes simple solutions such as the one that worked here are called for. We still don't know a lot about older sexuality and few older adults seek help when they have sexual problems, believing that it's all about aging and nothing can be done to help. Perhaps as the number of older men and women increases and a new openness develops as people live longer that more older adults will seek help. Certainly doctors, who more often work with older adults than human service professionals can help matters by discussing sexual problems and, when appropriate, refer people for help."

6.6 LOVE IN A TIME OF OLDER ADULTHOOD: A PERSONAL STORY

We were in our middle fifties when we met by Internet dating – "One and Only"! Of course, neither of us knew it then because we were both lying about our ages and had subtracted a neat ten years for purposes of the introductory bio.

Each of us thought that the qualities of vitality, sensuality and sexuality might only be found in someone in that younger decade.

Both David and I had given a lot of thought to our search for a partner … for "into the golden years."

Casualties of earlier failures, we had both been married and divorced twice. I had been single for five years after concluding a ten-year second marriage that I cheerfully described as "lousy," and David had been out of a marriage for about three years but was still jointly raising two pre-teen children. He had a less than cordial relationship with his children's mother.

Looking back, I think we had both made similar earlier mistakes in choosing a mate. Certainly, I had opted for physical attraction and sexual activity – not grasping that a lack of complementarity of intellectual and emotional styles would give rise to the later ever- widening abyss of non-communication in almost every aspect of daily life. My ex and I really didn't have that much in common, and while we still thought of one another as pretty nice people, we had no real interest or reason to be together. Tired of the emptiness of daily individual pursuits, we parted.

In David's case, he had married a young woman almost 19 years his junior. Over time she seems to have grown up – and away – in much the same fashion as I had experienced, until they were yoked together in a dry, frustrating monotony of daily non-connection. Ultimately they parted with pain and rancor and two children to raise in a newly non-conventional family situation.

Each in our own way still yearned for a "final partner." And, in that person we hoped for compassion, intellect, friendship, mutual values, similar goals and especially the capacity for a deep trusting bonding on which to rely. That list was really headed by the unspoken "I really want to feel excited and sexy (but I don't want to pay the price again for a poor choice)."

For my own part I'd taken a year off to be with my mother during her waning days and was feeling sad and hurt at her loss. I'd parted ways with a serviceable boyfriend who just wasn't available to make the leap to committed loving.

So, for a year, after a friend showed me about internet dating, I dated. I met a lot of very nice men but not anyone who "turned me on." I realized then that in addition to the more abstract qualities for which I was searching, there was that drop-dead essential component called "chemistry." Additionally, I reviewed my past relationships and con-cluded that all had been begun only on the basis of this "chemistry," and look where they were now!

Later, when David and I had already met and began exchanging thoughts, he too recognized that something in his selection process had also failed similarly. Of course, he gets handicap points for just being a man and being so much more visually stimulated, but nonetheless our processes were very similar.

By the time our paths crossed, David too had been dating for over a year and was really jaded. He's a jock kinda guy, once described as a man's man, who doesn't cook for himself and mopes when not in a relationship that gives him the opportunity to live out a number of role activities by which he defines himself, such as caretaking, supporting, and sharing the popcorn at the occasional movie. He had seen my bio on the dating site but wrote me off as GU (geographically undesirable).

He told me later that he'd thought me attractive, but was just too tired and was going to let the ad lapse and spend the rest of his life in a monastic moue.

But I contacted him! I'd decided that not only did this man's bio indicate some of the right things, I liked his looks!

Aha, there was that chemistry thing again, but this time I wanted to see if I could have it all – attraction together with stability, maturity, and character. This was a package I earnestly believed I could deliver, and I was confident that if it was explored in a conscious, persistent pattern, it was definitely possible.

David and I exchanged e-mails, then phone calls. But both of us wanted to have an in-person meeting as soon as possible. He did the gentlemanly thing and drove the 40 minutes to my neighborhood. Yes, I know, GU is something that is generally measured in state lines and international boundaries, but this was one fatigued knight errant, and the distance between our little communities looked more like the stretch across the great plains than a pleasant tootle along the Southern California coast.

He made it, parking in front of my little house on a Sunday afternoon while I was watering the roses awaiting his arrival. We rushed into one another's arms, pledged our undying troth and have lived happily ever after.

Well, not exactly.

David parked in front of my little house, strolled laconically up the drive and commenced an hour of being aloof and standoffish. First he was unfriendly at my pleasant welcome, simply shrugging and maintaining a distance. Then, after entering my house, he looked around and offered, "So? You rent here?"

Sure, I was surprised and somewhat baffled by this diffidence. But patience is a virtue that I'd grown into and I immediately decided to wait a bit and depend on the earlier long-distance conversations we had shared to show their true colors. I've lived all my life with animals, large and small, and I know that once injured, any animal with any sense is cautious and tentative in returning to try again.

Since that original meeting we've been together almost 24/7. We did spend the requisite time with beach walks and talks, candlelit dinners and hand holding at the movies, but we also almost immediately started meeting real-life issues head-on. These issues had previously triggered old, established patterns in each other which had led to less than happy results in the past.

David had children marching quickly into teen-angst. His parenting skills were limited, and mine were nonexistent as I had never raised children of my own. We clashed on beliefs about conflict resolution and emotional style. We both fell back into patterns, on his part consisting of angry outbursts, and on my part consisting of flight. After awhile I just kept a bag packed. This hurt us both and threatened to break a bond we both wanted to keep. We had periods of comfort and pleasure in one another's company, finding ever more areas in which we shared similar or complimentary interests and enjoyments, and devastating eruptions of emotional lava in areas of disagreement.

Finally we got the message. We're TOO OLD FOR THIS!

By this time we were no longer in our middle fifties – we were both approaching 60. We had to admit to ourselves and to one another that time was running out.

So we sat down and decided to combine our styles in an effort to attain our mutual goal – happiness together.

We looked at the "big picture," that we each continued to be attracted to one another intellectually, emotionally and sexually. We affirmed that it is the big picture – the company of one another – that is most important, and that continuing devastating conflict will so damage our little ship of state that it might sink. NOT ACCEPTABLE.

So then, what and how to fix? Well, we looked at what we were DOING. David was doing anger and I was doing flight. Both activities drove the other crazy. We looked at where these practices had originated – not new to our relationship! David was repeating a pattern learned in early childhood in which his mother had modeled nastiness and vituperation, taking no-prisoners attack verbiage as her expression of frustration or disappointment. I was still trying to run away from an angry and violent father as I had done when I was a toddler. So, we made a conscious decision to declare them "old baggage," didn't matter exactly from where – just doesn't work here. In fact, hurts more than it helps.

David agreed to modify his pattern of anger by not lashing out at me and I agreed to put away my suitcases and to call for a sit-down discussion of any "problem."

Now, when either of us flips back into some old emotional pattern of disgruntlement, we are committed to immediately recognizing it, acknowledging that it is a pattern, and breaking away from it so as not to damage the other person or the relationship. We simply promised ourselves and one another that we would not allow the old misunderstandings of how to treat a significant other to kill our love.

In this way we are affirming, as constantly as possible, our belief in and commitment to the other person and to the relationship that we enjoy.

And we DO ENJOY.

In every way, as we are kinder to, more entertained by, and accepting of our partner. We are so enriched and comforted by the friendship that continues to grow.

Unexpected fallout from our venture is that sensuality and sexuality has been enhanced.

By knowing David better every day, by letting down my own barriers and defenses, I feel safer and less "different" from him. And consequently I spend more time feeling that we are interacting facets of a "whole," so touching, sex, listening to each other, and sharing space all become moments of fulfillment and contentment. – CJR

6.7 SUMMARY

This chapter explores the issues of love and intimacy in older adulthood. Data are provided showing that many older adults maintain robust sexual lives. Physical and emotional issues that may interfere with love and intimacy are provided along with a case study exploring an older couple whose love life has become troublesome with a treatment intervention and a personal story of older love.

6.8 QUESTIONS FROM THE CHAPTER

1. Isn't it a little, well, disgusting to think about really old people making love?
2. People fall in love in their 70's and 80's? That seems pretty unlikely. Why would they do that?
3. It seems obvious that people who have been together a long time would begin to find their attraction to a spouse or mate diminished. What attracts us early in life often shifts as we age. Don't you agree?
4. I thought you were supposed to get wiser as you age. Why would there be old people out there who are as crazy when they love someone as they were when they were young?
5. The personal story certainly makes older love look awfully complicated. Shouldn't love be easier the older you get because you're wiser and you have more life experience?

REFERENCES

Bancroft, J. H. J. (2007). <http://cas.umkc.edu/casww/sa/Sex.htm>. *Sex and Aging.*

Clinical Effectiveness Group (The association of Genitourinary Medicine and Medical Society of the Study of Venereal diseases). (2005). National Guidelines for the management of the viral Hepatitides A, B and C. www.bashh. org/guidelines/2005/hepatitis

Erikson, E. H. (1963). *Childhood and Society* (2nd ed.). New York: Norton.

Genevay, B. (1999). Intimacy and older people: Much more than sex. *Dimensions, 6*(3).

Huffstetler. (2006). Sexuality in older adults: A deconstructionist perspective. *ADULTSPAN Journal, 5*(1), 4–14.

Kaas, M. J. (1981). Geriatric sexuality breakdown syndrome. *International Journal of Aging and Human Development, 13*, 71–77.

The National Council on the Aging. (1998). *Healthy Sexuality and Vital Aging. Executive Summary*, pp. 1–3 (September).

Perman, D. (2006). The changing face of romance in 2006: Are valentines just for the young?. *Intimacy and Aging: Tips for Sexual Health and Happiness. UBC Reports, 52* (2) (February 2).

Stein, R. (2007, Aug. 23). Elderly staying sexually active. *Washingtonpost. com*. <http://www.washingtonpost.com/wp-dyn/content/article/2007/08/22/AR2007082202000_pf.html>.

Walsh, F. (1988). The family in later life. In B. Carter & M. McGoldrick (Eds.) *The changing family life cycle* (pp. 311–332) (2nd ed.). New York: Gardner.

Zernike, K. (2007). Still many-splendored: Love in the time of dementia *NYTimes.com* (Nov 18). <http://www.nytimes.com/2007/11/18/weekinreview/18zernike.html>.

Chapter seven

Work, Retirement, and Ageism in the Workplace

7.1 INTRODUCTION

Because of better health that allows many people to continue working, forced layoffs because of age discrimination that stereotypes older workers as less competitive, and financial problems that prevent some workers from early retirement, many older adults face workplace issues that are confusing, difficult to resolve, and at times, filled with workplace bias and ageism. As Mor-Barak and Tynan (1993) argue, "Despite this interest in continued employment by employers and older adults, older workers are more likely to lose their jobs than younger workers in instances such as plant closings and corporate mergers (Beckett, 1988)" (p. 45). The authors go on to point out that many businesses can't or won't deal with life events faced by older workers such as "widowhood and caring for ailing spouses, and as a result many older workers are forced to retire earlier than planned" (p. 45).

Writing about the loss of work and its impact on older men, Levant (1997) says that as men lose their good-provider roles, the experience results in "severe gender role strain" (p. 221) that affects relationships and can be disruptive to the point of ending otherwise strong marriages. Because older adults are more likely to lose high-level jobs due to downsizing and ageism, social contacts decrease and many otherwise healthy and motivated workers must deal with increased levels of isolation and loneliness. Schneider (1998) points out that many Americans are workaholics and that when work is taken away or jobs are diminished in complexity and creativity, many older adults experience a decrease in physical and mental health. And while early retirement is touted as a way to achieve the good life at an early age, the experience is a complex and even a wrenching one, in which older adults who are financially able to retire often have little ability to handle extra time, have failed to make sound retirement plans, and find out quickly that not working takes away social contacts, status, and a way to organize time.

Heller (1993) reports that the loss of roles when older adults no longer work can be devastating: "A major problem is that individuals lose institutional roles with age (e.g., forced retirement at age 65) and find that their contribution to society is devalued, not on the basis of personal attributes or behavior but because age has moved them to the role of a non-participant in society" (p.125). Heller (1993) suggests that "[t]he challenge for society will be to find ways for elderly citizens to perform useful social roles in mediating structures of neighborhood, family, and voluntary social organizations – roles that convey a contin- ued sense of competence and esteem" (p. 125).

For many healthy, work-oriented, and motivated older adults, volunteer and civic roles are not at all what they are looking for. They want to continue to work, to contribute, and to receive the status and benefits related to work. The fact that social security has a benefit scale based on birth date will make it unlikely for many workers in their forties and fifties to retire early. Current economic problems that have reduced savings and pensions also suggest that older workers will continue to work well past their mid-sixties. But continued work beyond retirement age has negative ramifications for workers who have worked at physically and emotionally demanding jobs and have seen their bodies and nervous systems wear out. For many of them, working well into their seventies may be difficult if not impossible. Many older adults who work at menial jobs to supplement social security benefits and savings find the experience unenlightening, demeaning, and physically draining.

Zedlewski and Butrica (2007) report that more than 10 million healthy older adults without care-giving responsibilities, who would like to work or volunteer, are engaged in neither even though more than half are under the age of 75 and 90% have some paid work experience. Engagement in work or volunteerism improves health and mortality through increased cognitive activity, exposure to stimulating environ- ments, and social interactions (Hultsch et al., 1999; Kubzansky et al., 2000). Additionally, enhanced social status (Thoits and Hewitt, 2001) and greater access to social, psychological, and material resources can also be positively affected by work and volunteerism (Wilson, 2000).

Zedlewski and Butrica (2007) believe that many older workers would enjoy a paid work or volunteer position. The authors argue that funding for training programs that target low-income older adults and broader communication networks that connect older adults to available volunteer and work opportunities are needed. The author's write,

> Policymakers must understand the payoffs of keeping older adults engaged. Longer careers increase retirement incomes, generate greater tax revenue, and reduce net Social Security payouts. Increased volunteerism improves physical and mental health, potentially reduces public health care costs, and benefits those receiving the services older adults provide. Investments in training older adults for new work and volunteer opportunities will have large personal, community, and national economic rewards. (Zedlewski and Butrica , 2007, p. 8)

7.2 RETIREMENT STRESS

Mor-Barak and Tynan (1993) suggest that retirement at a specific age is an "artifact of the Social Security laws that has acquired certain conveniences, leading to its perception and adoption as 'normative'" (p. 49) and that it "enables employers to dispense with the services of older workers gracefully, avoiding the administrative difficulties of selectively firing often 'faithful' workers" (p. 49) while allowing older workers to "salvage" self-respect because retiring at a specific age means you a member of a class of workers who were let go by mandate from the workforce rather than being individually removed. However,

> [T]hese conveniences do not mean that the current retirement system is beneficial for everyone. Retirement, which was once seen as a great achievement for the worker, is now viewed as an obstacle by people who feel they can and want to continue participating in the work force. Improved health and longer life expectancy prolong the period in which older adults can be productive in society. In addition, the larger variety of jobs not demanding physical strength enables more older people to continue working. These changes call for policy alterations to provide older adults with options and real choices with respect to work and retirement. (Mor-Barak and Tynan, 1993, p. 49)

It is often assumed that retirement is a pleasant experience, and for many people it is, but the process itself can be daunting and the decision itself can be so difficult to make that approximately 30% of all retirees perceive it as being very stressful (Atchley, 1975; Bossé et al., 1991; Braithwaite et al., 1986). If 30% of adults over the age of 65 perceive retirement as a very stressful event, that means that currently more than 10 million people have experienced stress when making the decision to retire. This figure may grossly underestimate retirement stress because many people retire before age 65.

Factors that have been associated with retirement stress include forced retirement, worker burnout and job unhappiness, a belief that a new job will be just as unrewarding and stressful as a current position, early retirement, retirement because of ill health, and financial difficulties. Forced retirement or retirement where workers are given strong messages that they are unwanted have been associated with greater difficulties adjusting (Atchley, 1982; Walker et al., 1981), lower satisfaction with retirement (Isaksson, 1997), adverse psychological reactions (Sharpley and Layton, 1998), and increased stress (Isaksson, 1997; Sharpley and Layton, 1998).

Workers who retire early have been found to be less satisfied with their lives than people who continue to work well into their sixties and seventies (Palmore et al., 1984). Individuals who are forced to retire because of ill health predictably report lower levels of morale (Braithwaite et al., 1986), higher stress scores (Bossé et al., 1991), and are at greater risk for emotional difficulties (Sharpley and Layton, 1998). Martin et al. (1988) found that the lower the socioeconomic status of men, the more negative the impact of retirement overall. Individuals who experience a substantial loss of income during retirement tend to experience poor morale (Richardson and Kilty, 1991) and poor adjustment (Palmore et al., 1985). Many people who find their retirement plans changed because companies no longer honor pension plans or have grossly changed pension plans also report lower satisfaction with retirement and greater levels of stress.

Reeves and Darville (1994) found that well-adjusted retirees report more social support than retirees who are less well-adjusted (Reeves & Darville, 1994). Fletcher & Hansson (1991) report that retirees who expected to have very little personal control over their lives during retirement not only had more negative views of retirement but also feared the event. Glamser (1976) found that those who expected retirement to be a positive experience held a positive attitude about retirement, while those expecting retirement to be a negative experience held negative attitudes about their retired lives.

The issue of early retirement is one in which substantial involvement of helping professionals should exist. Early retirement is a complex issue for many older adults who may feel diminished and mistreated at work and see retirement as a way of coping with low morale and stress. Often it isn't a good solution since many early retirees have not thought through retirement as a life style change and may still desire to work, although in new organizations, but may believe that their age makes new employment unlikely. Financial incentive plans for early retirement that seem lucrative may in fact offer a person less financial security in the long run and reduced social security and pension benefits. Work is important to most people since it offers status and a daily schedule. When those two important factors are taken away, many early retirees feel unimportant and confused about how they plan to spend the day. As a nurse told a colleague when he mentioned his plan to retire early, "You have 30 good years ahead of you," she said, "What are you going to do with yourself?" He immediately forgot about early retirement and decided to handle his current job unhappiness by going elsewhere, and it worked.

Atchley (1999) propose six phases of retirement consisting of the following:

1. In the pre-retirement phase, workers become aware that retirement is approaching and in the years prior to retirement, save money, dream of life after retirement, and begin to gradually prepare for this change in life.
2. The honeymoon phase takes place immediately after the actual retirement event and is characterized by enjoyment of free time and the ability to do everything the retiree has wanted to do for years.
3. The disenchantment phase occurs when the retiree completes activities, trips and time with family, activities they had always wanted to do, and now feels depressed because there is a lack of new activities to remain engaged in and excited about, and boredom and unhappiness then set in.
4. The disenchantment period leads to a reorientation phase during which the retiree begins to develop a more realistic attitude toward the use of time, and priorities are set that contribute to the next phase.
5. In the stability phase, a retirement routine is developed that may include work, recreational activities, new learning opportunities and other activities that keep the retiree content and involved.
6. The terminal phase or the end of retirement occurs when illness or disability prevents the retiree from actively caring for himself or herself.

7.3 BEST EVIDENCE FOR WORK WITH RETIREMENT-RELATED STRESS

Because of the stressful nature of retirement, Nuttman-Schwartz (2007) suggests that helping professionals involve family members in retirement planning. The researcher writes, "The results [of his study] showed family perceptions' contribute to postretirement adjustment. Thus, in order to help the retirees to accept their retirement transition, it suggests that the pre-retirement intervention should focus on the family as a whole, especially when retirees plan their future" (p. 192). According to the author, pre-planning with family is particularly important when the retiree shows signs of loneliness and depression before retirement, because those emotional states may continue and even worsen after retirement.

Carpenter et al. (2006) found that adult children sometimes know their parents' preferences for retired life but are often unaware of many important issues, particularly those issues that pertain to achieving a high quality of life. The researchers suggest that families engage themselves in discussions of late-life issues and find out parental preferences. The authors recognize that families may not have these discussions "because of time constraints, discomfort bringing up topics that imply eventual impairment, or simply because families lack the tools to have productive discussions about preferences" (p. 562). The authors suggest a family process to reevaluate and accommodate the changing needs and preferences of older adults as they consider and move into retirement. The researchers conclude by saying that "[b]ecause most children inevitably play some role in guiding the psychosocial care of their parents, it is imperative to find ways to improve their knowledge about parent preferences and values" (p. 562).

Smith and Moen (2004) interviewed over 400 retired couples. Although 67% of the individual spouses said they were satisfied with retirement, 59% of the couples surveyed said they were jointly satisfied. Those couples most likely to report joint retirement satisfaction were retired wives whose husbands were not influential in their retirement decision. When a spouse retired and the other spouse was expected to stop work and move to a new locale as part of the overall retirement plan, satisfaction with retirement decreased as did marital satisfaction. Understandably, retirement should be a joint decision and both partners should have an equal say in how retirement might affect their lives.

Bakalar (2006) reports on a study of 280 socially disadvantaged men with low-level jobs who were interviewed about life satisfaction from adolescence until an average age of 75. The researchers found that happiness in retirement didn't depend on good health or having a large income in this group of men. Men who found retirement satisfying were more than twice as likely to report enjoying relationships, volunteering, and having hobbies among their favorite activities than were those who found retirement unrewarding. Men who were unhappily retired said that they occupied their lives with what the researchers called "autistic activities" such as watching television, gambling, or caring for themselves. Forty-three percent of the happiest retirees said they found purpose in community service, while only seven percent of those who found retirement unsatisfying did so. The researchers concluded that many of the issues that contribute to satisfaction after retirement are quite different from those that assure a contented and economically secure middle age.

Gellene (2007) reported a study done at Rush Medical Center in Chicago, which found that loneliness often precedes dementia in subjects over the age of 80. The study found that the risk of dementia increased 51% for every one-point increase on a five-point scale of loneliness. The same study found that in men and women aged 50–67, subjects who rated themselves as very lonely had blood pressure readings fully 30-points higher than subjects in the study who didn't rate themselves as being lonely. Although rates of loneliness among older adults might be higher than other age groups because of the death of loved ones and health problems, loneliness is a problem for older adults who were either lonely before they retired or who find that the loss of work reduces their network of friendships. This may be even truer among those who relocate after retirement and find it difficult to make friends.

EVIDENCE-BASED PRACTICE WITH JOB DISSATISFACTION IN AN OLDER ADULT: A CASE STUDY

Jason Stewart is a 63-year-old professor of counseling at a third-tier public university in the Midwest. He has been feeling burned out and unhappy about his job, believing that the students he trains are quite inferior, and that most students have lost their idealism and only want to be private practitioners and make a great deal of money. He chose counseling as a career to help others and to make the world a better place, ideas that seem old fashioned in the current climate of cynicism and narcissism he finds among the students he teaches. His feelings of burnout and unhappiness have been gaining in strength since Jason was passed over for the chairmanship of his department five years-ago. He is now wondering if he should quit work completely or seek another job, and has come for treatment to help him decide on a course of action. Jason has no hobbies other than reading mysteries, watching films, and writing articles and books. He admits that he thinks therapy is "nonsense" and wants the worker to use a brief problem-focused approach to resolve his problem, consistent with the notion of life coaching. Glicken (2005, p. 127) describes life coaching as follows:

1. Life coaching focuses on here-and-now problems. It doesn't assume that a problem has its origins in the past, and it tries to find quick and logical solutions.
2. Life coaching is very practical. It uses advice, homework, and searching for answers in the literature and on the Internet. Personal coaches often suggest that clients keep logs or write down ideas that are then shared with the coach (or therapist). This technique seems efficient for many men who believe that taking personal responsibility for change will speed up the process.
3. Life coaching encourages the use of behavioral charting to analyze a problem and to track success. Charting is a way of problem solving that is often familiar to men.
4. Coaching assumes that clients are emotionally healthy and functioning well but just need some practical and supportive assistance with problem-solving. Compare this to therapy that assumes dysfunction, describes people in unhealthy ways, and often uses labels. Whether people are emotionally healthy or not is something no one can tell for certain at the start of treatment. It should soon become apparent whether problems need deeper and more long-term approaches as the client tries to use coaching and finds that it either doesn't help or the material focused on is difficult for the client to apply to his life.
5. Coaching is very positive and optimistic. It believes that problems can be resolved in a short period of time and that the client has the necessary inner resources and skills to resolve the problem with just a little direction from the coach. Compare this to descriptions of therapy as an often long-term, painful, in-depth process, and you can see why many men would prefer coaching.
6. Coaching seems very much like the social encounters men have in their daily lives.
7. Everyone understands the term "coaching," while therapy is still a term with many misconceptions and, among some cultures and men, negative connotations.

Jason's therapist has used this type of brief, problem-focused treat-ment with a few clients and has found it superficial at best. Still, it seemed only fair that he take into consideration what Jason wanted and to work with him. The initial sessions went very well. Jason was highly motivated, did a great deal of reading about early retirement and older adult burnout, and found that it wasn't unusual for people in the human services to feel burned out and unhappy with their jobs after many years of tough, loyal, and successful work without very much financial or emo-tional payoff. As Jason read, talked to the therapist, and made behav-ioral charts, he began to complain about feeling depressed. "I still don't know what to do," he said, and wondered if the worker had any sugges-tions. He did. Why not enter the job market and see if he could find a job where his skills could be put to better use and where the students were academically stronger?

Jason did just that and, much to his surprise, he was a finalist for several very high-level positions in tier 1 universities. He spoke to the worker about the experience. "I wanted something better, but now I'm scared. I don't think I want to work that hard, and I'm worried that having been in a medi-ocre university makes me unprepared to deal with high-level faculty and students. The thought of moving makes me feel old and tired."

The worker listened to Jason for several sessions as he discussed his confusion and concern about his job possibilities. She told him that it seemed as if the pull to stay was stronger than the pull to leave. Was there a way he could stay at his university and perhaps change what he was doing and begin to work less? Jason explored these options and came back with an idea:

"I found out that we have an early retirement plan where you can get your pension and social security and still work for five years up to 50% of the time and get paid part-time using your current salary and benefit lev-els as a base. At the end of the five-year period, you can work part-time but at a lower salary rate. I think I could do that and perhaps it would help me deal with retirement. The problem is that I don't want to keep teaching, so I went to my chair and discussed the plan. He wants me to spend the 50% creating new curriculum and trying to deal with the prob-lems of poor students. He doesn't think we have enough diversity and he wants to see if we can admit more idealistic students and hire more idealistic faculty. Everyone was feeling the same way I did, he told me, which was a great surprise to me. He said that the reason I was passed over for the chair's position had nothing to do with me or the faculty. The faculty wanted me but the administration wanted someone younger. It pissed me off to find out about ageism, but I thought it was because they didn't like me. Five years to ease myself into retirement would give me time to write books and to do some traveling. I live alone and maybe it's time to find someone who can offer companionship and intimacy. I've put off those needs since I divorced 20 years ago and I feel very lonely at times."

The worker thought his idea was a good one and wondered how he might find someone to be in his life. "I was reading a mystery novel by the Swedish writer Henning Mankell called *Firewall* (1998)" he said, "and his main character, a cop called Kurt Wallander, is like me: lonely and set in his ways but in need of someone in his life. The detective uses a dating service and finds someone. I started thinking about women who have given me some indication that they are interested in me. Maybe I'll just follow up and see if I can find someone that way. I don't think I could ever use a dating service at my age, but we'll see. And I need to start going to our national conferences. I met my wife that way and we did pretty well for almost 20 years; not bad in this day and age."

Discussion

The therapist shared the following remarks about her client: "Jason is a healthy man. There's nothing wrong with getting burned out on a job or feeling unhappy about it. He tested the waters and decided he didn't want to take a job with even more potential for burnout and stress. Having made that decision, he found an alternative position. We don't know whether or not it will work but it seems like a good alternative to moving and dealing with even more stress than he has in his life now. Did I feel comfortable using the parameters he set down initially for treatment? Sure. Clients have to be invested in what they do and coaching, or at least his read on coaching, seemed feasible to me. Why assume that there are larger problems in his life when a brief, problem-focused approach might work? Using charts and reading is Jason's way to problem-solve. But as he found out, there's a difference between problem-solving and dealing with inner turmoil. You can know what to do logically but it can still make you anxious and uncertain. I have confidence in my clients to do what's best for them. Therapy is a process, and part of that process is to go through a series of steps to determine what to do about a problem so that you arrive at a point where the client does what he or she thinks is right for them now. My job is to facilitate the process and see that the client doesn't avoid any of the necessary steps.

"Has Jason done well? I spoke to him several weeks ago. He's been out of therapy for a year and called to chat. He said that he's happy that he went to work half-time and likes the time off. He isn't terribly happy about the work he's doing and finds that he just isn't interested in counseling anymore. His writing is going well and he may just focus on writing, but he isn't certain. He's been dating, but hasn't found anyone special. He sounds happier than when I first saw him, but he still has his down days. I asked if he wanted to come back and see me, but he said that he was OK with where we left things and that it had helped. He just didn't think the problems he was having warranted more therapy since the best thing for him now was to keep testing the waters to find the right solutions. He also said that our work together helped him a great deal. He was stuck then and now he wasn't.

"Do I think Jason has made substantial movement? I do. Could he have made more movement had he stayed in therapy longer? I don't think so since clients usually leave therapy when *they* feel ready, not when the therapist does. Are there underlying issues to deal with that could make him more successful as he ages? I don't know. Jason grapples with life in his own way, and in therapy with older adults you have to be careful not to step over the line. The line is that point when therapy becomes aversive because the subject matter either strays from what the client wants or because it causes more unhappiness. We focused on his many strengths. By doing this Jason ended treatment understanding several things: (1) there is nothing wrong with becoming tired of the work you do; (2) that he has many skills; (3) that he has options; (4) his personal life is very important and perhaps working on it might improve his overall happiness; (5) he could go to other jobs if he wanted; and, (6) not wanting to add to one's stress level by moving and taking on new responsibilities is perfectly fine. It seems to me that's quite a bit to gain from treatment, and my view is that he did quite well and should he need additional help, he'll get it."

7.4 BRIDGE JOBS BETWEEN LONG TERM CAREERS AND TOTAL RETIREMENT

According to Zedlewski and Butrica (2007) research evidence increasingly shows that older adults who regularly work after retirement enjoy better health and live longer, thanks to stimulating environments and a sense of purpose. In support of this position, Calvo (2006) found that paid work at older ages reduces morbidity and improves health. Tsai et al. (2005) followed a sample of early retirees for 30 years and found that they experienced higher morbidity rates than workers who retired later. Dhaval et al. (2006) indicate that complete retirement takes a toll on physical and mental health. The reasons why work improves health and mortality suggest increased cognitive activity, exposure to stimulating environments and social interactions (Kubzansky et al., 2000), enhanced social status (Thoits and Hewitt, 2001), and greater access to social, psychological, and material resources (Wilson, 2000). Some work activities help older adults develop knowledge and skills that boost their self-images and mental outlooks (Harlow-Rosentraub et al., 2006).

Once older adults reach age 65, most will opt for retirement (Ekerdt, 1998). Although some individuals move from full-time work to full-time leisure, a substantial number remain in the labor force (Hansson et al., 1997). Many of these working "retired" adults are in bridge-type jobs, which act as transitions between long-term career positions and total retirement (Feldman, 1994; Mutchler, Burr et al., 1997). Because of downsizing, employers have been offering incentives to induce or force costly older workers into early retirement so that many older adults have left the labor force before reaching retirement age ("Business: The jobs challenge," 2001). By the late 1990s, early retirements accounted for more than 80% of total retirements (Seymour, 1999). A significant number of these early retirees participate in some form of bridge employment (Feldman, 1994).

Bridge jobs may be part-time work, self-employment, or temporary work and often involve a combination of fewer hours, less stress or responsibility, greater flexibility, and fewer physical demands (Feldman, 1994). Bridge jobs offer possible remedies to older adults who are concerned about their financial security and to employers who face a labor shortage. Increased life expectancy, the high level of dependence on Social Security, and the increased number of workers not covered by pension plans contribute to the financial insecurity of older workers (Committee for Economic Development, 1999). To maintain desired incomes in retirement, older Americans have to save more during their working years and/ or retire later in life, including taking bridge employment.

Ulrieh and Brott (2005) studied the following strategies made by retirees to transition into bridging jobs:

1. The majority of the participants planned for their financial future but did not consider what they wanted to do after they retired and they failed to take advantage of their community's career and job search resources.
2. Some individuals did not have to start over again because they were able to build on their past career experience, marketable skills, reputations, and personal skills.
3. Participants discovered that a bridge job sometimes introduced unwanted changes, such as lower pay, lack of career advancement,

difficulties in forming close work relationships, separation from former career fields, and loss of responsibilities.

4. Without sufficient planning or reaching out to available resources, many participants found it difficult to switch to a new career. They had a hard time moving into a new job if the job titles did not match their long-term career titles or if they defined their occupational field too narrowly.

5. Many did not fully investigate a job opportunity before they accepted employment and were disappointed after a period of time on the job.

6. Participants were reluctant to move into new jobs because they lacked the appropriate technological skills or they questioned their ability to learn these new skills.

7. Taking employment-related tests was viewed as an unpleasant experience for these older adults.

8. At the end of their long-term career or during their transition to a bridge job, many participants speculated that their careers and their transition efforts were affected by subtle age discrimination, such as younger employees questioning their capabilities.

9. Regardless of these challenges, participants benefited greatly from their bridge jobs. They credited their bridge jobs for making them feel better about themselves, giving them a more balanced life, and helping them enjoy their work. They felt better about themselves because they continued to learn, make a difference to others, had an opportunity to demonstrate their competency, and felt healthy.

Ulrieh and Brott (2005) indicate a need for clinicians to address the unique needs of older workers who are redefining retirement through bridge employment. The challenges for clinicians are twofold: how to encourage older workers to take advantage of career counseling services, and how to effectively help older workers with the decision to continue working full-time, take bridge employment, or fully retire. Ulrieh and Brott (2005) suggest the following strategies clinicians could consider for encouraging older workers to seek career services: (a) develop a targeted message when presenting to community and employee groups; (b) establish relationships with individuals and organizations that provide retirement and financial planning; (c) seek opportunities to present at retirement planning events; and, (d) network with employers who sponsor retirement planning workshops.

7.5 PERSONAL STORY: WORKING AFTER RETIREMENT

"I drive two hours each way from my home to teach courses each semester at a major university. Driving down the mountain from my house in the Arizona backcountry is stunning. You go by Dead Bug Wash, Black River Canyon, Horse Thief Canyon, and vistas that make you want to hug the scenery. It's a little like you felt as a kid watching a John Wayne movie only you have a cup of coffee with you and you're listening to a tape by Alison Krauss so beautiful and touching that you want to play it for your students when you see them.

"On the way to class I stop at the factory outlet stores outside of Phoenix for coffee and find myself buying clothes I need but would never buy because… well. because I never thought of myself as some-one who wanted to look especially good for others. Academics are just not into clothes. Now that I have some decent clothes to wear I find myself enjoying the pleasure of dressing well (sort of well, anyway). I've lost a lot of weight so the pleasure is that much better.

"Once I get to campus I have a Starbucks coffee in the library, check my e-mail before class, and notice the serious working class students at a bank of computers. School is no picnic and most of them work second jobs, sometime full-time, to pay their tuition. It's hard to think that many of them have parents affluent enough to pay their university expenses, yet here they are. It makes me feel optimistic about the future to see such hard working young people.

"I go to my classes, and while I don't feel I'm as good as I could be because I'm a bit tired from the drive, the students are happy to see me. They've begun to realize that I spend much more time with them than their full-time teachers, and that I respond to e-mails and grade their papers very quickly. Several students have told me they never get responses from their teachers, and when I respond as soon as they send an e-mail, it's startling, but in a nice way.

"To help me remember lecture material I audiotape my lectures, play a bit of what I've recorded in class, and then expand on the material. It seems like a good approach and the students don't appear to mind. I record my lectures the day before classes in the morning when I'm fresh and then listen to them in the car while driving to teach. Many times I tell jokes when I record and find myself laughing at the puns and bad jokes I tell students.

"I've become very good at using the academic Internet program *Blackboard* and spent a few days with the help of an IT person learning the mysteries and benefits of that great teaching tool. Because of the long drive, I've decided to offer the occasional Internet class so that certain assignments and examinations can be done on line. The students like the freedom and their work is much improved.

"I make a paltry sum of money for teaching, but the money goes for the frivolous things I never felt comfortable buying before: clothes, a new tennis racquet, better tennis shoes, hiking gear so I can hike these beautiful Arizona mountains, particularly the many hiking trails in and around Sedona. I feel rich with the extra money, and it makes me very generous. I figure that what I make is play money because I get such pleasure from it, so why shouldn't other people benefit?

"I've tried to volunteer but I'm still tied to the notion that you should be paid for your labor if you are to be valued. I've begun consulting for a new university in my town that will offer a first year of college to young adults in recovery. The money is nice, the work is very interesting, and I feel valued. Between all of that and the books I write, my plate is full. I have time to work out, to hike, and to go to political and social events, but the work sustains me and makes me feel that, although I'm retired, I'm really still working but for myself and not the large organizations that treat older adults so badly. It's a wonderful feeling, one I dreamed of when I was working full-time at stressful jobs.

"I think work is a necessary part of the aging process. I don't think volunteer work has the same emotional value as paid work, but that's me. And it's not the amount of money you make, it's the fact that you can now focus on what you love doing. There is no amount of money that can equal the feeling of complete independence to pick and choose what excites you.

"It isn't growing old that worries us older people, it's the fear we'll grow old and be bored. To have work that still excites you, that's one of the best rewards. That, and someone who loves you without reservation." – MDG

7.6 SUMMARY

This chapter discusses issues pertaining to work, retirement and ageism in the workplace. Many older men and women would like to continue working, but at jobs that utilize talents and dreams and are different than the jobs they've held much of their lives. For many older adults, work after retirement is not a choice but a necessity caused by limited income after retirement. Data are provided showing that older adults do better if they work or volunteer in measures of physical and emotional health. A case study and a personal study explore some of the complicating factors, positive and negative related to work for older adults.

7.7 QUESTIONS FROM THE CHAPTER

1. Shouldn't older people retire and leave work to young people? If older people keep working where are the jobs going to be for young men and women?
2. Older people should volunteer but they should be able to do work that they're prepared and trained to do without having to go through the hoops of licensure and state certification. Do you agree?
3. Ageism is one of those politically correct terms that liberals use to describe conditions they think are unfair, but isn't it the job of business to prefer young people who have stamina and good health? Let's face it, older workers aren't as strong, energetic or willing to work long hours as young people. Don't you agree?
4. When I retire I'm going to take it easy and travel. I don't get why anyone who's worked all their life at hard jobs would want to continue working. Would you?
5. I have a professor who must be in his seventies and he falls asleep and can't remember anyone's name. Sometimes he forgets what he's talking about. I just think people should be made to retire when they can't do the job anymore. What do you think?

REFERENCES

Atchley, R. C. (1975). Adjustment to the loss of job at retirement. *International Journal of Aging and Human Development, 6*, 17–27.

Atchley, R. C. (1982). Retirement: Learning the world of work. *Annals of the American Academy of Political and Social Sciences, 464*, 120–131.

Atchley, R. C. (1999). Continuity and adaptation in aging. Baltimore: Johns Hopkins University Press.

Bakalar, N. (2006). Retirement contentment in reach for unhappy men http://www.nytimes.com/2006/04/04/health/psychology/04reti.html. *NewYorkTimes.com* (April 4).

Beckett, J. O. (1988). Plant dosing: How older workers are affected. *Social Work, 33*, 29–33.

Bossé, R., Aldwin, C. M., Levenson, M. R., & Workman-Daniels, K. (1991). How stressful is retirement? Findings from the normative aging study. *Journal of Gerontology, 46*, 9–14.

Braithwaite, V. A., Gibson, D. M., & Bosly-Craft, R. (1986). An exploratory study of poor adjustment styles among retirees. *Social Science and Medicine, 23*, 493–499.

Brewington, J. O., & Nassar-McMillan, S. (2000). Older adults: Work-related issues and implications for counseling. *The Career Development Quarterly, 49*, 2–15.

Business: The jobs challenge. (2001) (July 14). *The Economist, 360*, 56–57.

Calvo, E. (2006). *Does working longer make people healthier and happier? Work opportunities for older Americans brief,* series 2. Chestnut Hill, MA: Center for Retirement Research, Boston College.

Carpenter, B. D., Katy Rickdeschel, M. D., Van Haitsma, K. S., & Feldman, P. H. (2006). Adult children as informants about parent's psychosocial preferences. *Family Relations, 55,* 552–563.

Committee for Economic Development. (1999). *New opportunities for older workers.* New York: Author.

Dhaval, D., Rashad, I., & Spasojevic, J. (2006). The effects of retirement on physical and mental health outcomes. NBER Working Paper 12123. Cambridge, MA: NBER.

Ekerdt, D. (1998). Workplace norms for the timing of retirement. In K. Schaie & C. Schooler (Eds.), *Impact of work on older adults* (pp. 101–123). New York: Springer.

Feldman, D. C. (1994). The decision to retire early: A review and conceptualization. *The Academy of Management Review, 19,* 285–311.

Fletcher, W. L., & Hansson, R. O. (1991). Assessing the social components of retirement anxiety. *Psychology and Aging, 6,* 76–85.

Gellene, D. (2007). Loneliness often precedes elder dementia, study finds (Feb. 10). *Los Angeles Times,* A11.

Glamser, F. D. (1976). Determinants of a positive attitude toward retirement. *Journal of Gerontology, 31,* 104–107.

Glicken, M. D. (2005). Working with troubled men. A contemporary practitioner's guide. mahwah, N.J: Lawrence Erlbaum Associates, Inc.

Hansson, R. O., DeKoekkoek, P. D., Neece, W. M., & Patterson, D. W. (1997). Successful aging at work: Annual review, 1992–1996: The older worker and transition to retirement. *Journal of Vocational Behavior, 51,* 202–233.

Harlow-Rosentraub, K., Wilson, L., & Steele, J. (2006). Expanding youth service concepts for older adults: AmeriCorps results. In L. Wilson & S. Simson (Eds.), *Civic engagement and the baby boomer generation: Research, policy and practice perspectives* (pp. 61–84). New York: Haworth Press.

Heller, K. (1993). Prevention activities for older adults: Social structures and personal competencies that maintain useful social roles. *Journal of Counseling & Development, 72*(2), 124–130.

Isaksson, K. (1997). Patterns of adjustment to early retirement. Reports from the Department of Psychology (No. 828). Stockholm, Sweden: Stockholm University pp. 1–13.

Kubzansky, L. D., Berkman, L. F., & Seeman, T. E. (2000). Social conditions and distress in elderly persons: findings from the MacArthur Studies of Successful Aging. *Journals of Gerontology: Psychological Science, 55B*(4), 238–246.

Levant, R. F. (1997). The masculinity issue. *The Journal of Men's Studies, 5*(3), 221–229.

Mankell, H. (1998). *Firewall*. New York: The New Press.

Martin Matthews, A., & Brown, K. H. (1988). Retirement as a critical life event. *Research on Aging, 9*, 548–571.

Mor-Barak, M. E., & Tynan, M. (1993). Older workers and the workplace: A new challenge for occupational social work. *Social Work, 38*(1), 45–55.

Mutchler, J. E., Burr, J. A., Pienta, A. M., & Massagli, M. P. (1997). Pathways to labor force exit: Work transitions and work instability. *Journal of Gerontology: Social Sciences, 52B*, S4–S12.

Nuttman-Schwartz, O. (2007). *Men's Perceptions of Family During the Retirement Transition Families in Society, 88*(2), 192–202.

Palmore, E. B., Fillenbaum, G. G., & George, L. K. (1984). Consequences of retirement. *Journal of Gerontology, 39*, 109–116.

Reeves, J. B., & Darville, R. L. (1994). Social contact patterns and satisfaction with retirement of women in dual-career/earner families. *International Journal of Aging and Human Development, 39*, 163–175.

Richardson, V. E., & Kilty, K. M. (1991). Adjustment to retirement: Continuity vs. discontinuity. *International Journal of Aging and Human Development, 33*, 151–169.

Schneider, K. J. (1998). Toward a science of the heart: Romanticism and the revival of psychology. *American Psychologist, 53*(3), 277–289.

Seymour, L. (1999). Robust economy sends early retirements soaring to 81% of 1998 retirements. *Employee Benefit Plan Review, 54*, 50–51.

Sharpley, C. F., & Layton, R. (1998). Effects of age of retirement, reason for retirement and pre-retirement training on psychological and physical health during retirement. *Australian Psychologist, 33*, 119–124.

Smith, D. B., & Moen, P. (2004). Retirement satisfaction for retirees and their spouses: Do gender and the retirement decision-making process matter? *Journal of Family Issues, 25*, 262.

Thoits, P. A., & Hewitt, L. N. (2001). Volunteer work and well-being. *Journal of Health and Social Behavior, 42*(2), 115–131.

Tsai, S. P., Wendt, J. K., Donnelly, R. P., de Jong, G., & Ahmed, F. S. (2005). Age at retirement and long-term survival of an industrial population: prospective cohort study. *BMJ, 331*, 995.

Ulrich, L. B., & Brott, P. E. (2005). Older workers and bridge employment: Redefining retirement. *Journal of Employment Counseling, 42*, 159–170.

Walker, J., Kimmel, D., & Price, K. (1981). Retirement style and retirement satisfaction: Retirees aren't all alike. *International Journal of Clinical Psychological, 41*, 58–62.

Wilson, J. (2000). Volunteering. *Annual Review of Sociology, 26*, 215–240.

Zedlewski, S. R., & Butrica, B. A. (2007). Are we taking full advantage of older adults' potential? THE RETIREMENT PROJECT: Perspectives on productive aging. The Urban Institute No. 9 (Dec. 2007).

Chapter eight

Evidence-Based Practice with Older Adults Experiencing Social Isolation and Loneliness

8.1 INTRODUCTION

We often think of aging as a time of increased loneliness and isolation. Spouses have sometimes passed away or become too frail to offer companionship, and adult children are involved in their own lives and haven't time to be with parents. It is not uncommon in our society for older adults to have a limited role, and aging brings with it the isolation of not having family or family nearby. Illness often prompts an additional sense of isolation and aloneness, and romance and intimacy are sometimes increasingly limited. According to the literature, these conditions often lead to loneliness in older adults.

Estimates of the prevalence of loneliness range from 7% to 84% in studies where older people are asked if they feel lonely (Wenger, 1983; Sheldon, 1984). Prince et al. (1997) found that available studies of adults over age 65 indicate that 5% to 15% report frequently feeling lonely and an additional 20% to 40% report occasional feelings of loneliness. However, 50% of adults aged 80 or over often feel very lonely. Because of the tendency to give positive answers when the

159

opposite may be true, we should interpret these findings cautiously and accept that rates of loneliness may be higher than those found in surveys.

In explaining the reasons for loneliness and the large number of lonely older adults, Seligman and Csikszetmihalyi (2000) note that Americans "live surrounded by many more people than their ancestors did, yet they are intimate with fewer individuals and thus experience greater loneliness and alienation" (p. 9). Ostrov and Offer (1980) suggest that American culture emphasizes individual achievement, competitiveness, and impersonal social relations, and that loneliness may be quite pronounced in the face of such socially alienating values. Saxton (1986) argues that in contemporary American society there is a decline in the face-to-face, intimate contacts with family members, relatives, and close friends, which were much more prevalent several decades ago. Mijuskovic (1992) views American society as highly mechanized with "impersonal institutions, disintegration of the family as a result of a high divorce rate, high mobility rates with its impact on family and community ties; the fast-paced living and self-centeredness of the culture interferes with people's ability to establish and maintain fulfilling relationships" (RokAch, 2007, p. 184).

Martin Seligman (2002) worries that Americans have become so caught up in a personal sense of entitlement that even helping professionals have gone along with, and in fact encouraged, "The belief that we can rely on shortcuts to happiness, joy, rapture, comfort, and ecstasy, rather than be entitled to these feelings by the exercise of personal strengths and virtues, which results in legions of people who, in the middle of great wealth, are starving spiritually" (ABCNews.COM, 2002, online). Seligman argues that "Positive emotion alienated from the exercise of character leads to emptiness, to inauthenticity, to depression, and, as we age, to the gnawing realization that we are fidgeting until we die" (ABCNews.COM, 2002, online).

Robert Putnam (Stossel, 2000) believes that this focus on self is producing a country without a sense of social connectedness where, "Supper eaten with friends or family has given way to supper gobbled in solitude, with only the glow of the television screen for companionship" (p. 1). According to Putnam,

> Americans today have retreated into isolation. Evidence shows that fewer and fewer contemporary Americans are unionizing, voting, rallying around shared causes, participating in religious services,

inviting each other over, or doing much of anything collectively. In fact, when we do occasionally gather – for twelve-step support encounters and the like – it's most often only as an excuse to focus on ourselves in the presence of an audience. (Stossel, 2000, p. 1)

Putnam believes that the lack of social involvement negatively affects school performance, health and mental health, increases crime rates, reduces tax responsibilities and charitable work, decreases productivity, and "even simple human happiness – all are demonstrably affected by how (and whether) we connect with our family and friends and neighbors and co-workers" (Stossel, 2000, p. 1).

Commenting on the importance of understanding culture and the way cultures organize family life, belief systems, and closeness to others as factors in creating loneliness, RokAch (2007) writes,

Loneliness research tends to focus on individual factors, that is, either on personality factors or on lack of social contacts (Jylha and Jokela, 1990). However, loneliness could be expressive of an individual's relationship to the community. It is conceivable, then, that the difference between cultures and the ways in which social relations are organized within them will result in cross-cultural variations in the way people experience loneliness. The difference of the social tapestry, interpersonal interactions and the support networks which are available to individuals in various cultures are bound to affect the causes of loneliness. (p. 174)

Although loneliness in older adults may have social and cultural antecedents, many lonely people report feeling lonely and rejected by others from a very early age, and even in the presence of others. Among lonely older people who have experienced loneliness from an early age, the absence of social contacts as they age creates a sense of despair that should not be confused with depression. The loneliness they experience is a feeling of separateness and not fitting in that sometimes worsens with age. This type of loneliness may have its roots in failure to bond with parents or parental rejection. A case later in the chapter describes the treatment for this type of loneliness.

8.2 DEFINITIONS AND CAUSATION OF LONELINESS AND ISOLATION

Murphy (2006) describes loneliness "as a condition with distressing, depressing, dehumanizing, detached feelings that a person endures when there is a gaping emptiness in his or her life due to an unfulfilled social and/or emotional life" (p. 22). Uruk and Demir (2003) define loneliness as "an unpleasant experience that occurs when a person's network of social relationships is significantly deficient in either quality or quantity (Peplau and Perlman, 1984)" (p. 179). The authors add that loneliness is "the psychological state that results from discrepancies between one's desire for and one's actual composition of relationships" (p. 179). Young (1982) defines loneliness as the "perceived absence of satisfying social relationships, accompanied by symptoms of psychological distress that are related to the perceived absence" (p. 380) while Sermat (1978) defines loneliness "as an experienced discrepancy between the kinds of interpersonal relationships the individuals perceive themselves as having and the kind of relationships they would like to have" (p. 274). A second aspect of the definition of loneliness is the distinction between issues that may serve as catalysts for loneliness, such as the loss of friends, spouses and family members, and dispositional factors such as shyness, introversion, or high expectations and demands that make individuals more vulnerable to loneliness.

Uruk and Demir (2003) report a strong correlation between parents who have little time to spend with their children or fail to form attachments with their children, and the development of loneliness in adolescence that often continues into adulthood and later life. Joiner et al. (1999) believe that loneliness stems from a lack of pleasurable engagement and, as a result, a painful disconnection from trying to engage. The authors call this the "bedrock" of loneliness. Similarly, Jones and Carver (1991) believe that loneliness affects "one's opinion about people, life, and society in a manner suggesting that lonely people subscribe to negativistic, apathetical, and pessimistic views" (p. 400).

Weiss (1973) distinguishes loneliness due to emotional isolation from loneliness due to social isolation. Emotional isolation appears in the absence of a close emotional attachment (often related to a lack of parental attachment), while social isolation appears in the absence of an engaging social network (often related to a lack of peer support, friendships, and close social networks). Relationships with parents and peers constitute two different social contexts in which loneliness develops. Rubin and Mills (1991) believe that loneliness develops when a pattern made up of social anxiety, lack of dominance, and social isolation results in peer rejection and negative self-perception. Olweus (1993) reports that when children blame their own incompetence for negative social experiences with peers, which result in rejection, the end effect is often social withdrawal, feelings of isolation, and depression. Rotenberg et al. (2004) found considerable evidence that loneliness correlates highly with lack of trust, particularly in young women. The author's note,

> As we expected, the relationship between loneliness and trust is stronger for girls than it is for boys. The trust measures accounted for 57% of loneliness for girls but only 18% of loneliness for boys. These patterns are consistent with the hypothesis that if girls do not believe or rely on their same-gender peers to keep intimacies confidential and to fulfill promises then they are cut off from their preferred and prevalent form of interaction (i.e., same-gender close-peer networks) and therefore are highly prone to loneliness. Finding this pattern with girls and not with boys also is consistent with the notion that girls are more inclined to establish a network of close peers than are boys. Close peer networks may be normatively expected for girls, and thus they may be distinctly at risk for loneliness because they demonstrate both low trust beliefs in same-gender peers and low levels of reciprocal trusting behaviors with peers. (p. 235)

Rotenberg et al. (2004) report that these findings have implications for social functioning during adulthood. "Women have larger intimacy networks than do men and, therefore, the observed association between loneliness and trust beliefs in same-gender peers may be stronger for women than for men during adulthood as well" (p. 235).

Ekwall (2005) believes that it is important to differentiate social isolation from loneliness. Social isolation by choice is defined as aloneness, and can be understood as the desire to live in a way isolated from others. Social isolation without choice is defined as loneliness, and can best be understood as a desire to have contact with others, but because of social, emotional, or geographic barriers, an inability to do so. McWhirter (1990) suggests that older adult loneliness can take place in both the presence and absence of social contact. Akerlind and Hornquist (1992) believe that social support research emphasizes external factors and the availability of social support while loneliness research emphasizes internal negative emotions about relationships or deficits in relationships. Regardless of the reason, loneliness and social isolation in older adults have been shown to be major negative influence on psychosocial well-being.

8.3 THE IMPACT OF LONELINESS ON OLDER ADULTS

Russell (1996) found a relationship between loneliness, chronic illness, and lower self-rated health status in older adults. McWhiter (1990) found links between loneliness and suicide and suicidal ideation. Older adult loneliness has been found to increase alcohol abuse (Akerlind and Hornquist, 1992) and depression (Russell, 1996). Copel (1988) suggests that loneliness can reduce a sense of self-worth and inhibit the ability to develop and maintain interpersonal relationships. Peters and Liefbroer (1997) found that older adults not involved in a partner relationship were lonelier than older adults with a partner and that the loss or lack of a partner affected males more than females. Men rely on their spouses for social support, suggesting the absence of a multifaceted social network when compared to that of women. The dependence on spouses for support and companionship can lead to extreme loneliness when spouses die, prolonging bereavement, and widowed men remarrying at a much higher rate than women. Martikainen and Valkonen (1996) found that the death of a spouse affected everyday tasks such as housecleaning, preparing food, and taking needed medication. Anderson and Diamond (1995) found that older widowed men experienced difficulties in everyday tasks such as cooking and meal planning. Many of the widowed men in this study who thought they were good cooks found it difficult to cook or even plan a meal.

Gellene (2007) reports a study done at Rush Medical Center in Chicago that found loneliness often preceded dementia in subjects over the age of 80. The study found that the risk of dementia increased 51% for every one-point increase on a five-point scale of loneliness. Interestingly, the study found that subjects who indicated high rates of loneliness often did so when there were people around them, suggesting that perceptions of loneliness have a much stronger impact than the actual existence of social networks. Autopsies of subjects with dementia indicated no sign of strokes or Alzheimer's disease. The same study found that in men and women ages 50–67, subjects who rated themselves as very lonely had blood pressure readings fully 30 points higher than subjects in the study who didn't rate themselves as being lonely. High blood pressure contributes to cardiovascular problems associated with heart attacks and strokes.

The Brown University Long-Term Care Quality Advisor (1998) reports that elderly individuals who indicated a high degree of loneliness tended to be admitted to nursing homes sooner than those who are not as lonely. The researchers interviewed 3,763 rural Iowans – all over age 65, none of whom were living in a nursing home at the time of the first interview. Contact was maintained with the members of the group once a year for four years, and nursing home admission was noted. The report noted that

> One of the values of this study [is] that loneliness was determined before people went to a nursing home. Loneliness did not occur because the people became "sick or couldn't get around," says one of the authors, Dr Robert Wallace, a University of Iowa professor of preventive medicine. "It suggests that loneliness may be a precursor to mental and physical deterioration. It also suggests that interventions to prevent loneliness should be explored in order to keep older people independent." (p. 3)

In a study of over 600 older adults in two rural counties of western Arizona, Adams (2007) reports that almost one-third (29.6%) of the respondents reported that they felt lonely, sad, empty or depressed for two weeks or longer in the last 12 months. To a question about the best part of aging, almost 80% of those surveyed said, "there is no best part."

Bennett (1980) reports that social isolation among older adults has long been recognized as a problem that diminishes their well-being because of its association with problems of low morale, poor health, and the risk of premature institutionalization. Sorkin et al. (2002) found that social isolation and loneliness compromised immune functioning and have been linked to cardiovascular disease. Additionally, lonely people are more likely to suffer from cardiovascular disease because their lifestyles may include little or no exercise, unhealthy eating habits, alcohol abuse, and the lack of a support network. Feeling love and support from others helps encourage lonely older adults to maintain physical health (Blazer, 2002).

Blazer (2002a) reports that loneliness may be a risk factor for the low-level, sub-clinical depression that continues to be a leading mental health problem for older adults. Cohen (2000) suggests that loneliness in later life may be thought of as a "near-depression" and advises mental health professionals to reconsider the research and interventions used to treat loneliness. Blazer (2002b) indicates that loneliness may lead to depression when there are "age-related losses or challenges" or the at-risk experiences noted earlier in the chapter (p. 316).

However, in a meta-analysis of the research on loneliness and aging, Pinquart and Sörensen (2001) found that loneliness, at least among the young-old adults (those below 75), is not as great as stereotypes of aging suggest. When it did exist, it was associated with the following risk factors: a reduction in the quality and quantity of social contacts; limitations imposed by health problems; institutionalization; and lower income. The older one is, the more these risk factors increase loneliness because social contacts become difficult to sustain. The authors did not find a strong correlation between loneliness and the quality of social contacts with children, or what has been called "intimacy at a distance." The authors believe that preventing loneliness in older adults can be accomplished by providing transportation so that social contacts can be maintained, and by encouraging long-held relationships to continue, even if only by telephone and e-mail.

8.4 TREATING LONELINESS

It is natural to assume that depression and loneliness may be interrelated since most depressed people also experience feelings of severe loneliness and social isolation. Powell et al. (2001) studied the effectiveness of treatment with clients experiencing long-term mood disorders. They concluded that self-help groups were very important providers of positive management of mood disorders because social support forces otherwise lonely and isolated people to interact with others, often at a fairly intimate level. In considering demographic issues as a predictor of the ability to cope with mood disorders, the researchers failed to find any specific indicator other than the level of education which, the authors believe, is an important aspect of dealing with the disorder. Surprisingly, daily functioning was inversely related to the number of out-patient contacts, suggesting that, as people improve, they see less need for professional help. Support from families and friends also failed to predict outcomes.

Since early detection of depression is essential in learning to cope with feelings of loneliness and depression, Duffy (2000) reports several important predictors of depression:

A family history of major affective disorder is the strongest, most reliable risk factor for a major affective illness. Other factors associated with affective disorders include female sex (risk factor for unipolar illnesses), severe life events and disappointments, family dysfunction, poor parental care, early adversity, and personality traits.

Based on the current state of knowledge, emphasis on identifying and treating mood disorders as early as possible in the course and particularly early-onset (child and adolescent) cases and youngsters at high risk (given a parent with a major mood disorder) is likely to be an effective strategy for reducing the burden of illness on both the individual and society. (p. 345)

Duffy (2000) also reports beginning evidence that brief, family-based psycho-educational interventions decrease the negative impact of parental mood disorders in children and improve family functioning in mood-disordered children. Individual treatment and family psycho-educational interventions in adult bipolar patients often decrease relapse rates and improve overall family functioning. Duffy notes that while early identification of children at risk of mood disorders is necessary, "the most effective strategy for reducing the burden of illness on individuals and society is not clear" (p. 346). However, the serious impact of mood disorders on the individual and their families, and the high risk of suicide, justify a need to develop new and more effective interventions. In the meantime, early interventions that utilize education, identification of family members at risk, and family interventions, may decrease the seriousness of the condition and reduce fears and misconceptions among family members. Harrington and Clark (1998) indicate that early intervention through the use of appropriate medications and mood disorder therapies may actually reduce the severity and reoccurrence of mood disorders.

Adams et al. (2004) studied loneliness in retirement communities and discovered that while "residence in congregate facilities affords social exposure, it does not guarantee access to close relationships, so that loneliness may be a result" (p. 475). The authors did find that when retirement communities sponsored social and leisure activities to keep older adults from being lonely and used strategies to keep them engaged with family and friends living outside the community, such activities could indirectly prevent more serious health and mental health problems. The strategies mentioned by the authors included "sending reminder notes to designated family and friends encouraging them to call or visit, holding social events where residents may invite a guest, and regularly offering informal support or informational groups at the facility for close friends or family members of residents" (p. 483). Blazer (2002b) suggests the establishment of support groups designated for those who are most likely to be lonely, including residents who have recently relocated, the bereaved, or those who are shy or lack social skills. Andrews et al. (2003) suggest the use of "befriending schemes" where volunteers meet weekly with lonely elderly persons. All of these efforts have potential to help lonely and isolated older adults, according to the literature.

Studying the importance of educational achievement, Hobfoll (2002) suggested that people who experience difficulty or failure in school early in life come to devalue education and may choose to discontinue advanced levels of training that may, as a consequence, lead to vulnerability to stressors and negative psychological outcomes.

Lazarus and Folkman (1984) found that people who appraise situations as potentially threatening do so because they fail to acquire sufficient resources often resulting in negative psychological outcomes. Consequently, education may represent an important resource contributing to positive well-being in later life.

It is often assumed that loneliness is directly related to social support and that having an intimate relationship with a spouse or loved one inhibits feelings of loneliness. Bishop and Martin (2007) studied the emotional well-being of 227 older adults ages 65–94 living independently in the community who had never been married, divorced or widowed to determine the psychological impact of educational achievement. They found a direct relationship between educational attainment and positive well-being including reduced feeling of loneliness. The authors report that

> Three key outcomes emerged from the present study. First, past educational attainment appeared to directly reduce vulnerability to neuroticism and stress. Second, greater expression of neurotic personality traits and feelings of stress directly increases susceptibility to loneliness, whereas greater social support directly decreases loneliness. Third, past educational attainment indirectly reduces feelings of loneliness. Each of these findings provides support for educational attainment as a relevant factor of subjective wellbeing and warrant further discussion relative to unmarried marital status. (p. 910)

8.5 THE INTERNET AS A WAY OF COPING WITH LONELINESS

The use of the Internet has dramatically increased in older adults. Kadlec (2007) reports that in adults over the age of 50, 54% use the Internet and 24% have high-speed hookups. That's up sharply from 38% and 5% in 2002. Almost everyone who goes on line (87%) uses e-mail, although there is a big dropoff at present in adults over the age of 70. Kadlec (2007) reports that retired people are online an average of nine hours a week and that the numbers and amount of time spent on the Internet will increase as computer-savvy adults age.

White et al. (2002) believe that the Internet and, more specifically, e-mail, has the potential to increase social support and the emotional well-being of older adults in the following ways: they can use computers to communicate often, cheaply, and easily with family, friends, and others who have computers; they can get information about a variety of issues, particularly health and financial issues on the Internet; they can explore hobbies and find out information about their community; and they can meet new people and broaden their support system through chat rooms and bulletin boards. The authors write, "In essence, relatively isolated and disabled older adults can reconnect, strengthen and broaden their connection with the outside world by incorporating computer technology into their lives" (p. 214).

In a study done by White et al. (2002) to teach lonely frail older adults with a mean age of 71 to use the Internet, the authors report that 60% of the total sample and 74% of those who completed the nine-hour training course were using the Internet weekly within five months. Because of problems with the testing instruments used, a statistically significant relationship between using the Internet and a decrease in feelings of loneliness was not found. However, the authors write, "Looking only at the intervention group and comparing users to non-users there were trends toward decreased loneliness and depression" (p. 219). In summary, the author's noted that

> [T]he Internet is an exciting new technology with much potential for enriching the lives of many older adults. As a source of information, social activity, and interpersonal communication, the Internet may expand the constrained boundaries of congregate housing, retirement communities, and even skilled care nursing facilities. Depending on the older user, this expansion may include more frequent contacts with family and friends, new opportunities to pursue former interests, as well as avenues to meet new friends and to "travel" to places no longer accessible due to health limitations. (p. 220)

USING EVIDENCE-BASED PRACTICE WITH LONELINESS AND ISOLATION: A CASE STUDY

What happens when older adults who have been successful in many aspects of their lives are unable to shake severe feelings of loneliness when they retire? The following case study deals with that issue and begins with a 70-year-old male discussing life-long feelings of loneliness and how he's coping with those feelings following retirement. Thanks to Sage Publications for permission to reprint this case first found in Glicken (2006, p. 176–178).

Dr Jacob Goldstein is a divorced 70-year-old former English professor who has just retired to a community of scholars and researchers built by a large research university in the southwest to help retired university faculty and administrators continue their scholarly work and to have social and professional contacts with other scholars. Dr Goldstein chose the community because he thought the university affiliation would make the people similar to those he'd worked with all of his life. He spoke to the author about what he describes as life-long loneliness and how he is coping with it in retirement. He told me:

"I think people who grow up in very troubled families never quite get the hang of intimate relationships. In my family, we were so busy surviving poverty and the illness of my mother that none of us really mastered the ability to be loved or to love someone in return. My father's favorite saying was that it was better to be home by yourself reading a good book than to be out with bad friends. Of course, he considered all my friends to be bad so I spent my childhood reading books, pretty much alone.

"People sometimes think I'm arrogant because I'm so stand-offish, but I'm really very shy and introverted. I don't think people react well to me. I'm never invited to dinner by colleagues, or asked out for coffee, or any of the things that tell me others find me appealing. Sometimes it's very hurtful. Even so, I've been successful at work and wrote several well-received scholarly books and several less well received novels and books of poetry before retiring from an Ivy League college as a full professor. Before I retired, and even now, I experience loneliness when I'm not working on books. It can be a killer. I've tried everything including going to as many social function as possible to fill my time, but I feel even more alone and isolated when I'm with people I don't know. It's hard to explain being lonely when you're around people.

"I've gone for therapy, of course, but most of the time it's so superficial and completely misses the mark that it ends up hurting me more than helping. You go to a therapist and it's like falling in love. You have high expectations, and when they're not met and you've put in so much time and energy to get another person to listen, to maybe even *like* you a little and they don't, it hurts.

"Every once in a while I meet a lady and we enjoy a brief moment or two before the relationship ends. I'm seeing someone now and, knowing it's going to end sooner or later, I take the nights we spend together and I think of them as a collection of fine wines, or beautiful paintings, or wonderful memories; her mature body silhouetted against the moonlight, the strength of her legs, the loveliness of the nipples on her breasts. I know she's going to see me for what I really am and get rid of me. And then, instead of having the warmth of her companionship, I'll be alone again.

"I fight feeling down all the time. I force myself to get up in the morning and write or go to coffee at the community center where there are some guys like me who are single and want to kibitz a bit. I don't find it satisfying and I haven't made any friends since I've been here. I joined the tennis club, but I play with people who don't seem to want to develop a social relationship. Because of the heat for much of the year, we play at 6:00 a.m. and, when we're done, I go home to my empty condo. My girlfriend comes over at night after work, but I feel lonely with her as well. We haven't much to say so we watch TV in silence. I always experience a feeling of mild despair. I wouldn't call it a depression, but it's always there.

"I'm seeing a therapist now to help me with the adjustment to not working. It's helping, I think. She's been working on the origins of my loneliness and I'm astonished at how powerful it is to review the events in my life through fresh eyes. Knowing more about myself now, I've come to believe that I have to fight the urge to give up and to keep trying my best. My therapist has done a good job of getting me to continue going to social events even though I feel like giving up. I have to admit it's paying off some. I have a tendency to assume that other people I don't know don't like me when, perhaps, I'm distancing myself from them. So I practice not doing that. It's helping me have social contacts I would not have been patient enough to develop before I went into therapy. My therapist has urged me to read about loneliness and to join Internet chat rooms of other lonely people. It's an eye opener to find out that other people feel the same way I do, many of them even more successful than me.

"My therapist also urged me to join a self-help group. At first I thought it was a dumb idea. All I could think was that it would be like AA: 'Hi, my name is Jake and I'm lonely.' It wasn't like that at all. I've met some very nice people. We go to concerts and movies together. A few of the men and I meet for dinner once a week and, after talking about loneliness, we started talking about us. It was amazing to find such nice but hurting people. I've never really had a good and true friend but the guys feel that way to me. Who would have guessed?

"My therapist is a very gentle person but under the gentleness she's firm and direct. I was very touched to find out that she read one of my novels. We talked about it and used it in therapy because there were many themes of isolation and loneliness in the book. She had perceptions of it I didn't even have. I've always had a low opinion of therapy until this experience and now I think it's just great because we have this equal relationship and she really wants to hear what I think. I've been an educator all my life and what she's doing sort of feels like very sophisticated mentoring. I don't even know what kind of therapist she is, she's just awfully good.

"I don't think there's an easy answer to loneliness other than to keep on working at it. You keep on trying, you don't allow yourself to feel too sorry for yourself, and you take each day as it comes. I know those are clichés, but sometimes there is truth in a cliché. As someone who was raised on the messages my mother got from the radio soap operas, I believe that sometimes the Tooth Fairy takes your lost dreams and replaces them with gold."

Discussion with the Therapist

Dr Goldstein's therapist told me the following: "People who have lifelong problems with loneliness have a bit of paranoia about other people. They expect the worst and, when it happens, they're not surprised. When he called for an appointment and told me he was having trouble fitting in with others in the retirement community, I did a lot of reading about retirement and loneliness. I also tried to imagine how difficult it would be to retire after a long work life and to come somewhere and resettle all by myself. That takes a lot of energy and positive thinking. I also read one of Dr Goldstein's novels. It was a wonderful novel about lonely people. It told me a lot about him. I mentioned I'd read his novel and he was thrilled. He wanted to know if it told me anything about him. I told him it did and the discussion was really a breakthrough. He was much more open to the suggestions I made and worked very hard at dealing with shyness and a sense that others don't like him. It's tough work because it's almost a habit for him to think that social events will end badly and that people won't like him. He was the professor of the year for three years at a very prestigious university and yet he thinks others don't like him and avoid him. He's begun to see the signals he gives others to stay away and they, of course, do. Now he's giving off positive messages and, much to his amazement, people are reaching out to him. Intimacy is still a problem. His relationship with his lady friend feels very rigid and unemotional. He doesn't like it and they've begun to talk about coming for relationship therapy. All in all, I think he's a very lonely and isolated man, but he's trying and the results are paying off. Will they continue? I think they will. I plan on doing a lot of follow-up after he leaves treatment. Lonely people have spent many years practicing being lonely. In some ways it's satisfying to retreat inside their homes rather than face social challenges. But we live in hope and I have a good sense that Dr Goldstein will handle this challenge much as he's handled other: with inner resolve, dignity, and great effort."

8.6 A PERSONAL STORY: ISOLATION FROM AN ADULT CHILD

The following letter was written by an older mother (63) to her adult daughter (38) asking why the daughter seemed to be leaving her mother out of her life. The mother is feeling very lonely and had felt that an important contact as she aged would be her daughter's family. She now finds that isn't the case and wrote this letter to share her distress with her daughter. The correspondence continues with her daughter's reply and then a short response, not sent to her daughter, by her mother.

THE MOTHER'S LETTER

Dear Leah:

I hope you don't mind if I send you email at work. I do it partly because you don't seem to check your email at home very often, and also because you share that email address with John.

Some months ago I decided, as I told you, that I would try to make a point of calling you every Sunday. Most of the time when I call, you either aren't there or no one answers, in which case it is often several days before you return my call. Also, I try to call after I think Molly (5) is in bed, but before you are in bed. When that might be is just a guess on my part. I try to call when Molly isn't around, not because I don't want to talk to her, but because it seems to be difficult for you to talk on the phone when she is there and awake. She seems to demand your attention while you are on the phone, and it makes it tough for you and I to chat.

Anyway, in my trying to figure out when the best time might be to call, it seems in my mind that I see a rather narrow window. Consequently, because of what I see as that narrow window, and my admitted propensity to simply forget, I haven't been calling you as often as I intended, and would have liked.

Now, when I do think about calling, although I tend to think about it at the "wrong time," I find myself ruminating about why you never seem to call me. I imagine that if I were to ask you that question, you would tell me you are simply too busy. In my imaginary conversation with you, I would then protest that you *can't* be so busy in your life that you never have time to call your mother.

Then I find myself rather shocked that I seem to have become the kind of mother who whines that "her kids never call!" But, here I am, doing just that.

I occasionally look back on the days when you lived with me while you were in graduate school, and how we spent so much time together, going to the theater, to the coffeehouse on Sunday mornings, taking walks in the neighborhood, going on 5 K and 10 K runs, and lots of other things. I know we both have our own very different lives now, as it should be, but I truly do miss those days. We were very close, and I loved being with you, and I was, and am, exceedingly proud to have you as my daughter.

During the few years after Molly was born and before I met David, I was out at your house almost every other weekend, partly I suppose because I loved being with Molly and you, and partly because it seemed I had no other life. Toward the end of that time, I wondered whether I was coming out too often – if I was becoming a pest to you. I had visions of you groaning and rolling your eyes at the prospect of mom coming out there AGAIN.

Anyway, at the risk of being a whining mother, I wanted to tell you how I feel, that it is rather hurtful to me that you rarely pick up the phone to call. If it is merely because your life is too busy, perhaps you need to reassess your life, and consider the possibility that you may have too much on your plate. Or, more importantly, if you are angry at me, I would very much like for us to talk about it.

I couldn't bear for us to be estranged or for you to be angry with me.

Love,

Mom

THE DAUGHTER'S RESPONSE (AS TOLD TO THE AUTHOR BY THE MOTHER)

"Leah wrote me back and said she always calls me back as soon as she can. She said that starting a new business had taken all of her time. She reminded me that she also works 30 hours a week and has a 5-year-old daughter who has school, activities, homework, etc. She said she usually doesn't even sit down until 8:30 p.m. and because she doesn't have a desk job where she can check e-mails or call back right away it sometimes takes a few days before she can call or write back.

"She said that as soon as David came into my life that I stopped coming to see her. She said that happy as she was for me that I had someone in my life, it was me who disappeared, not her and that it was me who created the distance. The importance that she and Molly had in my life has changed and Molly hardly knows who I am because I'm not around much.

"She also said the reason she doesn't call more often is that she doesn't really know what to say and because by the time she rests, she's exhausted. She always wants to talk to me but her personal space window is not wide and that when she calls she tries to do it when she can provide quality time."

THE MOTHER'S RESPONSE (NOT SENT TO HER DAUGHTER BUT SHARED WITH THE AUTHOR)

"I guess Leah's response made me angry and hurt. I thought what I wrote was straightforward, asking that we resolve whatever issues were between us. What I got instead was a blaming letter. It was my fault and not hers. I know other parents who have done the same thing and gotten the same response. I wanted to try and work things out but I guess the best thing to do is to ignore her letter and get on with my life. It's pretty hurtful, and I haven't given up, but for the time being maybe it's just best for us to have some distance and maybe it'll work itself out.

"I guess you have to give children space, even adult children, and maybe I expect more than she's willing to give, but I'd be lying if I said it didn't hurt. David has had similar problems with his daughter but over the years he's managed to deal with it and his relationship with his daughter is much better now. He said he'd tried to make changes by being very positive and by focusing on her rather than him. I guess when this has blown over that's really what I'll do. Maybe I've taken too much for granted. You're a mother and you expect a child to be sensitive to you. Maybe the best thing to do is deal with my sense of loss and loneliness for the old relationship we had and do what I need to do to expand my close relationships. I've actually begun to do that and it feels pretty wonderful. I joined a tennis club, play 2–3 times a week, and have made a very dear friend. Maybe it does one a favor to have children distance themselves from you because it forces you to get on with your life knowing that you might have to do it without the close involvement of your children." – PHF

8.7 SUMMARY

This chapter about loneliness provides reasons for social isolation that sometimes leads to depression in older adults. Internal and external reasons for loneliness are explored and a case is presented of a lonely older man and the EBP treatment he receives for loneliness and why it seems to be helping him. A personal story explores the complicated relationship of a mother and daughter whose relationship is causing the mother to feel lonely and isolated from her family.

8.8 QUESTIONS FROM THE CHAPTER

1. In the letters the mother and daughter exchanged, I agree with the daughter. I think parents should let their kids grow up and, once they're grown, let us live our own lives without expecting that kids will be a big part of their parent's lives. It's called letting go. Don't you agree?
2. The lonely people I know are always complaining about other people snubbing them. I think it's paranoid and I think the main problem that lonely people have is that they imagine people behaving in ways that just aren't true. What do you think?
3. How can anyone be lonely when there are so many places to go and things to see? Maybe if they just realized how good life is they'd feel less lonely. Do you agree?
4. I think lonely people are just depressed. Isn't one of the symptoms of depression loneliness? Maybe we should eliminate the word lonely and substitute depressed and then we'd be able to help them better. What do you think?
5. I know people who like being by themselves. Don't we make too big a deal out of expecting people to be social when lots of people just aren't and prefer it that way?

REFERENCES

ABCNews.com. (2002). Authentic happiness: Using our strengths to cultivate happiness. Retrieved October 14, 2002 from the World Wide Web: <http://abcnews.go.com/sections/GMA/GoodMorningAmerica/GMA020904Happiness_feature.html>.

Adams, S. (2007). Results of community assessment: Pathways to caring communities. *Western Arizona Council on Government, Area Agency on Aging.*

Adams, A. K. B., Sanders, S., & Auth, E. A. (November 2004). Loneliness and depression in independent living retirement communities: Risk and resilience factors. *Aging and Mental Health, 8*(6), 475–485.

Akerlind, I., & Hornquist, J. (1992). Loneliness and alcohol abuse: A review of evidence of an interplay. *Social Science and Medicine, 34*(4), 405–414.

Anderson, K., & Diamond, M. (1995). The experience of bereavement in older adults. *Journal of Advanced Nursing, 22*, 308–315.

Andrews, G. J., Gavin, N., Begley, S., & Brodie, D. (2003). Assisting friendships, combating loneliness: Users' views on a 'befriending' scheme. *Aging and Society, 23*, 349–362.

Bennett, R. (1980). *Aging, isolation, and resocialization*. New York: VanNostrand Reinhold.

Bishop, A. J., & Martin, P. (2007). The indirect influence of educational attainment on loneliness among unmarried older adults. *Gerontology, 33*(10), 897–917.

Blazer, D. G. (2002). Self-efficacy and depression in late life: A primary prevention. *Aging and Mental Health, 6*(4), 315–324.

Blazer, D. G. (2002a). *Depression in late life* (3rd edn.). New York: Springer.

Blazer, D. G. (2002b). Self-efficacy and depression in late life: A primary prevention proposal. *Aging and Mental Health, 6*(4), 315–324.

Cohen, G. D. (2000). Loneliness in later life. *American Journal of Geriatric Psychiatry, 8*(4), 273–275.

Copel, L. C. (1988). Loneliness. *Journal of Psychosocial Nursing, 26*(1), 14–19.

Duffy, A. (2000). Toward effective early intervention and prevention strategies for major affective disorders: A review of risk factors. *Canadian Journal of Psychiatry, 45*(4), 300–349.

Ekwall, A. (2005). Loneliness as a predictor of quality of life among older caregivers. *Journal of Advanced Nursing, 49*(1), 23–32.

Gellene, D. (2007). Loneliness often precedes elder dementia, study finds (Feb. 10). *Los Angeles Times*, A11.

Glicken, M. D. (2006). *Learning from resilient people: Lessons we can apply to counseling and psychotherapy*. Thousand Oaks, CA: Sage.

Harrington, R., & Clark, A. (1998). Prevention and early intervention for depression in adolescence and early adult life. *European Archives of Psychiatry in Clinical Neuroscience, 248*, 32–45.

Hobfoll, S. E. (1989). Conservation of resources: A new attempt at conceptualizing stress. *American Psychologist, 44*, 513–524.

Joiner, T. E., Jr., Catanzaro, S., Rudd, M. D., & Rajab, M. H. (1999). The case for a hierarchical, oblique, and bidimensional structure of loneliness. *Journal of Social and Clinical Psychology, 18*, 47–75.

Jones, W., & Carver, M. (1991). Adjustment and coping implications of loneliness. In C. R. Snyder (ed.), *Handbook of social and clinical psychology*. New York: Pergamon Press.

Kadlec, D. (2007). Senior netizens (Feb. 12). *Time, 169*(7), 94.

Lazarus, R. S., & Folkman, S. (1984). *Stress, appraisal, and coping*. New York: Springer.

Loneliness may predict nursing home admission. (1998) (May). *Brown University Long-Term Care Quality Advisor, 10*(5), 3.

Martikainen, P., & Valkonen, T. (1996). Mortality after the death of a spouse: Rates and causes of death in a large Finnish cohort. *American Journal of Public Health, 86*(8), 1087–1093.

McWhiter, B. (1990). Loneliness: A review of current literature, with implications for counselling and research. *Journal of Counselling and Development, 68*(4), 417–422.

Mijuskovic, B. (1992). Organic communities, atomistic societies and loneliness. *Journal of Sociology and Social Welfare, 19*(2), 147–164.

Murphy, F. (June 2006). Loneliness: A challenge for nurses caring for older people. *Nursing Older People, 18*(5), 22–25.

Olweus, D. (1993). Victimization by peers: Antecedents and long-term outcomes. In K. H. Rubin & J. B. Asendorpf (Eds.), *Social withdrawal, inhibition and shyness in childhood* (pp. 315–341). Hillsdale, NJ: Erlbaum.

Ostrov, E., & Offer, D. (1980). Loneliness and the adolescent. In J. Hartog, J. R. Audy, & Y. Cohen (Eds.), *The anatomy of loneliness* (pp. 170–185). New York: International University Press.

Peplau, L. A., & Perlman, D. (1984). Loneliness research: A survey of empirical findings. In L. A. Peplau & S. E. Goldston (Eds.), *Preventing the harmful consequences of severe and persistent loneliness* (pp. 13–47). Rockville, MD: National Institute of Mental Health.

Peters, A., & Liefbroer, A. C. (1997). Beyond marital status: Partner history and well-being in old age. *Journal of Marriage and the Family, 59*(3), 687–699.

Pinquart, M., & Sörensen, S. (2001). How effective are psychotherapeutic and other psychosocial interventions with older adults: A meta-analysis. *Journal of Mental Health and Aging, 7*, 207–243.

Powell, T. J., Yeaton, W., Hill, E. M., & Silk, K. R. (2001). Predictors of psychosocial outcomes for patients with mood disorders. *Psychiatric Rehabilitation Journal, 25*(1), 3–12.

Prince, M. J., Harwood, R. H., Blizard, R. A., & Thomas, A. (1997). Socialsupport deficits, loneliness and life events as risk factors for depression in old age: The gospel oak project VI. *Psychological Medicine, 27*, 323–332.

RokAch, A. (2007). The effect of age and culture on the causes of loneliness. *Social Behavior and Personality, 35*(2), 169–186.

Rotenberg, K. J., MacDonald, K. J., & King, E. V. (2004). The relationship between loneliness and interpersonal trust during middle childhood (September). *Journal of Genetic Psychology, 165*(3), 233–249.

Rubin, K. H., & Mills, R. S. L. (1991). Conceptualizing developmental pathways to internalizing disorders in childhood. *Canadian Journal of Behavioral Science, 23*(3), 300–317.

Russell, D. (1996). ULCA loneliness scale (version 3): Reliability, validity, and factor structure. *Journal of Personality Assessment, 66*(1), 20–40.

Saxton, L. (1986). *The individual, marriage and family*. Belmont, CA: Wadsworth Publishing.

Seligman, M. E. P., & Csikszetmihalyi, M. (2000). Positive psychology: An introduction. *American Psychologist, 55*(1), 5–14.

Sermat, V. (1978). Sources of loneliness. *Essence, 2*, 271–276.

Sheldon, J. (1984). *The social medicine of old Age: A report of an enquiry in Wolverhampton*. Milton Keynes: Open University Press.

Sorkin, D., Rook, K. S., & Lu, J. L. (2002). Loneliness, lack of emotional support, lack of companionship, and the likelihood of having a heart condition in an elderly sample. *Annals of Behavioral Medicine, 24*(4), 290–298.

Stossel, S. (2000). Bowling alone (Sept. 21). *Atlantic Unbound*.

Uruk, A. C., & Demir, A. (2003). Loneliness. *Journal of Psychology, 137*(2), 179–194.

Weiss, R. S. (1973). *Loneliness: The experience of emotional and social isolation*. Cambridge, MA: MIT Press.

Wenger, G. (1983). Loneliness: A problem of measurement. In D. Jerome (Ed.), *Ageing in modern society*. London: Croom Helm.

White, H., McConnell, E., Clipp, E., Branch, L. G., Sloane, R., Pieper, C., & Box, T. L. (2002, August). A randomized controlled trial of the psychosocial impact of providing internet training and access to older adults. *Aging & Mental Health, 6*(3), 213–221.

Young, J. E. (1982). Loneliness, depression, and cognitive therapy: Theory and applications. In L. A. Peplau & D. Perlman (Eds.), Loneliness. A sourcebook of current theory, research and therapy (pp. 379–405). New York: Wiley.

Chapter | nine

Evidence-Based Practice and Older Adults Experiencing Elder Abuse and Neglect

9.1 INTRODUCTION

As the following data indicate, the abuse and neglect of older adults is a very serious and growing problem. The National Center on Elder Abuse Incidence Study (2005) estimated that in 2004, 565,747 elderly persons, age 60 and over, experienced abuse, neglect and/or self-neglect in domestic settings compared to 472,813 reports documented in the 2000 APS Survey. This represents a 19.7% increase in total reports. There were 461,135 investigations for adults of all ages in the 2004 study, representing a 16.3% increase from the 2000 Survey when states reported 396,398 investigations. For the 2004 study, 191,908 reports of abuse were substantiated for victims of all ages. This compares to 166,019 substantiated reports in 2000. Of the 42 states that could provide both the number of reports investigated and substantiated, the substantiation rate was 46.2%. This percentage is very similar to the 48.5% substantiation rate from the 2000 Survey. The median substantiation rate individual states was 35.1%.

According to The National Center on Elder Abuse Incidence Study (2005) neglect of the elderly was the most frequent type of elder maltreatment (48.7%); emotional/psychological abuse was the second (35.5%); physical abuse was the third (25.6%); financial/material exploitation was the fourth (30.2%); and abandonment was the least common (3.6%). Adult children comprised the largest category of perpetrators (47.3%) of substantiated incidents of elder abuse; spouses followed second by 19.3%; other relatives were third at 8.8%; and grandchildren followed last with 8.6%. Three out of four elder abuse and neglect victims suffer from physical frailty. About one-half (47.9%) of the substantiated incidents of abuse and neglect involved elderly persons who were not physically able to care for themselves, while 28.7% of victims could marginally care for themselves.

Levine (2003) believes that over 80% of all incidents of elder abuse go unreported because of fear of abandonment, institutionalization, and severe repercussions from the abuser (Cyphers, 1999). Welfel et al. (2000) report that a large number of older adults are unaware of the availability of services, or their rights, and that in some communities, services are almost nonexistent. The problem of proper reporting is complicated by the fact that many abusing caretakers were themselves abused by the older adult when they were children and are now seeking revenge. Knowing this, some older adults find it difficult to report abuse by the very people they abused, believing that child abuse trumps elder abuse. In fact, caregiver resentment is the strongest predictor of potentially harmful caregiver behavior (Shaffer et al., 2007).

Abuse and neglect in nursing homes and other care facilities is also a serious problem, one that increases in severity as growing numbers of older adults suffer from Alzheimer's and dementia. Clearly substandard care needs to be reported and improved, and human service professionals should be very clear regarding their obligation to enforce high standards on all facilities caring for elderly patients.

9.2 LEGAL DEFINITIONS OF ADULT ABUSE AND NEGLECT

The following definitions come from The 2004 Survey of State Adult Protective Services: Abuse of Adults 60 Years of Age and Older (2006, pp. 27–30):

Abandonment: The desertion of an elderly person by an individual who has assumed responsibility for providing care for an elder, or by a person with physical custody of an elder.

Abuse: The infliction of physical or psychological harm or the knowing deprivation of goods or services necessary to meet essential needs or to avoid physical or psychological harm.

Emotional/psychological/verbal abuse: The infliction of anguish, pain, or distress through verbal or nonverbal acts. Emotional/psychological abuse includes, but is not limited to, verbal assaults, insults, threats, intimidation, humiliation, and harassment. In addition, treating an older person as an infant; isolating an elderly person from his/her family, friends, or regular activities; and enforced social isolation are examples of emotional/psychological abuse.

Financial or material abuse/exploitation: The illegal or improper use of an older person's or vulnerable adult's funds, property, or assets. Examples include, but are not limited to, cashing an older/vulnerable person's checks without authorization or permission; forging an older person's signature; misusing or stealing an older person's money or possessions; coercing or deceiving an older person into signing any document (e.g., contracts or will); and the improper use of conservatorship, guardianship, or power of attorney.

Neglect: The refusal or failure to fulfill any part of a person's obligations or duties to an elder. Neglect may also include failure of a person who has fiduciary responsibilities to provide care for an elder (e.g., pay for necessary home care services) or the failure on the part of an in-home service provider to provide necessary care. Neglect typically means the refusal or failure to provide an elderly person/vulnerable adult with such life necessities as food, water, clothing, shelter, personal hygiene, medicine, comfort, personal safety, and other essentials included in an implied or agreed-upon responsibility to an elder.

Self-neglect: An adult's inability, due to physical or mental impairment or diminished capacity, to perform essential self-care tasks including (a) obtaining essential food, clothing, shelter, and medical care; (b) obtaining goods and services necessary to maintain physical health, mental health, or general safety; and/or (c) managing one's own financial affairs. Choice of lifestyle or living arrangement is not, in itself, evidence of self-neglect.

Vulnerable adult: A person who is either being mistreated or in danger of mistreatment and who, due to age and/or disability, is unable to protect himself or herself. Though most adult protective service (APS) programs serve vulnerable adults regardless of age (based either on their age or incapacity), some serve only older persons. A few programs serve only adults aged 18–59 who have disabilities that keep them from protecting themselves. Interventions provided by APS include, but are not limited to, the following: receiving reports of adult abuse, neglect, or exploitation; investigating these reports; assessing risk; developing and implementing case plans; monitoring services; and evaluating the impact of intervention. Further, APS may provide or arrange for a wide selection of medical, social, economic, legal, housing, law enforcement, or other protective emergency or supportive services (NAAPSA, 2001).

9.3 INDICATORS OF ELDER ABUSE

Older adult victims of abuse and neglect often suffer from depression, hopelessness, unhappiness, shame, and guilt (NCEA, 1998). Dyer et al. (2000) found that abused and neglected older adults had significantly higher scores on the Geriatric Depression Scale when compared with those who had not experienced abuse. Consistent with signs of depression, The National Center for Elder Abuse (1998) reports that the most likely indicators of elder abuse include continual and unexplained crying and nonspecific fears about the home they live in and the people they live with. The NCEA report says that indications of physical abuse include "bruises, welts, lacerations, rope marks, broken bones and fractures, untreated injuries, broken eyeglasses, laboratory findings of medical overdose, and reports of being hit, slapped, kicked, or mistreated" (The National Center for Elder Abuse, 1998, The Basics Section, p.1).

Additional indicators of possible abuse are a sudden change in the older person's behavior or a caregiver's refusal to permit visitors. Signs of sexual abuse include "bruises around the breast or genitals, unexplained venereal diseases, unexplained vaginal or anal bleeding, and torn or bloody clothing" (NCEA, 1998). Examples of emotional abuse include non-responsiveness, sucking, biting, or rocking behavior. Neglect and self-neglect are often evidenced by "dehydration, malnutrition, untreated bedsores, poor hygiene, unattended health problems, unsafe living conditions, or unsanitary living conditions" (NCEA, 1998). Indications of financial exploitation include sudden changes in banking practices, the inclusion of additional names on an elder's banking card, unauthorized withdrawals, abrupt changes in the will, the unexplained disappearance of funds or valuables, unexplained transfers of funds to family members, and forged signatures on financial documents (NCEA, 1998).

Marshall et al. (2000) warn that abuse is not always obvious. Clues that something might be wrong include client stories that appear rehearsed and clients who seem cautious and fearful when sharing information. Frequent hospitalizations may also indicate recurrent abuse (Marshall et al. 2000). Cyphers (1999) analyzed Adult Protective Services statistics and found that women had a higher incidence of physical, emotional, and sexual abuse than men and a much greater probability of financial abuse and self-neglect.

Not surprisingly, Jogerst et al. (2000) found that elder abuse was much more likely to occur in older adults with high rates of poverty who lived with families that had histories of violence, substance abuse, and mental illness. Quinn and Tomita (1997) found that older adults living with spouses or relatives were three times more likely to be abused. Relatives who were dependent on the victim for financial support or housing were often at greater risk of becoming abusive (Levine, 2003; Wolf, 1998) and that the onset of new cognitive impairments in an elder increased the likelihood of abuse.

9.4 ABUSIVE CARETAKERS

Ramsey-Klawsnik (2000) believes that there are five types of abusive caretakers: Overwhelmed, impaired, narcissistic, bullying, and sadistic offenders. The author defines each type of abuser as follows:

1. **Overwhelmed caretakers** commonly want to give adequate care but discover that the care needed goes beyond their abilities and may lead to verbal and physical abuse. Overwhelmed caregivers are often aware of their abusive behavior but may find it difficult to seek help, often because they fear the loss of the financial assistance they receive for taking care of the older adult. Other reasons include lack of sleep and limited leisure or personal time. Older adults who are demanding and the lack of medical supplies, financial resources, and assistance also increase stress for caretakers.

2. **Impaired caretakers** may mean well but they have physical and emotional problems that make caretaking problematic. Unlike the overwhelmed caretaker, the impaired caretaker may be unaware

of how badly they are treating the older adult in their care and tend to be neglectful or do a poor job of administering medication (Ramsey-Klawsnik, 2000). An educationally oriented intervention may help impaired caretakers, along with assistance in some of the services they provide plus a good deal of support that focuses on their positive caretaking accomplishments.

3. **Narcissistic offenders** are only "interested in exploiting the older person and his or her assets. The mistreatment in which they engage tends to be chronic, escalates over time, and takes the form of neglect and financial exploitation" (Thompson and Priest, 2005, p. 120).

4. **Bullying offenders** mistreat older adults because they have power over them and feel justified in abusing others. Because their victims are often frightened of the bully's behavior they go to extremes to placate them. Frequently used forms of abuse include sexual abuse, physical and emotional abuse, financial abuse, and neglect.

5. **Sadistic caretakers** humiliate, terrify, and harm older adults in their care and lack remorse or guilt for their behavior.

Ramsey-Klawsnik (2000) believes that impaired and overwhelmed caretakers are the most responsive to help. Narcissistic, bullying, and sadistic caretakers often don't want to give up control or take responsibility for their behavior and are therefore unmotivated for treatment. To complicate the caretaking picture, Cyphers (1999) found that adult children were responsible for more than 50% of substantiated cases of domestic violence, abuse and neglect of their parents and grandparents. While the proportion of abusive caretakers by gender is almost equal (Cyphers, 1999; Marshall et al., 2000), women tend to neglect older victims while men are more likely to use physical, sexual, or emotional abuse and to engage in financial exploitation (Cyphers, 1999; NCEA, 1998).

9.5 INTERVENTIONS WITH CARETAKERS

Typically, when caretaker abuse is discovered, the victims are removed from the home and placed in more stable settings. This is true of more obvious forms of abuse, but when caretakers are tired or stressed out and aren't doing a fully competent job, there are a number of interventions that can help. Certainly giving caretakers time out and assistance in the form of others helping the caretaker reduces some of the stress. Better financial supports may also relieve some of the economic drain. Family interventions, which include the older adult, and training in caretaking could also be an aide to overwhelmed caretakers. The strengths approach might work well with caretakers who want to do a good job but just lack the time, energy, and sometimes, the ability.

In explaining the strengths perspective Van Wormer (1999) notes that, "[a]t the heart of the strengths perspective is a belief in the basic goodness of humankind, a faith that individuals, however unfortunate their plight, can discover strengths in themselves that they never knew existed" (p. 51). Van Wormer (1999, pp. 54–56) goes on to suggest the use of the following strengths techniques with clients:

1. Seek the positive in terms of people's coping skills, and you will find it. Look beyond presenting symptoms and setbacks and encourage clients to identify their talents, dreams, insights, and fortitude.
2. Listen to the personal narrative. Through entering the world of the storyteller, the practitioner begins to grasp the client's reality, at the same time attending to signs of initiative, hope, and frustration with past counterproductive behavior that can help lead the client to a healthier outlook on life. The strengths therapist, by means of continual reinforcement of positives, seeks to help the client move away from what van den Bergh (1995, p. xix) calls "paralyzing narratives."
3. In contradistinction to the usual practice in interviewing [abusive caretakers], which is to protect yourself from being used or manipulated, this approach would have the practitioner temporarily suspend skepticism or disbelief and enter the client's world as the client presents it, showing a willingness to listen to his or her own explanations and perceptions. This approach ultimately encourages the emergence of the client's truth.
4. Validate the pain where pain exists. Reinforce persistent efforts to alleviate the pain and help people recover from the specific injuries of oppression, neglect, and domination.
5. Don't dictate: collaborate through an agreed upon, mutual discovery of solutions among helpers, families, and support networks. Validation and collaboration are integral steps in a consciousness-raising process that can lead to healing and empowerment.

Moxley and Washington (2001) suggest that the advantage of using the strengths perspective with chemically dependent clients, some of whom are abusive, is that it provides an alternative to labeling which has dubious validity or value, and that it doesn't blame the client or focus on the client's deficiencies. "Labeling, diagnosis, and blaming the victim can introduce into the process of treatment and into the treatment relationship itself a cynicism about the potential for change that can contaminate the thinking of both helpers and recipients and, as a consequence, limit their willingness to engage in the transformational process of change the practice of recovery demands" (Moxley and Washington, 2001, p. 251).

Brun and Rapp (2001) report that quantitative studies suggest positive outcomes when strengths-based case management is used with people who have substance-abuse problems. Substance abuse is often associated with physical and sexual abuse, particularly domestic violence. Those outcomes reported by the authors include lessened drug use, retention in treatment programs, and improved functioning at work.

Sherman and Newman (1979) suggest that prevention is the best way to stop elder abuse. In their study, considerable effort was placed on helping caretakers before the burden became great by offering training and advice in the early stages of the older adult's stay with caretakers. Most of the caretakers (70%) in their study had no experience helping the elderly, particularly elderly clients with multiple physical and emotional problems. The authors found that training, follow-up visits, and supportive help kept most placements stable and that from the caretakers' points of view the quality of the follow-up rather than the quantity was most helpful. By helpful, caretakers reported that workers who offered support, advice, and encouragement, and were available to them by phone, were far more helpful than workers who were only interested in whether health and nutritional standards were being met.

9.6 TREATING ABUSED OLDER ADULTS: EFFECTIVE INTERVENTIONS

Even when older adults are referred because of their abuse, the range of treatment options seems limited. Thompson and Priest (2005) complain that "little attention has been paid to treating elder abuse; consequently, a dearth of interventions and preventions exists" (p. 123). The authors believe it is imperative that we develop more effective ways of helping abused older adults. Because of the dramatic increase in the number of older adults and their extended life spans, many families with limited resources find it difficult to provide adequate care. As the economic realities of caring for older adults increases, and with it the pressures on family life, the authors believe that elder abuse will increase.

While effective approaches for working with older adult victims of abuse are limited, several seem to offer some hope. In a general discussion of treatment, Papadopolous and LaFontaine (2000) suggest that intervention should involve a combination of individual therapy, family therapy, and relationship counseling that focuses on behavioral skills training, cognitive restructuring, and emotional control. The authors also suggest that we attempt to empower caregivers by recognizing their needs and working with them to help older family members. Browne and Herbert (1997) emphasize positive reminiscences as an approach for enhancing compassion and attachment between the caregiver and the older adult. Wolf (1998), however, believes that we need to acknowledge and address the depression, sadness, shame, and guilt experienced by victims of elder abuse by focusing on enhancing the strengths and life skills of victims.

Reay and Browne (2002) applied an education and anger management intervention by first assessing conflict, strain, depression, anxiety, and the cost of caring in 29 caretakers who abused and neglected older relatives. The educational intervention was done in a single 90-minute session with a psychologist who gave comprehensive information about the victim's illness, the services and resources available, and the nature of caring for older individuals. The anger management component was also done in a single 90-minute session by a psychologist and focused on the nature, stages of anger, and anger management skills. Pre-test, post-test, and a 6-month follow-up showed a reduction in strain, depression, anxiety, and conflict tactics. However, the study lacked a control group and the sample size was small.

Davis and Medina-Ariza (2001) report a field study to reduce repeat incidents of elder abuse. Randomly selected public housing projects (30 of 60) in New York City received educational material about elder abuse, while others did not. Some households that reported elder abuse to the police were selected by lottery to receive a follow-up home visit from a police officer and a domestic violence counselor. Data on post-report abuse were collected at 6 and 12 months periods after the initial report to the police. According to the authors, the interventions were difficult to implement because of delays in services and lack of cooperation of victims or their caretakers. Only 50% of targeted households received full home visits, on average 56 days after the initial call to police, and only 6% of the elderly residents at targeted housing projects attended educational presentations. The interventions showed no measurable effects on the victim's knowledge of elder abuse issues or of available social services. Nonetheless, households that received home visits and were in housing projects that received public education called the police significantly *more* often, and also reported significantly *higher* levels of physical abuse to research interviewers than control households. Households that received home visits only (but were not in projects receiving public education) also called the police *significantly more* often than control households, but did not report more abuse to interviewers. These increased calls to police were found 6 months after the trigger incident but disappeared by 12 months.

The authors offer several explanations for the findings. The most plausible may be that the combined interventions incited abusers rather than deterring them (the study did not provide direct evidence on this point, however, because abusers were not interviewed). The researchers speculate that elder abuse victims are often dependent on their abusers in multiple ways and when compared with domestic violence victims, may have even less hope of gaining independence from their abusers.

The National Center on Elder Abuse (2005) studied the impact of a counseling program serving abused elders that used intensive brief psychotherapy. In the evaluation, both the clients who participated in the Elder Abuse Counseling Program and the counselor were asked to assess the impact of program participation on mental health status, behavior, co-morbidities, and risk status. Data analyses revealed significant improvements in all areas that were assessed. In addition, client satisfaction was high for both individual and group counseling sessions. These results suggest that an intervention program involving counseling for elder abuse victims can bring about positive results.

In agreement with Thompson and Priest (2005), the study noted that material on treating abused elders was seriously lacking. For reasons that may have to do with dismissing abused elders as unable to benefit from interventions other than changes in their living situation and better health care, the authors suggests that the following beliefs must be operable among human service professionals before clinical interventions can be developed:

1. A belief that abused elders have emotional reactions to their abuse and can benefit from clinical interventions. The idea that elderly people can't benefit from clinical help is untrue.
2. A belief that older abused adults want to discuss their lives and, in particular, their abuse. Often the abusers are their own children. The opportunity to resolve problems with children could lead to better long-term relationships with family.

3. Abused older adults may have many years to live. Helping to resolve the emotional effects of their abuse can result in great benefit for longer, healthier, and happier lives.

4. When caretakers are the children of older adults, abused older adults may not have treated their caretakers well as children and the children are gaining revenge on older relatives for their treatment as children. The opportunity to resolve long-standing problems can help both victims and caretakers.

5. We have a growing body of research on the effectiveness of several types of therapy with depression, bereavement, and anxiety in older adults. Many of these treatments can be used with abused elders and are discussed in detail in following chapters.

6. The lack of best evidence to help abused elders is a type of ageism all too common in our society. It points to a belief that older people don't have the same needs, feelings, desires, hopes, and dreams as younger people. The lack of concern for elders is a way of negating their existence and, in many ways increases the probability that abuse will take place.

7. Workers need to begin identifying effective interventions and share them with colleagues. Small pieces of research and research with single subject designs would be ideal for this type of endeavor.

EVIDENCE-BASED PRACTICE WITH AN ABUSED OLDER ADULT: A CASE STUDY

Loretta Bascom is an 82-year-old former accountant who lives with her daughter Mildred (52), son-in-law Jim (53), and grandson Alec (19). Loretta was living independently when her hip broke and surgical complications extended her stay beyond the 100 days covered by Medicare. With a very long recuperation awaiting her and no funds for a continued stay in a rehabilitation facility, Loretta was forced to live with her only relative, her daughter Mildred.

The stay has been fraught with problems, not least of which are Mildred's unwillingness to help her mother bathe, exercise, and have clean clothes and bedding as well as Loretta's son-in-law's attempt to take over Loretta's finances. Loretta pays her daughter $1,000 a month, which is most of her social security check, leaving Loretta with only a few hundred dollars for medication and medical supplies.

Loretta was seen by the hospital social worker when she developed bedsores and her daughter began to worry that the infection would spread to her family. Loretta cried when the social worker saw her. She could not understand why she was being treated so badly by her daughter and son-in-law, believing that she had been a good mother and had helped her daughter on a number of occasions when her daughter was in financial difficulty. Loretta maintained that she had always been respectful of the need to allow her daughter and family space to live their own lives without her "meddling."

In reporting her history with her daughter, Loretta said that Mildred had made many mistakes in her life and had abused drugs and alcohol as a teenager and young adult. Loretta had often helped her out of legal difficulties and paid a small fortune for legal help. She recognized Mildred's limitations as a caretaker but could not think of an alternative because of her limited finances and lack of friends who could help her. She admitted that she had been feeling too depressed to do much of anything and wondered if the worker could help.

The worker said that the first thing to understand was that Mildred's lack of care was indicative of neglect and that the unhappy living situation would certainly interfere with her recovery. She strongly urged Loretta to consider other living arrangements and wondered if Loretta had a preference for where she would like to live. Loretta had found an assisted living facility that she thought would be ideal but the cost was in excess of her social security check. The worker wondered if Loretta would like her to check into financial arrangements with the facility as well as other forms of financial help. Loretta said that would be a good idea and thanked the worker.

The worker said that it might also be important to discuss, in more detail, Mildred's behavior since it had, in the worker's opinion, a great deal to do with Loretta's depression. Loretta cried a bit and said, "I can't say I'm surprised, I'm just hurt. Mildred has never been one to help others and she certainly hasn't been helpful to me as I age. I knew better than to live with her but being hospitalized, hurting so much, and then not having money to go elsewhere, I asked Mildred for help and, to my surprise she said yes."

"It must have been tough to ask," the worker replied.

"It was, but what else could I do? I thought I'd figure something out and be out of Mildred's house soon enough, but then I got depressed and I just couldn't figure anything else to do."

The worker thought it might be a good idea to discuss Loretta's options and said that perhaps having the doctor talk to her about depression might be helpful since he might have a suggestion for medication. Loretta agreed that she would like some help with medication but asked if the worker could talk to her about the situation with Mildred and her family. She always felt that she was a pretty normal person. She knew about Mildred's deficiencies and accepted them but couldn't understand why they were bothering her so much now. The worker promised she would see Loretta the next day and made an appointment for an hour session.

After the initial meeting the worker went to the literature and found that Gallagher-Thompson et al. (1990) had followed elderly clients for two years after completion of treatment for depression and found that 52% of the clients receiving cognitive treatment, 58% of the clients receiving behavioral treatment, and 70% of the clients receiving brief dynamic treatment had no return of depressed symptoms two years after treatment. The authors reported that these rates of improvement were consistent with a younger population of depressed clients.

Believing that Loretta was asking for help in understanding Mildred's behavior, the next meeting was spent in a discussion of the relationship between mother and daughter. As they delved into the relationship, it became clear that Mildred had always resented her mother's support and acceptance and that Mildred's sense of failure was such that her mother's positive behavior wasn't thought to be genuine. Many times over the years Mildred had complained that her mother was covering up her negative feelings about Mildred. As much as her mother denied this, Mildred persisted. It also became clear that Mildred believed that her choice of husbands was poor and that her mother tacitly agreed.

As they continued the discussion over several sessions, Loretta seemed to have closure on the subject and began to ask for help in finding a new living arrangement. "Why stay in a place where I'm not wanted?" she asked. "I love my daughter, but I'm also sure if I stay there it'll be the end of me and I still have some living to do."

The worker was able to arrange for Loretta to receive assistance to go to the assisted living facility she had found. A social worker on staff continues to work with Loretta and they often discuss the mother–daughter relationship and other life issues Loretta finds necessary to understand. With the worker's help, she has discovered a wealth of information on the Internet about aging and mother–daughter relationships. She has also joined a self-help group on the Internet for abused elders and corresponds daily with several members of the group who have similar problems with their daughters. The members come from all over the world and it's exciting for Loretta to have such diverse friends.

After six months in the assisted care facility, Loretta has been able to find a small apartment where she lives independently with weekly visits from the public health nurse and a public health social worker. She continues to discuss her daughter and reports that Mildred has been very conciliatory about her mother's leaving the home but Loretta guesses her daughter just misses the $1,000 a month. In any event she has a good relationship with her grandson who visits often and, in Loretta's words, "More than makes up for my daughter's shortcomings."

Discussion

I spoke to the worker who explained her choice of treatment approaches. She told me that "while I consider myself someone who does very brief behaviorally-oriented work, from her work success and past absence of any emotional problems, Loretta seemed able to make life changes without much direction from me. She wanted to find out why her daughter was being so neglectful and why their relationship had been so difficult. This seemed important to her, and while I found several studies supporting the use of behaviorally or educationally oriented approaches, I used the brief form of dynamic therapy discussed by Plopper (1990) who found that brief dynamic treatment was as effective as cognitive or educationally-oriented approaches with older adult clients suffering from depression. I thought the following discussion of brief dynamic therapy by Landreville and Gervais (1997) was very helpful:

> [T]here is evidence to suggest that brief psychodynamic psychotherapy is as effective as behavioral or cognitive therapies for treating depression in the elderly (Thompson et al., 1987). Psychodynamic treatment, which aims at providing clients with both support and a personal understanding of their current difficulties, emphasizes the importance of interpreting the patient's emotional experience through the therapeutic relationship. As stated by Rodin et al. (1991), this relationship can be helpful to medical patients not only by alleviating depression but also by facilitating relationships with other caregivers (i.e., physicians, occupational therapists, nurses, etc.). These authors describe three phases in the psychodynamic treatment of depression in the medically ill which are also relevant to disabled older adults: (a) the facilitation of grief and mourning; (b) the provision of meaning; and (c) the achievement of a sense of mastery over the feelings associated with the physical disorder. (p. 203)

"I thought this would be something I could accomplish over the several weeks Loretta was hospitalized and before she was transferred to a rehabilitation setting, and it seemed to work. Listening to what the client wants from us is particularly important. I think workers often discount older adults and communicate with them as if they were talking to children. Although she's in a difficult situation, Loretta is a bright, attentive, and assertive woman with a great deal of self-motivation and direction.

Finding out more about her relationship with her daughter was just what she needed to help her move away from a very difficult situation.

"I should add that I spoke to Mildred and told her that the medical staff was concerned that her mother was being neglected and that she would move elsewhere. Mildred blamed her mother and said that she was lazy and unwilling to do things for herself. I felt her behavior defined her as a narcissistic caretaker only 'interested in exploiting the older person and his or her assets. The mistreatment in which they engage tends to be chronic, escalates over time, and takes the form of neglect and financial exploitation' (Thompson and Priest, 2005, p. 120). As a mandated reporter I contacted the county department of aging with a formal report, but by the time it reached the department and action was taken, Loretta was living elsewhere. However, Mildred and her husband received a severe written reprimand and were told that they would not be allowed to care for older adults in the future. I explained my actions to Loretta who seemed saddened by it all but accepting."

9.7 COMMUNITY SERVICES

Treatment alone is not the only answer to elder abuse or to its prevention. Elder abuse needs to be addressed on a broader level and community-based educational interventions should be offered to both older adults and potential caregivers focusing on issues associated with their care and the possibility of abuse. With this knowledge, caregivers will be better equipped to decide if they are capable of caring for older relatives. Kosberg and Garcia (1995) believe that understanding potentially aversive consequences may deter older family members from choosing to live with relatives. Should this happen, it is important that affordable housing for older adults, foster care, and group living are available as substitutes to living with relatives. As important as the living situation is the ability to receive supportive services for caregivers. Such services may include day care, senior citizen centers, and home health services. Having other people to talk to is a necessary way to reduce stress and share solutions.

Reay and Browne (2002) suggest a three-stage approach to community-based services, which could also limit the frequency of elder abuse. In stage one, nursing and day residential services would be created or enhanced to provide caregivers with breaks and time outs. They also suggest the availability of overnight care and a confidential hotline to discuss problems in caring with older relatives. Stage one would also emphasize the rights, safety, and health of older people and the reduction of the stigmas of aging that stereotype older adults as senile, rigid, physically decrepit and slow. Reay and Browne (2002) believe that stereotypes about older adults often lead to elder abuse and neglect because they continue a societal bias against older men and women.

At stage two, Reay and Brown (2002) suggest increased screening and identification, noting that many older people are admitted to the hospital with physical injuries consistent with abuse or neglect that are not investigated. At stage three, interventions should involve a thorough assessment of the client's needs. Unfortunately, tertiary interventions for elder abuse commonly involve removing the older individual from home and placing him or her in a hospital or a residential facility, even though the older client would prefer to remain in the home. (Bergeron, 2000; Quinn and Tomita, 1997). Practitioners should understand that abusive behaviors are often learned and repeated in families, and caregivers may respond to elderly parents in the same abusive way their parents responded to them as children (Schwiebert et al., 2000). If this behavior cannot be changed, and often it can't, then the correct thing to do is to help clients find a safe place to live where the cycle of abuse will stop.

9.8 RESEARCH QUESTIONS

Bonnie (2002) believes that before we can successfully deal with elder abuse and neglect that we need strong research efforts aimed at older adults. Among the questions he believes we need to study are the following:

1. **The need to define elder abuse and neglect for policy, treatment, and prevention purposes.** Bonnie believes that legal definitions and responses should be grounded in empirical studies of conduct that pose the most serious risks to older adults. He wonders if we know enough about elder abuse to construct necessary treatment approaches with good outcome potential, and acknowledges the need for good longitudinal studies of vulnerable elders who have (and have not) been mistreated.
2. **The need to collect data in a systematic way that monitors occurrences of mistreatment in various settings, including emergency rooms and long-term care facilities.** Bonnie believes

that issues of definition and measurement need to be studied and resolved in order to implement useful surveillance systems.

3. **The need to identify elders who are being neglected or abused for the purpose of effective intervention and preventing further harm.** Bonnie suggests that a key to protecting vulnerable elders from mistreatment is careful screening and individual assessment. Two challenges arise with screening and case-identification. The first is to develop ways to identify hidden mistreatment, while the other is to differentiate natural conditions and illnesses associated with aging from mistreatment. While burns and ligature marks are often reliable indicators of mistreatment, fractures may not necessarily suggest maltreatment. Bonnie believes that mistakenly attributing nutritional deficiencies to an illness when it is in fact a sign of neglect can prolong suffering. On the other hand, mistakenly identifying a spontaneous bruise or other injury as intentionally inflicted is an error that is likely to have legal implications and hurt innocent caretakers.

4. **Prevent mistreatment before it occurs or escalates in severity.** We need to study the effects of policies and programs to prevent elder mistreatment by prioritizing concerns about harmful nursing home care and the occurrence of mistreatment.

5. **Assessing cost-effective preventive and protective intervention.** Bonnie indicates that we should study programs to reduce morbidity and mortality, including Medicare and Medicaid, and that we begin now to lay a foundation to analyze data that might help us understand whether social and medical programs actually achieve a desirable end result.

9.9 SUMMARY

This chapter on elder abuse discusses the frequency of abuse, caretakers who abuse elders, and treatment interventions with caretakers and victims. The lack of research data on interventions with abused elders is noted and suggestions are given as to how points of view about aging need to change to prompt more research. A case study applying EBP is provided along with a discussion of the case by the worker. Legal definitions of elder abuse are also given, as well as research questions that need to be answered for the human services to reduce the frequency of abuse. Community and policy interventions are also provided.

9.10 QUESTIONS FROM THE CHAPTER

1. Given the large amount of elder abuse, do you think ageism is the primary reason for the lack of practice research and best evidence to treat elder abused? Provide other reasons.
2. It appears from the chapter that most abusive caretakers cannot be helped and only those who are stressed or lack knowledge stand much of a chance of changing their abusive behavior. Do you agree with this assessment? If so, why, and if not, why not?
3. Lack of training to be a caretaker seems to be a primary reason for neglect. What information, values and skills might be included in a training program for caretakers?
4. In the case study, the worker makes a quick decision that the daughter is a narcissistic person who won't change her neglectful behavior toward her mother. Provide information from the case study to indicate that the daughter is untreatable.
5. Would it be true to say that most human service professionals would prefer not to work with older adults (only 3% of all social work graduate students specialize in aging), and that working with abused elderly is the least likely type of work with older adults most human service professionals want to perform? Provide supportive evidence for your answer.

REFERENCES

Bergeron, R. L. (2000). Serving the needs of elder abuse victims. *Policy and Practice of Public Human Services, 58*(3), 40–45.

Bonnie, R. J. (2002). Elder mistreatment in an aging America: An urgent need for research. Statement before the Committee on Finance, US Senate (June).

Browne, K., & Herbert, M. (1997). *Preventing family violence*. London: Wiley.

Brun, C., & Rapp, R. C. (2001). Strengths-based case management: Individuals' perspectives on strengths and the case manager relationship. *Social Work, 46*(3), 278–288.

Cyphers, G. C. (1999). Out of the shadows: Elder abuse and neglect. *Policy and Practice of Public Human Services, 570*, 25–30.

Davis, R. C., & Medina-Ariza, H. (2001, September). Results from an elder abuse prevention experiment in New York City. *US Department of Justice, Office of Justice Programs, Institute of Justice*, 1–7.

Dyer, C. B., Pavlik, V. N., Murphy, K. P., & Hyman, D. J. (2000). The high prevalence of depression and dementia in elder abuse and neglect. *Journal of American Geriatrics Society, 28*, 205–208.

Gallagher-Thompson, D., Hanley-Peterson, P., & Thompson, L. W. (1990). Maintenance of gains versus relapse following brief psychotherapy for depression. *Journal of Consulting and Clinical Psychology, 58*, 371–374.

Jogerst, G. J., Dawson, J. D., Hartz, A. J., Ely, J. W., & Schweitzer, L. A. (2000). Community characteristics associated with elder abuse. *Journal of American Geriatrics Society, 48*, 513–518.

Kosberg, J. I., & Garcia, J. L. (1995). *Confronting the maltreatment of elders by their family*. Thousand Oaks, GA: Sage.

Landreville, P., & Gervais, P. S. (1997). Psychotherapy for depression in older adults with disability: Where do we go from here? *Aging & Mental Health, 1*(3), 197.

Levine, J. M. (2003). Elder neglect and abuse: A primer for primary care physicians. *Geriatrics, 5S*(10), 37–44.

Marshall, G. E., Benton, D., & Brazier, J. M. (2000). Elder abuse: Using clinical tools to identify clues of mistreatment. *Geriatrics, 55*(2), 47–50.

Moxley, D. P., & Washington, O. G. M. (2001). Strengths-based recovery practice in chemical dependency: A transpersonal perspective. *Families in Society, 82*(3), 251–262.

National Center on Elder Abuse. (1998). *National elder abuse incidence survey.* Retrieved 09.09.2004 <http://www.aoa.dhhs.gov/eldfam/Elder_Rights/Elder_Abuse/ABuseReport_Full.pdf/>

National Center on Elder Abuse. (n.d.). *NCEA: The source of information and assistance on elder abuse.* Retrieved 24.08.2005 <http://www.elderabusecenter.org/>

National Center on Elder Abuse Incidence Study. (2005). Summary of unpublished research. National Center on Elder Abuse. Grant No. 90-AM-2792. National Association of State Units on Aging, 1201 15th Street, NW, Suite 350, Washington, DC 20005 (March).

Papadopolous, A., & LaFontaine, J. (2000). *Elder abuse: Therapeutic perspectives in practice*. Bicester, UK: Winslow.

Plopper, M. (1990). Evaluation and treatment of depression. In B. Kemp, K. Brummel-Smith, & J. W. Ramsdell (Eds.), , *Geriatric rehabilitation* (pp. 253–254). Boston: College-Hill.

Quinn, M. J., & Tomita, S. K. (1997). *Elder abuse and neglect*. New York: Springer.

Ramsey-Klawsnik, H. (2000). Elder-abuse offenders: A typology. *Generations, 24*(2), 17–22.

Reay, G. A., & Browne, K. D. (2002). The effectiveness of psychological interventions with individuals who physically abuse or neglect their elderly dependents. *Journal of Interpersonal Violence, 17*, 416–431.

Rodin, G., Craven, J., & Littlefield, C. (1991). *Depression in the medically ill: An integrated approach*. New York: Brunner/Mazel.

Schwiebert, V. L., Myers, J. E., & Dice, G. (2000). Ethical guidelines for counselors working with older adults. *Journal of Counseling & Development, 78*, 49–67.

Shaffer, D., Dooley, K., & Willaimson, G. (2007). Endorsement of proactively aggressive caregiving strategies moderates the relation between caregiver mental health and potentially harmful caregiving behavior. *Psychology and Aging, 22*(3), 494–504.

Sherman, S., & Newman, E. S. (1979, July). The role of social work in adult foster care. *Social Work*, 324–328.

Thompson, H., & Priest, R. (2005). Elder abuse and neglect: Considerations for mental health practitioners. *ADULTSPAM Journal, 2*, 116–128.

van den Bergh, N. (Ed.). (1995). *Feminist practice in the 21st century*. Washington, DC: NASW Press.

Van Wormer, K. (1999). The strengths perspective: A paradigm for correctional counseling. *Federal Probation, 63*(1), 51–58.

Welfel, E. R., Danzinger, P. R., & Santoro, S. (2000). Mandated reporting of abuse/maltreatment of older adults: A primer for counselors. *Journal of Counseling & Development, 78*, 284–292.

Wolf, R. S. (1998) Clinical geropsychology. Washington, DC: American Psychological Association.

Chapter ten

Evidence-Based Practice with Depressed and Suicidal Older Adults

10.1 INTRODUCTION

Large numbers of depressed older adults often go undiagnosed and untreated because symptoms of depression are often thought to be physical in nature and professionals frequently believe that older adults are neither motivated for therapy nor find it an appropriate treatment. This often leaves many older adults trying to cope with serious depressions without adequate help. As this chapter will indicate, the numbers of older adults dealing with depression are considerable and growing as their numbers increase in the USA. Health problems, loss of loved ones, loss of status related to work, financial insecurities, lack of a support group, a growing sense of isolation and a lack of self-worth are common problems among the elderly that lead to serious symptoms of depression. Two case studies at the end of the chapter provide additional information about the causation and treatment of depression in older adults.

10.2 DEPRESSION IN OLDER ADULTS

While symptoms of depression are consistent across age groups, Wallis (2000) suggests that older adults may express depression through such physical complaints as insomnia, eating disorders, and digestive

201

problems. They may also show signs of lethargy, have less incentive to participate in the activities they enjoyed before they became depressed, and experience symptoms of depression while denying that they are depressed. Mild and transient depression brought on by situational events usually resolve themselves in time, but moderate depression may interfere with daily life activities and can result in social withdrawal and isolation. Severe depression may result in psychotic-like symptoms including hallucinations and a loss of being in touch with reality (Wallis, 2000). The DSM-IV (APA, 1994) does not distinguish depression in older adults from depression in the younger population, and the subtle as well as the overt signs of depression in the elderly are not discussed. This lack of differentiation of depression among age groups makes diagnosis more problematic and is one possible explanation of why depression is often not treated when elderly clients have co-existing medical problems. Whether the medical problem results in the depression or the depression contributes to the medical problem is difficult to determine and remains an area requiring more study. Clearly, however, older adults have intrusive health and mental health issues that may cause depressed feelings and may lead to changes in functioning.

Zalaquett and Stens (2006) believe that depression is often undiagnosed and untreated in older adults causing "needless suffering for the family and for the individual who could otherwise live a fruitful life" (p. 192). The authors point out that we have sufficient evidence that longstanding depression predicts earlier death while recovery leads to prolonged life. Suicide is a significant risk factor for older adult clients suffering from depression. Depression, according to the authors, may increase the risk of physical illnesses and disability. Unützer et al. (2003) report that depression affects between 5% and 10% of older adults who visit a primary care provider and is a chronic, recurrent problem affecting many older adults, especially those with poor physical health. The authors note that late life depression has been associated with substantial "individual suffering, functional impairment, losses in health-related quality of life, poor adherence to medical treatments and increased mortality from suicide and medical illnesses" (p. 505).

In a study of older adults living in a specific community, Blazer et al. (1987) found that 8% had symptoms of depression or other disorders serious enough to warrant treatment. Older adults in acute health care facilities had rates of depression of 5–15%, while residents of long-care facilities had symptoms, not captured in current descriptions of major depression, of 25% (Blazer, 1993). Wallis (2000) reports a depression rate of 6% among older adults, nearly two-thirds of who are women. Wallis notes that depression is more prevalent among an older population because of loss of loved ones, health problems, and the inability to live independently. According to Wallis, 75% of older adults in long-term care have mild to moderate symptoms of depression. Mills and Henretta (2001) indicate that more than two million of the 34 million older Americans suffer from some form of depression, yet late-life depression is often undiagnosed or under-diagnosed.

Casey (1994) reports a study that found rates of suicide among adults 65 and older almost double that of the general population, and that the completion rate for suicide among older adults was 1 in 4 as compared to 1 in 100 for the general population (Casey, 1994), suggesting that older adults are much more likely to see suicide as a final solution rather than a cry for help. Older adults who commit suicide often suffer from major depression, alcoholism, severe medical problems, and social isolation (Casey, 1994). Although adults aged 65 and older comprise 13% of the US population, they account for 18% of the total number of suicides that occurred in 2000. The highest rate of suicide (19.4 per 1,000) was among people aged 85 and over, a figure that is twice the overall national rate. The second highest rate (17.7 per 100,000) was among adults aged 75 to 84.

Hepner et al. (2007) found that primary care physicians do well in detecting and initiating treatment for depression but provide substantially "lower-quality care in terms of completion of a minimal course of treatment for depression (especially among elderly persons) or assessment and treatment of psychiatric co-morbid conditions" (p. 324). In addition, the researchers found little evidence of appropriate responses to suicidal ideations, low rates of referral to mental health specialists for complex patients, and low rates of completion of treatment even though 85% of the patients were open to receiving treatment (p. 327). The authors note that

> When patients did access mental health specialists, nearly half did not report receiving any elements of evidence-based (cognitive-behavioral) therapy, such as being helped to reduce negative thoughts. We found rates of treatment completion (46%) that were in the range reported by other investigators, such as Charbonneau and colleagues, who reported 45% completion of antidepressant treatment. (Hepner et al., 2007, pp. 326–327)

Older adults also have a considerably higher suicide completion rate than other groups. While for all age groups combined there is one completed suicide ending in death for every 20 attempts, there is one completed suicide ending in death for every four attempts among adults who are 65 and older (Beeler, 2004). The Centers for Disease Control (2005) reports that 14.3 of every 100,000 people age 65 and older died by suicide in 2004, higher than the rate of about 11 per 100,000 in the general population. Non-Hispanic white men aged 85 and older were most likely to die by suicide, with an astonishing rate of 49.8 suicide deaths per 100,000 persons in that age group.

10.3   REASONS FOR OLDER ADULT DEPRESSION

To determine whether there are factors other than generalized health problems or issues of isolation that cause depression, Mills and Henretta (2001) found significant differences along racial and ethnic lines. Many more Hispanics and African Americans over the age of 65 report that their health is only fair or poor as compared with non-Hispanic white elderly. Axelson (1985) reports that Mexican Americans tend to see themselves as "old" much earlier in life than other groups (e.g., at about age 60, as compared with age 65 for Black Americans and age 70 for White Americans). Axelson believes that attitudes and expectations about aging "may put the Hispanic elderly at increased risk of what has been called psychological death, meaning a giving up or disengagement from active involvement in life" (Found in Mills and Henretta, 2001, p. 133).

Social support networks for older adults are also a factor in positive health and mental health. Tyler and Hoyt (2000) studied the emotional impact of natural disasters on older adults who had pre-disaster indications of depression and found that subjects with consistent social supports had lower levels of depression before and after a natural disaster than depressed subjects without social supports. In describing why many older people who have been symptom-free and, indeed, are considered to be resilient in the face of serious traumas, Kramer (2005) believes that resilience may move into depression many years after a successfully coped-with trauma. "Depression," he writes, "is not universal even in terrible times. Though prone to mood disorders, the great Italian writer Primo Levi, who committed suicide at the height of his success at age 67, was not depressed in his months at Auschwitz" (p. 53). Kramer continues,

> I have treated a handful of patients who survived horrors arising from war or political repression. They come to depression years after

enduring extreme privation. Typically such a person will say: "I don't understand it. I went through____," and here he will name a shameful event of our time. "I lived through *that* and in those months, I never felt *this*." *This* refers to the relentless bleakness of depression, the self as hollow shell. Beset by great evil, a person can be wise, observant and disillusioned and yet not be depressed. Resilience confers its own measure of insight. (p. 53)

Not surprisingly, Mavandadi et al. (2007) found a strong relationship between negative social interactions with older adults, and physical pain and depression. The authors conclude that "negative exchanges with social network members may be sources of acute stress or chronic strain that could detract considerably from psychological well-being" (p. 815). Negative exchanges might include messages that convey displeasure and criticism, blaming the older adult for their pain and depression, making suggestions that appear critical and unlikely to help to the older adult, and a lack of concern about the pain they are in. The researchers urge treatment personnel to be aware of the relationship between pain, negative social interactions and depression, and report that when social interactions improve as a result of treatment, pain and depression subside.

10.4 BEST EVIDENCE FOR TREATING DEPRESSION IN ELDERLY CLIENTS

Gallagher-Thompson et al. (1990) followed elderly clients for two years after completion of treatment and found that 52% of the clients receiving cognitive treatment, 58% of the clients receiving behavioral treatment, and 70% of the clients receiving brief dynamic treatment had no return of depressed symptoms two years after treatment. The authors report that these rates of improvement are consistent with a younger population of depressed clients. However, Huffman (1999) reports high rates of recurrence of depression in older adults following treatment. In subjects over 70 who received psychotherapy and a placebo as an antidepressant, the recurrence rate for depression was 63% within a three-year period of time. For subjects 60–69, the recurrence rate was 65%. Subjects treated with just an antidepressant and scheduled office visits to check on their progress did least well, with a 90% recurrence rate for both age groups (Huffman, 1999).

Lebowitz et al. (1997) found that certain types of psychotherapy are effective treatments for late-life depression. For many older adults, especially those who are in good physical health, combining interpersonal psychotherapy with antidepressant medication appeared to provide the most benefit. The authors note that about 80% of older adults with depression recovered with this kind of combined treatment and had lower recurrence rates than with psychotherapy or medication alone. The authors report another study of depressed older adults with physical illnesses and problems with memory and thinking that showed combined treatment was no more effective than medication alone. Apparently, the more cognitively and physically healthy the client, the more likely that therapy will be beneficial.

Lenze et al. (2002) studied the effectiveness of interpersonal treatment in conjunction with antidepressives with depressed elderly clients. Not surprisingly, given the lack of awareness of late-onset depression in elderly clients, they report that, "[T]o our knowledge, this is the first report concerning social functioning in a controlled randomized study of elderly patients receiving maintenance treatment for late-life depression" (p. 467). The authors found improved social adjustment attributable to combined interpersonal psychotherapy and maintenance medication. While improvement in social functioning could not be related directly to therapy, maintenance of the gains made in social functioning seemed directly related to therapy. The most significant gains reported by the authors were in the areas of interpersonal conflict role transitions and abnormal grief.

Kennedy and Tannenbaum (2000) report compelling evidence that older patients experience a variety of emotional problems including depression, anxiety, caregiver burden, and extended bereavement. The authors believe that many elderly clients can benefit from psychotherapeutic interventions and suggest that adjustments for clinical practice with elderly clients should include consideration of "sensory and cognitive" problems, the need for closer collaboration with the clients' family and other care providers, and a belief by the clinician, shared with the elderly client and his or her family, that treatment will result in improved functioning and symptom reduction to offset stereotypes that elderly clients with emotional problems are untreatable or unlikely to improve. The authors suggest that work with elderly clients also requires skill with a variety of approaches, including work with couples, families, and groups and that the use of pharmotherapy may produce very positive results with late-onset social and emotional problems experienced by elderly clients.

Zalaquett and Stens (2006) believe we have "a great body of data supporting the use of medication and/or psychosocial therapy to help the person with [late life] depression return to a happier, more fulfilling life … and shorten the time to recovery" (p. 192). Pinquart and Sörensen (2001) suggest that using psychosocial therapy with older adults is valuable because it decreases depression and promotes general psychological well being. The National Institutes of Health's (NIH) Consensus Panel on Diagnosis and Treatment of Depression in Late Life (1992) found that there are many different treatments of depression in older adults that have been shown to be safe and effective.

O'Connor (2001) reports that older clients usually get better after their first episode of depression but that the relapse rate is 50%. Clients with three episodes of depression are 90% more likely to have additional episodes. O'Connor suggests that we need to accept depression as a chronic disease and that therapists must be prepared to "give hope, to reduce shame, to be mentor, coach, cheerleader, idealized object, playmate, and nurturer. In doing so, inevitably, we must challenge many of our assumptions about the use of the self in psychotherapy" (p. 508). O'Connor (2001) also suggests that depressed clients seek approval from therapists and that the effective therapist give such support warmly and genuinely through smiles, nods, and recognition that the client has "accomplished something difficult, an indication that you share the patient's valuation of what he/she has accomplished, an emotional mirroring of the patient's pride – these can have powerful impact on the depressed patient" (p. 522).

Plopper (1990) believes that brief and focused approaches to the treatment of depression are preferable to intensive psychodynamic psychotherapy. However, there is evidence to suggest that brief psychodynamic psychotherapy is as effective as behavioral or cognitive therapies for treating depression in the elderly (Thompson et al., 1987). Psychodynamic treatment, which aims at providing clients with both support and a personal understanding of their current difficulties, emphasizes the importance of interpreting the patient's emotional experience through the therapeutic relationship.

Roth and Fonagy (1996) report that group therapies with older adults experiencing depression showed promise of reducing symptoms of depression. In one study, psychodynamic group therapy and cognitive behavioral group therapy approaches were compared and found to be equally effective in reducing levels of depression. Another study reported by Roth and Fonagy (1996) evaluated the effectiveness of self-help books with mildly to moderately depressed older adults (Scogin et al., 1989). Participants were randomly assigned to a cognitive bibliotherapy group, a behavioral bibliotherapy group, or a delayed treatment control group. Participants in the cognitive bibliotherapy group received a cognitive therapy self-help book, and participants in the behavioral bibliotherapy group received a behavioral therapy self-help book. Participants were told to read the books and were contacted in four weeks with follow-up questions to determine the impact of the books on depression. The results suggested "a clinically significant change" in depression with both cognitive and behavioral therapy self-help books. Gains continued at six-month and two-year follow ups.

Table 10.1 (Zalaquett and Stens, 2006, p. 197) shows our current state of research-based knowledge about treatments that work best with older adults experiencing depression.

In summarizing treatment effectiveness with older clients experiencing depression, Myers and Harper (2004) report that many interventions have been found effective with older adults "diagnosed with subclinical or clinical depression. These include reminiscence; individual behavioral, cognitive, and brief psychodynamic therapies; group psychodynamic and cognitive-behavioral therapies; and self-help bibliotherapy" (p. 210).

Table 10.1 Psychosocial Treatments for Major Depression and Dysthymia in Older Adults

Therapy	Major depression	Dysthymia	Maintenance
CBT	Probably efficacious	Potentially useful/ helpful	Incomplete evidence
IPT	Incomplete evidence	Potentially useful/ helpful	Useful with medication
BCT	Probably efficacious	No data	No data
RT	Potentially useful/helpful	No data	No data
Family	Incomplete evidence	Incomplete evidence	Incomplete evidence
Group	Has been researched with incomplete evidence	Incomplete evidence	Incomplete evidence

Note: CBT = cognitive-behavioral therapy; IPT = interpersonal therapy; BDT = brief dynamic therapy; RT = reminiscence therapy

CASE STUDY: EVIDENCE-BASED PRACTICE WITH A DEPRESSED OLDER ADULT MALE AND AN EVALUATION OF TREATMENT EFFECTIVENESS

The following case study and discussion first appeared in Glicken (2005, pp. 227–231). The author thanks the publisher for granting permission to use this material.

Jake Kissman is a 77-year-old widower whose wife, Leni, passed away a year ago. Jake is emotionally adrift and feels lost without Leni's companionship and guidance. He has a troubled relationship with two adult children who live across the country and has been unable to turn to them for solace and support. Like many older men, Jake has no real support group or close friends. Leni's social circle became his, but after her death, her friends left Jake to fend for himself. Jake is a difficult man who is prone to being critical and insensitive. He tends to say whatever enters his mind at the moment, no matter how hurtful it may be, and then is surprised that people take it so badly. "It's only words," he says. "What harm do words do? It's not like smacking somebody." Before he retired, Jake was a successful salesman and can be charming and witty but, sooner or later, the disregard for others comes through and he ends up offending people.

Jake's depression shows itself in fatigue, feelings of hopelessness, irritability, and outbursts of anger. He doesn't believe in doctors and never sees them. "Look what the "Momzers" (bastards) did to poor Leni. A healthy woman in her prime and she needed a surgery like I do. They killed her, those butchers." Jake has taken to pounding on the walls of his apartment whenever noise from his neighbors upsets him. Complaints from surrounding neighbors have resulted in the threat of an eviction. Jake can't manage a move to another apartment by himself and someone from his synagogue contacted a professional in the community who agreed to visit Jake at his apartment. Jake is happy that he has company, but angry that someone thought he needed help. "Tell the bastards to stop making so much noise and I'll be fine. The one next door with the dog, shoot her. The one on the other side who bangs the cabinets, do the same. Why aren't *they* being kicked out?"

The therapist listens to Jake in a supportive way. He never disagrees with him, offers advice, or contradicts him. Jake is still grieving for his wife and her loss has left him without usable coping skills to deal with the pressures of single life. He's angry and depressed. To find out more about Jake's symptoms, the therapist has gone to the literature on anger, depression, and grief. While he recognizes that Jake is a difficult client in any event, the data he collected helped him develop a strategy for working with Jake. The therapist has decided to use a strengths approach (Weick et al., 1989; Saleebey, 1992; Glicken, 2004) with Jake. The strengths approach focuses on what clients have done well in their lives and uses those strengths in areas of life that are more problematic. The approach comes from studies on resilience, self-healing, and on successful work with abused and traumatized children and adults.

Jake has many positive attributes that most people have ignored. He was a warm and caring companion to Leni during her illness. He is secretly very generous and gives what he has to various charities without wanting people to know where his gifts come from. He helps his children financially and has done a number of acts of kindness for neighbors and friends, but in ways that always make the recipients feel ambivalent about his help. Jake is a difficult and complex man and no one has taken the time to try and understand him. The therapist takes a good deal of time and listens closely.

Jake feels that he's been a failure at life. He feels unloved and unappreciated. He thinks the possibility of an eviction is a good example of how people "do him in" when he is least able to cope with stress. So the therapist listens and never disagrees with Jake. Gradually, Jake has begun discussing his life and the sadness he feels without his wife who was his ballast and mate. Using a strengths approach, the therapist always focuses on what Jake does well and his generosity, while Jake uses their time to beat himself up with self-deprecating statements. The therapist listens, smiles, points out Jake's excellent qualities, and waits for Jake to start internalizing what the therapist has said about him. Gradually, it begins to work. Jake tells the therapist to go help someone who needs it when Jake's anger at the therapist becomes overwhelming. Jake immediately apologizes. "Here you're helping me and I criticize. Why do I do that?" he asks the therapist. There are many moments when Jake corrects himself or seems to fight an impulse to say something mean-spirited or hurtful to the therapist, who tells him, "Jake, you catch more flies with honey than you do with vinegar." To which Jake replies, "So who needs to catch flies, for crying out loud? Oh, I'm sorry. Yeah, I see what you mean. It's not about flies, it's about getting along with people."

Gradually, Jake has put aside his anger and has begun talking to people in the charming and pleasant manner he is so capable of. The neighbors who complained about him now see him as a "doll." Jake's depression is beginning to lift and he's begun dating again, although he says he can never love anyone like his wife. "But a man gets lonely. So what are you supposed to do, sit home and watch soap operas all day? Not me." The therapist continues to see Jake and they often sit and quietly talk about Jake's life. "I was a big deal once. I could sell an Eskimo an air conditioner in winter. I could charm the socks off people. But my big mouth, it always got in the way. I always said something that made people mad. Maybe it's because my dad was so mean to all of us, I got this chip on my shoulder. Leni was wonderful. She could put up with me and make me laugh. When she died, I was left with my big mouth and a lot of disappointments. You want to have friends, you want your kids to love you. I got neither, but I'm not such an "alte cocker" (old fart) that I don't learn. And I've learned a lot from you. I've learned you can teach an old dog new tricks, and that's something. So I thank you and I apologize for some things I said. It's hard to get rid of the chip on the shoulder and sometimes it tips you over, that big chip, and it makes you fall down. You're a good person. I wish you well in life."

Discussion

Most of the treatment literature on work with older depressed adults suggests the use of a cognitive approach. Jake's therapist felt that the oppositional nature of Jake's personality would reject a cognitive approach. Instead, a positive and affirming approach was used that focused on Jake's strengths because "[M]ost depressed patients acutely desire the therapist's approval, and it is an effective therapist who gives it warmly and genuinely" (O'Connor, 2001, p. 522). While much of the research suggests the positive benefits of cognitive therapy, the therapist found the following description of cognitive therapy to be at odds with what might best help Jake. Rush and Giles (1982) indicate that cognitive treatment attempts to change irrational thinking through three steps: (1) identifying irrational self-sentences, ideas and thoughts; (2) developing rational thoughts, ideas and perceptions; and (3) practicing these more rational ideas to improve self-worth and, ultimately, to reduce depression. While this approach might work with other older clients, the therapist believed that Jake would take offense and reject both the therapy and the therapist, finding them preachy and critical.

Instead, the therapist decided to let Jake talk, although he made comments, asked questions to clarify, and made connections that Jake found interesting and oddly satisfying. "No one ever said that to me before," Jake would say, shaking his head and smiling. "You learn something new everyday, don't you." The therapist would always bring Jake back to the positive achievements in his life which Jake would initially toss away with comments like, "That was then when I paid taxes, this is now when I ain't gotta penny to my name." Soon, however, Jake could reflect on his positive achievements and began to use those experiences to deal with his current problems. In discussing the conflict with one of his neighbors, Jake said, "Maybe I should bring flowers to the old hag. Naw, I can't bring flowers, but she's no hag. I've seen worse. What about flowers? Yeah, flowers. Down at Vons I can buy a nice bunch for a buck. So it costs a little to be nice. Beats getting tossed out on my keester." Or he would tie something he had done when he was working to his current situation. "I had something like this happen once. A customer complained to my boss, so I go over and ask her to tell me what she's mad about so I can fix it, and she does, and it gets fixed. Sometimes you gotta eat a little crow." As Jake made connections and as he began to trust the therapist, this process of self-directed change reinforced his sense of accomplishment and led to a decrease in his depression. It also led to a good deal of soul searching about how he had to make changes in his life now that his wife was gone. "So maybe I should stop feeling sorry for myself and take better care. What do you think?"

10.5 EVALUATING ONE'S OWN PRACTICE WITH OLDER DEPRESSED ADULTS

Because the literature on the treatment of older adult depression is somewhat limited, therapists are encouraged to individualize treatment by working cooperatively with the client to find an approach that works. It also makes sense to track client change and to set goals for treatment. Evaluating one's own practice is always important, but it's particularly important with older clients whose depressed feelings may have a highly negative impact on health and may increase the risk of physical deterioration and even suicide.

One way to evaluate practice effectiveness is through the use of goal attainment scaling with single subject design. In single subject research, we are only interested in studying one subject at a time. The following discussion explains single subject research and presents a goal attainment scale specifically developed for treating Jake's depression. A more complete discussion of single subject research and goal attainment scaling can be found in a book on social research by the author (Glicken, 2003).

10.6 SINGLE SUBJECT APPROACHES TO EVALUATE DEPRESSION IN OLDER ADULTS

10.6.1 Single subject research

Single subject research is only interested in determining how well a single client does in treatment. Unlike empirical designs that require a control group, in single subject research, subjects act as their own control groups. While generalizing findings to other clients or showing a cause–effect relationship between treatment and client change as a result of a single case is not possible in single subject research, if enough people using a similar treatment approach have similar results, it may be possible to show a link between treatment and improvement rates, but not a direct correlation. Correlations require stringent research methodologies that are not evident in single subject research.

10.6.2 AB Designs

The most common single subject design is the AB design which has the following steps:

1. A steady state is determined that indicates how long the condition we are treating has existed.
2. A baseline measure or pre-test is then taken before the treatment begins.
3. The treatment approach is agreed upon with the client.
4. A time line is determined indicating how long the treatment will last.
5. A post-test is given to measure change when treatment is completed.
6. Further post-tests might also be given to determine how long the change lasts after intervals of six months, 12 months and 24 months following the end of treatment.
7. If the steady state (how long the condition existed *before* treatment began) is long enough, it would suggest that changes taking place once treatment is initiated are the result of the treatment and not because of some intervening or capricious events. We can say this because change that does not occur over a long period of time before treatment (the steady state) and now changes with the onset of treatment, can logically be thought to have occurred because of the treatment. The longer a depression lasted before treatment begins, the more likely it is that any improvement is the result of the treatment.

10.6.3 Goal attainment scaling

Goal attainment scaling is used when the therapist and client agree on goals of treatment that are measurable and are then used to monitor progress in achieving those goals. Goal attainment scaling is only used for observable behaviors that are easy to measure and have relevance from the research literature. For example, much of the research literature on treating depression suggests that a goal of treatment should be an increase in social contacts. This would therefore be a logical and measurable goal of treatment. The amount of improvement we expect in our clients should be based on the length of time the client has experienced depression and the severity of the problem. The longer our treatment continues, the higher our expectation should be for change. While goal attainment scaling is often used with single subject designs in which we are only interested in the improvement rate of an individual client, evaluating a sufficient number of clients using a single subject design might suggest links between treatment for a specific type of problem and its effectiveness with similar clients.

10.6.4 Baseline measures

A baseline measure is a pre-test measuring the behaviors to be changed over the course of treatment. Baseline measures should be behavioral in nature. Some examples might be weight, blood pressure, grades, exercise regimens, and blood-alcohol content. Happiness, morale, or work satisfaction would all be examples of behaviors that are difficult to measure because they are so subjective in nature. Goal attainment scaling is concerned with changes in behavior that can be directly observed in a person's life and can therefore be measured. The client with a weight problem is weighed every session. The client who agrees to walk two miles a day must have a card signed by someone from a health facility who has observed the two-mile walk and will verify it on paper. Independent verification is always necessary in measuring change.

10.6.5 Post-tests

The same set of goals used at the beginning of treatment must be used to determine change when treatment ends. Post-tests following the end of treatment and taken several more times in an 18–24 month period of time will indicate the behavioral gains the client has made and maintained as a result of treatment.

10.6.6 Goals of treatment

Goals are done conjointly with the client in the first session of treatment. The goals must be easily measured with no reliance on subjective client feedback. They must also be directly related to the new behaviors the clients must practice to change the presenting problem. For example, diet, exercise and social activities may lead to lower rates of anxiety and depression.

10.7 A GOAL ATTAINMENT SCALE MEASURING IMPROVEMENT IN JAKE'S DEPRESSION

In the following goal attainment scale we might use with Jake, we are using the CES-D Instrument to measure depression (the dependent variable) and various behaviors we think will decrease his depression as independent variables. The four independent variables are positive social interactions with his neighbors, increased contact with his children, attending meetings and social events in his condo complex, and swimming as a form of exercise to decrease levels of depression. We've chosen swimming because of a nearby heated pool and because Jake likes to swim but avoids the pool since he must interact with people he dislikes. If the client exercises and improves the number of social contacts as a positive result of our treatment, then, hopefully, the dependent variables (the CES-D score) should improve. All four independent variables can be verified by talking to the lifeguard at the pool, checking his phone records for calls to his children, checking receipts at social events, and by talking to neighbors. More examples of Goal Attainment Scaling (GAS) may be found in Glicken (2003).

10.7.1 Directions for creating a sale: intervals and weightings

On a goal attainment scale, 0% represents the client's functioning at the start of treatment. Each increment of 25% represents our "hoped for" levels of improvement. For purposes of calculating improvement rates, the intervals between the percent of gain made must be equal. In the following goal attainment scale, intervals on the CES-D are five points, while intervals of the other variables included on the scale should be consistent with what is realistic, attainable, and will lead to a reduction in his depression. One hundred percent improvement is our agreed upon improvement rate when a goal has been fully achieved. "W" (weighting) is the importance of each variable. For computational purposes, total weightings cannot surpass 1.0. The CES-D is a depression instrument with good validity and reliability that should show improvement as the other four variables improve. Social contact and exercise should increase as the depression lessens. The dependent variable (the depression scale) has a higher weighting than the independent or treatment variables (exercise, calls to his children, social events, and positive social contacts). Indications that the depression is lifting are more significant than the treatment inputs but are, in and of themselves, an indication that the depression is decreasing in severity.

10.7.2 How to calculate the overall gain made on a goal attainment scale

To calculate the total rate of improvement as a result of our treatment of our depressed client Jake, some arbitrary improvement rates are provided for each variable on the goal attainment scale, followed by an interpretation of the meaning of the data.

1. **Improvement rate on the CES-D = 75%.** Multiply 0.075 by 0.5 = 37.5% gain.
2. **Improvement rate in positive social contacts with neighbors = 50%.** Multiply 0.050 by 0.2 = 10% gain.
3. **Improvement rate in contacts with his children = 50%.** Multiply 0.050 by 0.1 times = 5% gain.
4. **Number of laps per day = 25%.** Multiply 0.025 by 0.1 = 2.5% gain.
5. **Social events improvement rate = 75%.** Multiply 0.075 by 0.1 = 7.5% gain.

Add all the percentages of improvement together for a total improvement rate after six months of treatment for depression as follows:

CES-Dw= 37.5%
Social contacts with neighbors= 10%
Contacts with children = 5%
Swimming laps= 2.5%
Social events= 7.5%
Total = 62.5% of the contracted for goals were achieved after six months of treatment.

Table 10.2 A Goal Attainment Scale Measuring Success in Reducing Depression

CES-D score	Positive interactions with neighbors per day	Telephone contact with children per month	Swimming laps per day	Social events attended per week
(W = 0.5)	(W = 0.2)	(W = 0.1)	(W = 0.1)	(W = 0.1)
0% baseline score= 35 on the CES-D	0% = 0 positive interactions	0%= 0 contacts per month	0% = 0 laps per day	0% = 0 social events per week
25% improvement = 30 on the CES-D	25% improvement = 1 positive interaction per day	25% improvement = 1 contact per child per month	25% improvement = 4 laps per day	25% improvement = 1 social events per week
50% improvement= 25 on the CES-D	50% improvement = 2 positive interactions per day	50% improvement = 2 contacts per child per month	50% improvement= 8 laps per day	50% improvement= 2 social events per week
75% improvement= 20 on the CES-D	75% improvement = 3 positive interactions per day	75% improvement = 3 contacts per child per month	75% improvement = 16 laps per day	75% improvement= 3 social events per week
100% improvement= 15 on the CES-D	100% improvement = 4 positive interactions per day	100% improvement = 4 contacts per child per month	100% improvement = 24 laps per day	100% improvement = 4 social events per week

10.7.3 What this tells us

Jake has achieved more than a 60% gain in the goals we jointly set. There is a 75% improvement rate on the depression scale (the CES-D), but scores on psychological tests may be prone to the halo effect (the improvement that comes when any intervention is provided but rapidly decreases after treatment ends) and social desirability (the tendency to say you're less depressed than you actually are). The client has improved in all other areas. The swimming of four laps per day may be a realistic level for him. At the very least, he's going to the pool every day, which is certainly a good sign. He has improved in all other areas measured by the scale but, most specifically, in attending social events. This isn't surprising since he can attend an event and not interact with others. Still, all of his goals show progress, and given where he was functioning at the beginning of treatment, his improvement rate is significant. Post-tests at predetermined intervals will help us track whether his level of improvement is maintained or shows signs of deterioration. If deterioration is apparent, treatment should be reinitiated and goals of treatment reevaluated.

10.8 SUMMARY

This chapter on EBP with depressed older clients points out the frequency and severity of depression in older adults and the high rate of completion of suicide, particularly in aging men. The chapter also notes the efficacy of treatment with older depressed clients and shows how single subject research with goal attainment scaling can be a simple and effective way of evaluating treatment progress. Two case studies show the cause of depression in two older adult clients and the way EBP approaches best evidence for use in treatment decisions.

10.9 QUESTIONS FROM THE CHAPTER

1. Wouldn't the amount of depression in an older population be reduced if we had free health care, low-cost housing, and support groups for elders?
2. Why would a physician not refer an older adult client with depression for therapy? Do you think the same thing would happen to a younger client? Does the lack of referral for therapy suggest low esteem for therapy?

3. How can therapy possibly help older adults deal with deteriorating health and the diminished capacity to do physical activities that were so easy for them to do when they were younger, but are now so difficult?

4. The goal attainment scaling approach seems unlikely to show cause–effect relationships between treatment and client improvement. Can you think of some research approaches that might actually show a cause–effect relationship and would therefore be more useful in producing best evidence?

5. The case study describing Jake seems to suggest that we should not confront older adults who have self-destructive behaviors. How can we change their conduct if we don't let them know that it's harmful?

REFERENCES

American Psychiatric Association (1994). *Diagnostic and statistical manual of mental disorders* (4th ed.). Washington, DC: Author.

Axelson, J. A. (1985). *Counseling and development in a multicultural society.* Monterey, CA: Brooks/Cole.

Beerler, M. (2004, May 23). Aging and depression don't go hand in hand. *Oakland Tribune*. http://findarticles.com/p/articles/mi_qn4176/is_20040523/ai_n14575239.

Blazer, D. G., Hughes, D. C., & George, L. K. (1987). The epidemiology of depression in an elderly community population. *Journal of the American Geriatric Society, 27*, 281–287.

Blazer, D. G. (1993). *Depression in late life* (2nd ed.). St Louis, MO: Mosby.

Casey, D. A. (1994). Depression in the elderly. *Southern Medical Journal, 87*(5), 559–564.

Centers for Disease Control and Prevention. (2005). National Center for Injury Prevention and Control. Web-based injury statistics query and reporting system (WISQARS) [online]. Available from URL: <www.cdc.gov/ncipc/wisqars/> Accessed 31.01.2007

Charbonneau, A., Rosen, A. K., Ash, A. S., Owen, R. R., Kader, B., Spiro, A., 3rd, et al. (2003). Measuring the quality of depression care in a large integrated health system. *Med Care., 41*, 669–680.

Gallagher-Thompson, D., Hanley-Peterson, P., & Thompson, L. W. (1990). Maintenance of gains versus relapse following brief psychotherapy for depression. *Journal of Consulting and Clinical Psychology, 58*, 371–374.

Glicken, M. D. (2003). *A simple guide to social research.* Boston, MA: Allyn and Bacon/Longman.

Glicken, M. D. (2004). *The strengths perspective in social work practice: A positive approach for the helping professions.* Boston, MA: Allyn and Bacon/Longman.

Hepner, K. A., Rowe, M., Rost, K., Hickey, S. C., Sherbourne, C. D., Ford, D. E., Meredith, L. S., & Rubenstein, L. V. (2007). The effect of adherence to practice guidelines on depression outcomes. *Annals of Internal Medicine, 147*(5), 320–329.

Huffman, G. B. (1999). Preventing recurrence of depression in the elderly. *American Family Physician, 59*(9), 2589–2591.

Kennedy, G. J., & Tannenbaum, S. (2000). Psychotherapy with older adults. *American Journal of Psychotherapy, 54*(3), 386–407.

Kramer, P. D. (2005, April 17). There's nothing deep about depression. *New York Times Magazine*, 50–53.

Lawton, M. P. (1977). The impact of the environment on aging and behavior. In J. E. Birren & K. W. Schaie (Eds.), *Handbook of the psychology of aging* (pp. 276–301). New York: Van Nostrand Reinhold.

Lawton, M. P., & Nahemow, L. (1973). Ecology and the aging process. In C. Eisdorfer & M. P. Lawton (Eds.), *The psychology of adult development and aging* (pp. 619–674). Washington, DC: American Psychological Association.

Lebowitz, B. D., Pearson, J. D., Schneider, L. S., Reynolds, C. F., III, Alexopoulos, G. S., Bruce, M. L., Conwell, Y., Katz, I. R., Meyers, B. S., Morrison, M. F., Mossey, J., Niederehe, G., & Parmelee, P. (1997). Diagnosis and treatment of depression in late life. Consensus statement update. *Journal of the American Medical Association, 278*(14), 1186–1190.

Lenze, E. J., Dew, M. A., Mazumdar, S., Begley, A. E., et al. (2002). Combined pharmacotherapy and psychotherapy as maintenance treatment for late-life depression: Effects on social adjustment. *American Journal of Psychiatry, 159*(3), 466–468.

Mavandadi, I., Sorkin, D. H., Rook, K. S., & Newsom, J. T. (2007). Pain, positive and negative social exchanges, and depressive symptomatology in later life. *Journal of Aging and Health, 19*(5), 813–830.

Mills, T. L., & Henretta, J. C. (2001). Racial, ethnic, and socio-demographic differences in the level of psychosocial distress among older Americans. *Research on Aging, 23*(2), 131–152.

Myers, J. E., & Harper, M. C. (2004). Evidence-based effective practices with older adults. *Journal of Counseling & Development, 82*, 207–218.

NIH Consensus Panel on Diagnosis and Treatment of Depression in Late Life(1992). Diagnosis and treatment of depression in late life. *Journal of the American Medical Association, 268*, 1018–1024.

O'Connor, R. (2001). Active treatment of depression. *American Journal of Psychotherapy, 55*(4), 507–530.

Pinquart, M., & Sörensen, S. (2001). How effective are psychotherapeutic and other psychosocial interventions with older adults? A meta-analysis. *Journal of Mental Health & Aging, 7*, 207–243.

Plopper, M. (1990). Evaluation and treatment of depression. In B. Kemp, K. Brummel-Smith, & J. W. Ramsdell (Eds.), *Geriatric rehabilitation* (pp. 253–264). Boston: College-Hill.

Robert, S. A., & Li, L. W. (2001). Age variation in the relationship between community socioeconomic status and adult health. *Research on Aging, 23*(2), 233–258.

Roth, A. D., & Fonagy, E. (1996). *What works with whom? a critical review of psychotherapy research*. New York: Guilford Press.

Rush, A. J., & Giles, D. E. (1982). *Cognitive therapy: Theory and research in short term psychotherapies for depression*. New York: Guilford Press (pp. 143–181).

Saleebey, D. (1992). *The strengths perspective in social work practice*. White Plains, NY: Longman.

Scogin, F., Jamison, C., & Gochneaur, K. (1989). Comparative efficacy of cognitive and behavioral bibliotherapy for mildly and moderately depressed older adults. *Journal of Consulting and Clinical Psychology*, 57, 403–407.

Thompson, L. W., Gallager, D., & Breckenridge, J. S. (1987). Comparative effectiveness of psychotherapies for depressed elders. *Journal of Consulting and Clinical Psychology, 55*, 385–390.

Tyler, K. A., & Hoyt, D. R. (2000). The effects of an acute stressor on depressive symptoms among older adults. *Research on Aging, 22*(2), 143–164.

Unützer, J., Katon, W., Callahan, C. M., Williams, J. W., Hunkeler, E., Harpole, L., Hoffing, M., Della Penna, R. D., Noel, P. H., Lin, E. H. B., Vaillant, G. E., & Mukamal, K. (2001). Successful aging. *American Journal of Psychiatry, 158*(6), 839–847.

Wallis, M. A. (2000). Looking at depression through bifocal lenses. *Nursing, 30*(9), 58–62.

Weick, A., Rapp, C., Sullivan, W. P., & Kisthardt, W. (1989). A strengths perspective for social work practice. *Social Work, 34*, 350–354.

Zalaquett, C. P., & Stens, A. N. (2006, Spring). Psychosocial treatments for major depression and dysthymia in older adults: a review of the research literature Journal of Counseling & Development, 84, 192–201.

Chapter eleven

Evidence-Based Practice with Older Clients Experiencing Anxiety

11.1 INTRODUCTION

The prevalence of anxiety disorders has usually been thought to decrease with age, but recent findings suggest that generalized anxiety is actually a more common problem among the elderly than depression. A study reported by Beekman et al. (1998) found that anxiety affects 7.3% of an elderly population as compared to 2% for depression in the same population. Lang and Stein (2001) estimate that the total number of older Americans suffering from anxiety could be in excess of 10%. Since many anxious elderly people do not meet the criteria for anxiety found in a number of research studies, the prevalence of anxiety-related problems in the elderly could be as high as 18% and constitutes the most common psychiatric symptom for older adults (Lang and Stein, 2001). Anxiety and depression among older adults frequently co-exist with common physical manifestations including chest pains, heart palpitations, night sweats, shortness of breath, essential hypertension, headaches, and generalized pain. Because physicians often fail to diagnose underlying symptoms of anxiety and depression in elderly patients, the emotional component of the symptoms are frequently not dealt with. Definitions and descriptions of anxiety used to diagnose younger patients often fail to capture the unique stressors that older adults must deal with. Those stressors include the fragile nature of life while attempting to cope with limited finances, failing health, the death of loved ones, concerns about their own mortality, and a sense of uselessness and hopelessness as their roles as adults become dramatically altered due to age and retirement.

However, in a large sample of elderly subjects, Himmelfarb and Murrell (1984) found a low correlation between age, physical health, and anxiety. Wagner and Lorion (1984) found that "death anxiety" does not exist among all older adults but may be more prevalent among women, married people, African-Americans, less educated older adults, and less affluent elders. The reader is cautioned that both studies noted above are older studies and may not accurately reflect the way older adults currently react to physical health and fears of death. However, Smith et al. (1995) report that

> Community studies of the elderly have found that anxiety symptoms in primary care patient populations ranged from 5% to 30%. And many such patients suffer from co-morbid depression. Late life anxiety does exist, and it may have a variety of causes. Old age can be a time of "intense" anxiety resulting from feelings of loneliness, worthlessness, and uselessness. Ill health, the loss of friends and loved ones, and financial problems all can contribute to the development of anxiety symptoms. (p. 5)

Lang and Stein (2001) found that women have higher rates of anxiety across all age groups, and that older adults who have had anxiety problems in the past are more at risk of the problem worsening as they age. Agoraphobia may also be more likely to have late-life onset as a result of physical limitations, disabilities, unsafe neighborhoods, and other factors that make some older adults fearful of leaving home. Because anxiety in the elderly may have a physical base, or may realistically be connected to concerns about health, Kogan et al. (2000) provide some guidelines for distinguishing an anxiety disorder in the elderly from anxiety related to physical problems. A physical cause of anxiety is more likely if the onset of anxiety comes suddenly, the symptoms fluctuate in strength and duration, and if fatigue has been present before the symptoms of anxiety were felt. The authors identify the following medical problems as reasons for symptoms of anxiety: (1) medical problems that include endocrine, cardiovascular, pulmonary, or neurological disorders; and (2) the impact of certain medications, most notably stimulants, beta-blockers, certain tranquilizers and, of course, alcohol.

An emotional cause of anxiety is more likely if the symptoms have lasted two or more years with little change in severity and if the person has other co-existing emotional symptoms. However, anxiety may cycle on and off, or a lower level of generalized anxiety may be present which causes the elderly client a great deal of discomfort. Obsessive concerns about financial issues and health are common and realistic worries that trouble elderly clients. The concerns may be situational or they may be constant but not serious enough to lead to a diagnosis of anxiety; nonetheless, they cause the client unhappiness and may actually lead to physical problems including high blood pressure, cardio-vascular problems, sleep disorders, and an increased use of alcohol and over-the-counter medications to lessen symptoms of anxiety.

The Surgeon General's Report on mental health (1999) reminds us that some disorders such as anxiety that currently have lower rates of occurrence in older adults will very likely increase as veterans of the wars in the mid-east currently experiencing PTSD begin to age. As an explanation of the relationship between PTSD and later life anxiety, a study by McFarlane and Yehuda (1996) indicated a rate of 15% in symptoms of PTSD 19 years after combat exposure in Vietnam. In addition, research indicates that PTSD can manifest itself for the first time long after the traumatic event (Aarts and Op den Velde, 1996), raising the possibility that additional older adult clients with symptoms of anxiety will be identified in the future.

11.2 DIAGNOSING ANXIETY IN OLDER ADULTS

The DSM-IV (APA, 1994) defines 12 types of anxiety disorders in the adult population. They can be grouped under seven headings:

1. **Panic disorders with or without agoraphobia**. The chief characteristic of panic disorder is the occurrence of panic attacks coupled with fear of their recurrence. In clinical settings, agoraphobia is usually not a disorder by itself, but is typically associated with some form of panic disorder. Patients with agoraphobia are afraid of places or situations in which they might have a panic attack and be unable to leave or to find help. About 25% of patients with panic disorder develop obsessive-compulsive disorder (OCD). Agoraphobia is an abnormal anxiety regarding public places or situations from which the patient may wish to flee or in which he or she would be helpless in the event of a panic attack.

2. **Phobias.** These include specific phobias and social phobia. A phobia is an intense irrational fear of a specific object or situation that compels the patient to avoid it. Some phobias concern activities or objects that involve some risk (for example, flying or

driving), but many are focused on harmless animals or other objects. Social phobia involves a fear of being humiliated, judged, or scrutinized and manifests itself as a fear of performing certain functions in the presence of others, such as public speaking or using public lavatories.

3. **Obsessive-compulsive disorder (OCD).** This disorder is marked by unwanted, intrusive, and persistent thoughts or repetitive behaviors that reflect the patient's anxiety or attempts to control it. It affects between 2 and 3% of the population and is much more common than was previously thought. A compulsion is a repetitive or ritualistic behavior that a person performs to reduce anxiety. Compulsions often develop as a way of controlling or "undoing" obsessive thoughts. An obsession is a repetitive or persistent thought, idea, or impulse that is perceived as inappropriate and distressing.

4. **Stress disorders**. These include post-traumatic stress disorder (PTSD) and acute stress disorder. Stress disorders are symptomatic reactions to traumatic events in the patient's life.

5. **Generalized anxiety disorder (GAD)**. GAD is the most commonly diagnosed anxiety disorder and occurs in as many as 7% of healthy older adults in the community. GAD is characterized by difficulty relaxing, constant anticipation of the worst, and difficulty controlling this worry or concern. For GAD to be diagnosed, symptoms must be present for at least six months and occur more days than not. Psychological symptoms may include uncontrollable worry or nervousness, edginess, irritability, and difficulty concentrating. GAD manifests itself in physical symptoms including fatigue, low energy, muscle tension, restlessness, and difficulty sleeping.

6. **Anxiety disorders due to known physical causes**. These include general medical conditions or substance abuse.

7. **Anxiety disorder not otherwise specified**. This last category is not a separate type of disorder, but is included to cover symptoms that do not meet the specific DSM-IV criteria for other anxiety disorders.

All DSM-IV anxiety disorder diagnoses include a criterion of severity. The anxiety must be severe enough to interfere significantly with the patient's occupational or educational functioning, social activities or close relationships, and other customary activities.

Pingitore and Sansone (1998) suggest the following steps to diagnose an anxiety disorder in older adults:

1. Consider the possibility of a medical problem as the cause of the older adult's anxiety-related symptoms. If there is no evidence of a medical problem;
2. Consider the possibility of the role of substance use or drug interactions in the client's anxiety.
3. If this is not the case, determine if the symptoms are better explained by another psychiatric disorder such as adjustment disorder, depression, or manic symptoms.
4. If this is not the case, decide if the symptoms can be diagnosed using a "not otherwise specified" category. If the full criteria are met for "panic disorder without agoraphobia," for example, the category "anxiety disorder not otherwise specified" would not be considered.
5. Select the proper DSM diagnostic code.

11.3 BEST EVIDENCE FOR THE TREATMENT OF ANXIETY WITH AN OLDER ADULT POPULATION

Beck and Stanley (1997) and Stanley and Novy (2000) report positive results with anxious older clients using cognitive-behavioral therapy and relaxation training. Benefits for older clients experiencing anxiety appear as positive as they are with younger clients. Smith et al. (1995) have found that older adults respond well to psychotherapy for anxiety, "especially if it supports their religious beliefs and encourages life review that helps to resolve both hidden and obvious conflicts associated with specific events in the patient's life history" (p. 6). The authors recommend medications only after all options have been considered. Most anxiety problems in younger clients are treated with benzodiazepines but have only a "marginal efficacy for chronic anxiety and are especially bad for older adults because the body accumulates the drug and may produce excess sedation, diminished sexual desire, worsening of dementing illness, and a reduction in the general level of energy" (Smith et al., 1995, p. 6). The authors also warn that Prozac may actually cause anxiety as a side-effect and recommend pinpointing the cause of the anxiety problem before considering the use of medications.

Although the benefits of cognitive-behavioral approaches seem positive, Lang and Stein (2001) recommend that treatment of anxiety in older adults should be tailored to the individual needs and cognitive abilities of the client. Some older clients resent advice given by professionals younger than they are. They may find relaxation approaches inappropriate or childish. Systematic desensitization may be seen as unrelated to their situation or to the origins of their anxiety, and they may view changes in the way they are told to perceive life events as dangerous to their survival since long-held beliefs and behaviors have often served them well in the past. Being asked to view a situation with clarity and rationality may suggest to the older adult that workers believe they are lying about an event. Older adults may discount psychological explanations for their anxiety and prefer to think that it has a physical origin. All of these cautionary suggestions should be taken into account when working with anxious older adults or one runs the risk of having psychological treatments dismissed completely.

A suggestion to encourage better acceptance of any intervention is to give clients reading materials to help them understand the origins of their anxiety and the approach most likely to help relieve their symptoms. Testimonials from other clients might also be helpful, or suggestions made by other professionals they trust could help the client accept treatment. Keep in mind that older adults are like all of us. They may be suffering, but they also fear that accepting new ways of approaching life may actually increase their level of anxiety. However, as Lang and Stein (2001) report, there are harmful side effects to the long-term use of many anti-anxiety medications. While some of the cognitive-behavioral approaches used in the treatment of anxiety may not always fit an older adult's frame of reference, it's wise to let them know about medical treatments and the potential for harm as one way to acknowledge that medications have risks that should be considered, just as there are associated risks in doing nothing.

CASE STUDY: ANXIETY IN AN ELDERLY CLIENT

Irma Kolb is a 71 year-old resident of a 55-and-over condominium complex in San Diego, California. Irma's husband passed away four years ago, and since then Irma has experienced generalized but manageable anxiety. She takes a mild tranquilizer to help control her anxiety. Several weeks after the condo complex was sold to new owners, Irma discovered that the unit she and her husband had rented for almost 15 years was due for renovation. The condo company which owns the complex will move her, at its expense, to another unit, and when her unit is completed, the company will move her back at its expense and she will continue paying the very low rent she presently enjoys. The notification of a temporary move threw Irma into a severe anxiety state with panic attacks. Her friends have promised to help her pack, and several employees who know and like Irma have promised to pack dishes and other breakable items at no cost. Many of her friends are also experiencing anxiety because of the disruption in their lives brought on by the renovations, but Irma's level of obsessive worry and panic has become so overwhelming that she was hospitalized for a week to try to lower her anxiety level and to regulate suddenly severe chest pains and high blood pressure, neither of which have a somatic cause.

Irma's son and daughter live on the east coast. They have tried to speak to her by phone and to assure her that everything will be fine. They point out how lucky she will be to live in a nicer condo without having to pay higher rent, but she is convinced that this is the first step in an attempt to get rid of renters who pay low rents. Many of her friends feel the same way and the level of worry is high in the complex. Irma has begun to feel that she will be forced out of her home because of the high rents she believes will be initiated over the next few years, and that she will end up on the streets as a homeless person. Her social security pension allows her little more than her rent, and she lives a very limited but satisfying lifestyle surrounded by friends and good neighbors in a community with excellent weather and medical care she likes and uses easily.

Since her hospitalization, she is unable to do most of the activities she did before she was hospitalized, and sits at home obsessively worrying and unable to do the packing that needs to be done over the next week. When her friends come to help, she sits immobilized with anxiety and isn't able to give directions or instructions. The condo complex has given her notice that if she isn't ready to move in a week, she will be evicted from her home and lose her right to return when the renovations are completed.

Intervention: Case Management

One of Irma's friends who volunteers at a local family service agency in San Diego contacted the head of services for the elderly. This person immediately sent a case manager to Irma's home. The case manager confirmed that Irma was immobilized with anxiety, contacted her friends and the employees who had offered to help her move, and asked them to help organize the move. The agency has a fund for emergency help if anyone needs to be hired to help with the move. The case manager also called the utility companies and changed Irma's service and made other changes of address brought on by the move (her bank, social security, health care provider, etc.). She and Irma walked to the temporary unit and were happily surprised to see that it was exactly like her current unit. The case manager made a diagram of Irma's home so that she could place her furniture in exactly the same position as her current home. The case manager assured the condominium company that Irma would be moved in time and had them send a letter to Irma assuring her that she would be able to move back to her renovated unit at her current rent. The case manager had several retired volunteers who were licensed therapists spend time with Irma to offer support and any practical help with concerns that Irma may have had.

In the course of the successful move and in the months following the move, Irma shared with the volunteer therapists that her family had been evicted many times from homes in Germany before World War II because they were Jewish and, having nowhere to go, the family often lived on the streets. Irma was just a small child then but the fear of once again living on the streets was a painful reminder of life in Germany and the hardships her family endured. Those hardships included starvation, dealing with extreme cold, and taunts and beatings from the Germans who had so recently been their neighbors and friends. Irma's fears were enhanced when the condo company threatened to evict her.

The president of the condominium company personally met with Irma and her neighbors to apologize for the incident and to once again assure them that they would not have their rents raised. Their city councilman and representatives from the local television stations were also present. The apology and the meeting went a long way to help ease Irma's anxiety. When her condo unit was renovated, Irma returned to find it a lovely, modern unit. A formal letter guaranteed her current rent for a year with the promise that yearly raises would not exceed the 4% Irma and her neighbors had experienced in the past. The letter said the company hoped Irma would stay at the complex for as long as she wished and called her a good neighbor and a great renter.

Irma continues on in therapy with several of the volunteer therapists who use a supportive and positive approach with Irma. They praise her resilience in dealing with a difficult life event and her ability to cope with life after what she endured as a child in Germany. She continues using a more substantial anti-anxiety medication and sees her physician frequently to monitor any health problems. Her blood pressure is lower than it was when she experienced her first anxiety attacks but it is still too high and a beta-blocker is being used for her hypertension and to lower her level of anxiety. Her chest pains continue at a reduced level and while there is seemingly no physical reason for the pain, her doctor takes it seriously and wants Irma to see him often so they can be proactive if a problem arises. Irma has been encouraged by her doctor to exercise and diet, which she has done by joining a health group at her complex. She walks two miles every day and has lost 15 pounds. The benefit of her new health consciousness is a reduction in her blood pressure, reduction her level of anxiety, and fewer episodes of chest pain.

In discussing her work with Irma, the case manager, a licensed clinical social worker, said the following:

"Elderly people have many realistic reasons to worry. Finances, health problems, loneliness, family loss, and little sense of contribution are common concerns for older people. Unlike many other cultures, the elderly are not revered in America and have a limited role in life, even though they've had successful lives and have made major contributions. At our agency, we view clients like Irma and her response to the move as a serious sign of difficulty. We've found that direct intervention is often necessary before clients can mobilize their own coping skills. We believe strongly in using our retired volunteers, many of whom are licensed therapists. They visit clients in their homes and provide a high level of supportive help that serves to energize clients and allows them to better utilize their own coping skills. We advocate directly for clients but we only do for them what they can't do for themselves. We've found that with highly anxious elderly clients, managing the case requires interaction with everyone involved with the client, particularly the client's health care provider. As an agency, we often interact with other social, mental health, and health care agencies about the best care for elderly clients.

"What we've sadly discovered is that many professionals still think of the elderly as somehow less cognitively able than younger clients. Stereotypes about the elderly of having diminished capacities to cope with life are very common. Professionals often think that medication is the only answer and that therapy is inappropriate for older persons. However, many older clients have resilience, intelligence, and skills that haven't diminished at all over the years. What they often need is help in an emergency, and some honest concern for them once the emergency is over. We've tracked our case management clients for many years. An approach that utilizes immediate help in a crisis, some homemaker care when needed, direct advocacy when the client can't do certain things for themselves, supportive therapy, and a belief that older people have the motivation, intelligence, and ability to change when faced with problems has resulted in few of our elderly clients requiring nursing care or moving into states of dementia. We think that active people live longer, are healthier, and have happier lives. In return for our services, our clients who are able volunteer to help others. It's a *quid-pro-quo* that has resulted in extraordinary longevity and life meaning for our older adult clients."

11.4 A PERSONAL STORY ABOUT SOCIAL ANXIETY

"I'm 68 and I've been anxious in social situations for as long as I can remember. I don't feel anxiety when I do professional presentations or in my work life, but when it comes to meeting people at parties, I feel like that famous story about William Faulkner at a party in Hollywood who was so uncomfortable that he kept backing up toward the balcony of the home where the party was being held until he fell over the balcony and landed in the swimming pool. That's the way I feel at parties. It's agony. I avoid parties or social activities where I don't know people, and even if I *do* know them, I assume they'll ignore me or avoid me, which is even worse.

"My brother and sister both feel the same way, so I have to guess that these feelings of anxiety have much to do with our upbringing as Jewish people in a small anti-Semitic town where my immigrant parents moved from Eastern Europe in the 1920s. My parents didn't want us socializing with non-Jewish people, whom they said would never accept us. I think we all felt like outsiders. Even as a kid I didn't think people liked me much and I still feel that way. One of my friends says that I put up a shield that tells people to lay off. It might be true, but whatever I do, the end result is that social events are agony and I feel awful about myself when I go, and just as awful when I decide to avoid them.

"Maybe I'm an anxious person to begin with. I worry a lot, and I always seem to think the worst is going to happen. For several years in my mid-forties I was on medication for generalized anxiety that was so bad I went into therapy. It didn't help much and neither did the medication. Gradually, as I divorced and eliminated many of my responsibilities, I became a lot less anxious. I sleep well now and I'm productive, but until my early fifties I guess you could say I was pretty anxious.

"I also notice that I obsess about people and the slights I imagine they've done to me. I feel absolute blinding hatred for anyone who's critical of me. If I play golf and someone says something mean or obnoxious about the way I play, or look, or the clothes I wear, I think about it for weeks. It's all I can do not to wrap my nine iron around their head. Who knows where this hostility comes from? I don't, and I've been through enough therapy that I should know by now.

"I've concluded that life isn't a bowl of cherries and that Forrest Gump was wrong. It's tough, and you have to hang on tight or you'll just fly off into space and never be seen again. I guess I feel that way often – that I'm invisible and when I die, no one will even remember me. I don't know. You work hard, you try your best, you do the things no one else can do, and still you end up feeling unloved and unwanted. It's like a knife in your heart where your feelings live. The anxiety mystifies me. What am I anxious about? I don't know. Maybe magically something will happen and I won't care what other people say or think about me. Maybe I'll get it right when I'm 70. Two years to go. It can't happen soon enough." – HBF.

11.5 SUMMARY

This chapter discusses the serious problem of anxiety in older adults. Diagnostic suggestions are made to distinguish anxiety brought on by both physical and social causes. A case study using case management and a personal story explore older adult anxiety and the very real pain it causes older adults.

11.6 QUESTIONS FROM THE CHAPTER

1. Older men seem to be less anxious than older women. Doesn't that prove that men get smarter about life as they age than women?
2. The personal story sounds like the guy is lonely and anxious but still hopeful. Isn't a positive way of looking at life and being optimistic the best cure for anxiety? What could he possibly get out of treatment that he doesn't already know?
3. I'd worry a lot too if I were facing serious illness and the death of friends and spouses. Isn't it natural for older people to worry a lot?
4. Don't you think people worry more when they can't control their lives? Isn't that true of older people, too?
5. Doesn't it make sense that people who worry a lot probably use substances to help them stop worrying so much? Isn't that true of older adults who I hear drink a lot and use a lot of anti-anxiety drugs to calm themselves down? Shouldn't we be doing more to help older folks stop abusing substances?

REFERENCES

Aarts, P., & Op den Velde, W. (1996). Prior traumatization and the process of aging. In B. A. van der Kolk, A. C. McFarlane, & L. Weisath (Eds.), *Traumatic Stress: The Effects of Overwhelming Experience on Mind, Body and Society* pp. 359–377. New York: Guilford Press.

Beck, J. G., & Stanley, M. A. (1997). Anxiety disorders in the elderly: The emerging role of behavior therapy. *Behavior Therapy, 28,* 83–100.

Beekman, A. T., Bremmer, M. A., Deeg, D. J. H., et al. (1998). Anxiety disorders in later life: A report from the longitudinal aging study Amsterdam. *International Journal of Geriatric Psychiatry, 12*(10), 717–726.

Himmelfarb, S., & Murrell, S. A. (1984). Prevalence and Correlates of *Anxiety* Symptoms in Older Adults. *Journal of Psychology, 116*, 159–167.

Kogan, J. N., Edelstein, B. A., & McKee, D. R. (2000). Assessment of anxiety in older adults: Current status. *Journal of Anxiety Disorders, 14*(2), 109–132.

Lang, A. J., & Stein, M. B. (2001). Anxiety disorders. *Geriatrics, 56*(5), 24–30.

McFarlane, A. C., & Yehuda, R. (1996). Resilience, vulnerability, and the course of post-traumatic reactions. In B. A. van der Kolk, A. C. McFarlane, & L. Weisath (Eds.), *Traumatic Stress: The Effects of Overwhelming Experience on Mind, Body and Society,* pp. 155–181. New York: Guilford Press.

Pingitore, D., & Sansone, R. A. (1998, October 15). Using DSM-IV primary care version: A guide to psychiatric diagnosis in primary care. *American Family Physician, 58*(6).

Smith, S. S., Sherrill, K. A., & Celenda, C. C. (1995). Anxious elders deserve careful diagnosing and the most appropriate interventions. *Brown University Long-Term Care Letter, 7*(10), 5–7.

Stanley, M. A., & Novy, D. M. (2000). Cognitive-behavior therapy for generalized anxiety in late life: An evaluative overview. *Journal of Anxiety Disorders, 14*(2), 191–207.

Surgeon General's Report. (1999) Older Adults and Mental Health (Anxiety Disorders, Chapter 5) http://www.surgeongeneral.gov/library/mentalhealth/chapter5/sec5.html#anxiety

Wagner, K. D., & Lorion, R. P. (1984). Correlates of death anxiety in elderly persons. *Journal of Clinical Psychology, 40*, 1235–1241.

Chapter twelve

Evidence-Based Practice with Older Adults Who Abuse Substances

12.1 INTRODUCTION

This chapter discusses older adult substance abuse, best evidence for treatment effectiveness, and includes a case study showing the use of EBP with an alcohol-abusing older adult. Many of the myths about older adults and substance abuse are also discussed and dispelled.

Blow (2007) believes that the misuse of alcohol and prescription drugs among adults 60 and older is one of the fastest growing health problems facing the USA. He argues that "even as the number of older adults suffering from these disorders climbs, the situation remains underestimated, under-identified, under-diagnosed, and under-treated" (p. 1). Blow notes that substance abuse often has a serious impact on the health of older adults and writes:

> The reality is that misuse and abuse of alcohol and other drugs take a greater toll on affected older adults than on younger adults. In addition to the psychosocial issues that are unique to older adults, aging also ushers in biomedical changes that influence the effects that alcohol and drugs have on the body. Alcohol abuse, for example, may accelerate the normal decline in physiological functioning that occurs with age. In addition, alcohol may elevate older adults' already high risk for injury, illness, and socioeconomic decline. (p. 2)

Sorocco and Ferrell (2006) suggest that there are two widely-held myths regarding alcohol use among older adults: (1) that it is an infrequent problem; and (2) that when older adults have drinking problems, treatment success is limited. In fact, according to the authors, "alcohol abuse among older adults is one of the fastest-growing health problems facing this country and even a one-time brief encounter of 15 min or less can reduce nondependent problem drinking by more than 20%" (p. 454).

According to the National Institute for Alcohol Abuse and Alcoholism (NIAAA, 1997) roughly 49% of all adults aged 60 years and older drink alcohol. Among those aged 60–64 responding to a national survey on drug use and health sponsored by SAMHSA (2004), 50% used alcohol in the past month, and 35% of individuals aged 65 or older used alcohol in the past month. Seven percent of adults aged 65 or older reported binge drinking, and 1.8% reported heavy drinking. Binge drinking is defined as five or more drinks on the same occasion on at least one day in the past month. Heavy drinking is defined as five or more drinks on the same occasion on each of five or more days in the past 30 days.

Adams et al. (1996) report that among community-dwelling, non-institutionalized older adults, 2–15% have been shown to exhibit symptoms consistent with alcoholism. The estimated use of alcohol increases significantly for primary care patients where 10–15% of the older adult patients met the criteria for problem drinking. Oslin (2004) considers drinking problematic if it leads to physical, social, or emotional problems. Sorocco and Ferrell (2006) estimate that "a minimum of one in every 10 older patients in a medical setting most likely suffers from an alcohol problem" (p. 454) and predict that by 2030, when the population of older adults will exceed 70 million, that the problem will be much greater than it is at present.

Although the data on older adult alcohol abuse suggests a growing problem, Sorocco and Ferrell (2006) note how difficult it is to pinpoint alcohol abuse in this population. Even though a third of all heavy drinkers begin their patterns of alcohol abuse after age 60 (Barrick and Connors, 2002), many symptoms of problem drinking "mimic" physical problems common to this age group, including depression and dementia. Because of stereotypes of older adults by health care professionals, doctors are often unlikely to screen for alcohol problems, particularly in women and patients who are well educated or affluent. Because alcohol abuse is still considered a morally offensive problem, clients and their families may feel "ashamed" to discuss the problem with their physicians. As a result of stereotypes that older adults want to be left alone or have few opportunities for happiness, some clinicians believe that drinking is one of the few pleasures left to older men and women.

In a large-scale meta-analysis of errors made in diagnosing substance abuse by physicians, Banta and Montgomery (2007) found that regardless of the specialty, the elderly are less likely to receive substance abuse treatment. The authors suggest that "Substance abuse among older adults may be underestimated due to perceived stigma of abuse and the fact that its symptoms are similar to dementia and depression" (p. 587). The authors indicate that increased detection of older adult substance abuse may be found by using the screening tools for substance abuse developed and tested in primary care settings suggested by Nemes et al. (2004), which can be administered verbally, as pencil and paper tests, or as computerized screening instruments.

An additional finding of note in the study of the diagnosis of substance abuse by physicians is that African-Americans and Hispanics older adults

> were less likely than whites to have a substance abuse diagnosis which further corroborates national studies which found that African-Americans and Hispanics were more likely than Whites to have no access or delayed access to substance abuse and mental health treatment. Additionally African-American older adults were less likely than White adults to receive mental health counseling during outpatient visits. Potential under-treatment is of concern since ethnic minorities tend to experience worse health and social consequences from drinking. (Nemes et al., 2004, p. 587)

There are a number of negative consequences of older adult problem drinking. Oslin (2004) reports that even small to moderate amounts of alcohol can increase the risk of hypertension, sleep problems, and malnutrition. The risk of falls increases with alcohol consumption and significantly increases when 14 or more drinks are consumed per week (Mukamal et al., 2004). Older adults are quite vulnerable to the negative effects of alcohol because they take more medications than younger people and are therefore at risk for drug or alcohol interactions. Because of slower metabolic and clearance mechanisms, older people are also more likely to experience adverse drug and alcohol interactions. Slower metabolic and clearance mechanisms delay their resolution. Onder et al. (2002) studied alcohol consumption among a population of older adults 65–80 years of age and found that even moderate consumption of alcohol increased the risk of an adverse drug reaction by 24%.

12.2 DIAGNOSTIC MARKERS OF SUBSTANCE ABUSE

All adults aged 60 years or older should be screened for alcohol-use problems at their annual physical exam (SAMHSA, 1998). Patients younger than 60 should be screened if they are experiencing major life changes. Retirement issues, loss of work, divorce and empty nest syndrome are a few major life issues that can affect people in their fifties. Younger individuals exhibiting physical symptoms suggestive of an alcohol-use disorder should also be evaluated for alcohol use, particularly when blood pressure has increased or other signs of cardiovascular problems seem to have a sudden onset.

Sorocco and Ferrell (2006) report that certain clinical symptoms may suggest alcohol problems, including the following:

> [T]herapy that is not working for a normally treatable medical illness (e.g., hypertension); insomnia or chronic fatigue related to poor sleep; diarrhea, urinary incontinence, weight loss or malnutrition; complaints of anxiety (related to undiagnosed withdrawal), with frequent use of or request for anxiolytics, sedatives, or hypnotics; unexplained postoperative agitation, anxiety, confusion, or new-onset seizures (also suggestive of withdrawal). Among older adults, there also are several cognitive signs of alcohol abuse such as consistent intellectual deficits on tasks that involve frontal lobe activity, perceptual-motor deficits, and memory deficits—particularly, short-term memory impairment (SAMHSA, 1998). Most interesting, verbal and arithmetic skills generally remain unimpaired among older adults with alcohol-use problems. (p. 456)

The DSM-IV uses the following diagnostic markers to determine whether substance use is abusive. A dysfunctional use of substances causing impairment or distress within a twelve-month period as determined by one of the following:

1. frequent use of substances that interfere with functioning and the fulfillment of responsibilities at home, work, school, etc.;
2. use of substances that impair functioning in dangerous situations such as driving or the use of machines;
3. use of substances that may lead to arrest for unlawful behaviors; and
4. substance use that seriously interferes with relations, marriage, child-rearing and other interpersonal responsibilities (APA, 1994, p. 182).

Substance abuse may also lead to slurred speech, lack of coordination, unsteady gait, memory loss, fatigue and depression, feelings of euphoria, and lack of social inhibitions (APA, 1994, p. 197).

12.2.1 Short tests

Miller (2001) reports that two simple questions asked of substance abusers have an 80% chance of diagnosing substance abuse: "In the past year, have you ever drunk or used drugs more than you meant to?" and, "Have you felt you wanted or needed to cut down on your drinking or drug abuse in the past year?" Miller reports that this simple approach has been found to be an effective diagnostic tool in three controlled studies using random samples and laboratory tests for alcohol and drugs in the blood stream following interviews.

Stewart and Richards (2000) and Bisson et al. (1999) suggest that four questions from the CAGE questionnaire are predictive of alcohol abuse. CAGE is an acronym for Cut, Annoyed, Guilty, and Eye-Opener (see the questions below). Since many people deny their alcoholism, asking questions in an open, direct and non-judgmental way may elicit the best results. The four questions are:

1. **Cut:** Have you ever felt you should cut down on your drinking?
2. **Annoyed:** Have people annoyed you by criticizing your drinking?
3. **Guilty:** Have you ever felt guilty about your drinking?
4. **Eye-Opener:** Have you ever had a drink first thing in the morning (eye-opener) to steady your nerves or get rid of a hangover? (Bisson et al., 1999, p. 717).

Stewart and Richards (2000) write, "A patient who answers yes to two or more of these questions probably abuses alcohol; a patient who answers yes to one question should be screened further" (p. 56). Not everyone is certain that the CAGE instrument, developed in the late 1970s to distinguish heavy from moderate drinkers, is an effective diagnostic tool. Bisson et al. (1999) write: "If the CAGE had any utility as an instrument informing on the prevalence or incidence of heavy drinking within the population, it would have discriminated between heavy and non-heavy drinkers. Our results show that this is not the case" (p. 720). The authors think the instrument is less than accurate because many people have a new awareness of alcoholism and have tried to do something to limit their alcohol use. Additionally, the instrument asks about last year's alcohol consumption. Since subjects may have changed their alcohol-related behavior, the answers may be misleading. Alcohol consumption has also decreased somewhat nationally. Consequently, a direct series of questions answered truthfully may fail to distinguish those who drink heavily from those who drink moderately because the responses from both groups may tend to be the same. This finding supports the concern that short questions may not be accurate in diagnosing substance abuse and that diagnosis requires an in-depth social, emotional, and medical history in which the guidelines of the DSM-IV provide direction for the types of historical and medical issues one might look for. Perhaps this lack of an in-depth history is why Backer and Walton-Moss (2001) found that fully 20–25% of all patients with alcohol-related problems were treated medically for the symptoms of alcoholism rather than for the condition itself, and that a diagnosis of alcohol abuse was never made in almost one-fourth of all alcoholics seen for medical treatment.

Another instrument to assess alcohol use is The MAST-G (Blow et al., 1992), which was specifically developed for use with older adults. Questions on the instrument are all geared to life situations among older adults that may have acted as catalysts for excessive alcohol use. An example is item #20, which asks if drinking has increased after experiencing a loss. The MAST-G consists of 24 yes or no items which may take some older adults a long time to complete. The 10-item version Short Michigan Alcoholism Screening Test-Geriatric (SMAST-G) is also available. Two or more yes responses on the SMAST-G indicate an alcohol problem (Blow, 1991).

12.2.2 Psychosocial variables

A serious problem caused by the lack of a complete psychosocial history is that services are often withheld from elderly patients with substance abuse problems. Pennington et al. (2000) report that older patients referred to a psychiatric service with a diagnosis of alcohol abuse failed to receive the clinical assessment recommended by the American Geriatric Society. Rather than being treated for alcoholism as a primary problem, most elderly clients abusing alcohol (four out of five) were treated for depression or associated medical problems. The authors believe that the reason elderly patients are not adequately screened for alcohol abuse is that "some health professionals harbor a misguided belief that older people should not be advised to give up established habits, or they may be embarrassed to ask older patients personal questions about alcohol use" (Pennington et al., 2000, p. 183), even though those behaviors may be self-injurious and possibly dangerous to others.

Writing about female alcohol abuse, Backer and Walton-Moss (2001) report that, "Unlike men, women commonly seek help for alcoholism from primary care clinicians. Further, the development and progression of alcoholism is different in women than in men. Women with alcohol problems have higher rates of dual diagnoses, childhood sexual abuse, panic and phobia disorders, eating disorders, posttraumatic stress disorder, and victimization. Early diagnosis, brief interventions, and referral are critical to the treatment of alcoholism in women" (p. 13). The authors suggest the following diagnostic markers for female alcoholics: since women metabolize alcohol differently than men, women tend to show signs of becoming intoxicated at a later age than men (26.5 versus 22.7), experience their fist signs of a recognition of alcohol abuse later (27.5 versus 25), and lose control over their drinking later in life (29.8 versus 27.2). The mortality rate for female alcoholics is 50–100% higher than it is for men. Liver damage occurs in women in a shorter period of time and with lower amounts of intake of alcohol. Backer and Walton-Moss (2001) report that "female alcoholics have a higher mortality rate from alcoholism than men from suicide, alcohol-related accidents, circulatory disorders, and cirrhosis of the liver" (p. 15). Use of alcohol by women in adolescence is almost equal to that of male adolescents, suggesting equal rates of alcohol abuse in older men and women. Backer and Walton-Moss (2001) suggest that while men use alcohol to socialize, women use it to cope with negative moods and are likely to use alcohol in response to specific stressors in their lives.

12.2.3 Early abuse of substances

Grant and Dawson (1997) report that heavy use of alcohol in adolescence is a very strong predictor of life-long alcoholism and indicate that 40% of young adults aged 18–29 years who began drinking before the age of 15 were considered to be alcohol-dependent as compared to roughly 10% who began drinking after the age of 19. While Kuperman et al. (2001) suggest that early substance abuse is often predictive of alcoholism, the reasons for alcohol use offered by the authors (family and peer problems) are evident in adolescents who do not develop alcohol and drug problems and are common behaviors in a society where many adolescents are rebellious and partake in risky behaviors. Nonetheless, the wise clinician will be aware that early and frequent use of alcohol has a fairly high probability of leading to prolonged alcohol use and will understand its importance when screening clients.

12.2.4 Related medical problems

Stewart and Richards (2000) conclude that a number of older adult medical problems may have their origins in heavy alcohol and drug use. Head injuries and spinal separations as a result of accidents may have been caused by substance abuse. Because heavy drinkers often fail to eat, they may have nutritional deficiencies that result in psychotic-like symptoms including abnormal eye movements, disorganization, and forgetfulness. Stomach disorders, liver damage, and severe heartburn may have their origins in heavy drinking because alcohol destroys the stomach's mucosal lining. Fifteen percent of all heavy drinkers develop cirrhosis of the liver and many develop pancreatitis. Weight loss, pneumonia, muscle loss because of malnutrition, and oral cancer have all been associated with heavy drinking. Stewart and Richards (2000) indicate that substance abusers are poor candidates for surgery. Anesthesia and pain medication can delay alcohol withdrawal for up to five days postoperatively. "Withdrawal symptoms can cause agitation and uncooperativeness and can mask signs and symptoms of other postoperative complications. Patients who abuse alcohol are at a higher risk for postoperative complications such as excessive bleeding, infection, heart failure, and pneumonia" (Stewart and Richards, 2000, p. 58).

Stewart and Richards (2000, p. 59) provide the following blood alcohol levels as measures of the impact of alcohol in screening for abuse:

- 0.05% (equivalent to one or two drinks in an average-sized person) – impaired judgment, reduced alertness, toss of inhibitions, euphoria.
- 0.10% – slower reaction times, decreased caution in risk taking behavior, impaired fine-motor control. Legal evidence of intoxication in most states starts at 0.10%.
- 0.15% – significant and consistent losses in reaction times.
- 0.20% – function of entire motor area of brain measurably depressed, causing staggering. The individual may be easily angered or emotional.
- 0.25% – severe sensory and motor impairment.
- 0.30% – confusion, stupor.
- 0.35% – surgical anesthesia.
- 0.40% – respiratory depression, lethal in about half of the population.
- 0.50% – death from respiratory depression (p. 59).

12.3 BEST EVIDENCE FOR THE TREATMENT OF SUBSTANCE ABUSE

12.3.1 Short-term treatment

Herman (2000) believes that individual psychotherapy can be helpful in treating substance abusers and suggests five situations where therapy would be indicated:

1. as an appropriate introduction to treatment;
2. as a way of helping mildly or moderately dependent drug abusers;
3. when there are clear signs of emotional problems such as severe depression since these problems will interfere with the substance abuse treatment;
4. when clients progressing in 12-step programs begin to experience emerging feelings of guilt, shame, and grief; and
5. when a client's disturbed interpersonal functioning continues after a long period of sustained abstinence and therapy might help prevent a relapse.

One of the most frequently discussed treatment approaches to addiction in the literature is brief counseling. Bien et al. (1993) reviewed 32 studies of brief interventions with alcohol abusers and found that, on the average, brief counseling reduced alcohol use by 30%. However, in a study of brief intervention with alcohol abusers, Chang et al. (1999) found that both the treatment and control groups significantly reduced their alcohol use. The difference between the two groups in the reduction of their alcohol abuse was minimal. In a study of 175 Mexican-Americans who were abusing alcohol, Burge et al. (1997) report that treated and untreated groups improved significantly over time, raising questions about the efficacy of treatment versus natural recovery. In an evaluation of a larger report by *Consumer Reports* on the effectiveness of psychotherapy, Seligman (1995) notes that "Alcoholics Anonymous (AA) did especially well … significantly bettering mental health professionals [in the treatment of alcohol and drug related problems]" (p. 10).

Bien et al. (1993) found that two or three 10–15 minute counseling sessions are often as effective as more extensive interventions with older alcohol abusers. The sessions include motivation-for-change strategies, education, assessment of the severity of the problem, direct feedback, contracting and goal setting, behavioral modification techniques, and the use of written materials such as self-help manuals. According to

Fleming et al. (1997), brief interventions have been shown to be effective in reducing alcohol consumption, binge drinking, and the frequency of excessive drinking in problem drinkers. Completion rates using brief interventions are better for elder-specific alcohol programs than for mixed-age programs (Atkinson, 1995), and late-onset alcoholics are more likely to complete treatment and have somewhat better outcomes using brief interventions (Liberto and Oslin, 1995).

Miller and Sanchez (1993) summarize the key components of brief intervention using the acronym FRAMES: feedback, responsibility, advice, menu of strategies, empathy, and self-efficacy.

1. **Feedback:** includes an assessment with feedback to the client regarding the client's risk for alcohol problems, his or her reasons for drinking, the role of alcohol in the patient's life, and the consequences of drinking.
2. **Responsibility:** includes strategies to help clients understand the need to remain healthy, independent, and financially secure. This is particularly important when working with older clients and clients with health problems and disabilities.
3. **Advice:** includes direct feedback and suggestions to clients to help them cope with their drinking problems and with other life situations that may contribute to alcohol abuse.
4. **Menu:** includes a list of strategies to reduce drinking and help cope with such high-risk situations as loneliness, boredom, family problems, and lack of social opportunities.
5. **Empathy:** Bien et al. (1993)strongly emphasize the need for a warm, empathic, and understanding style of treatment. Miller and Rollnick (1991) found that an empathic counseling style produced a 77% reduction in client drinking as compared to a 55% reduction when a confrontational approach was used.
6. **Self-efficacy:** this includes strategies to help clients rely on their inner resources to make changes in their drinking behavior. Inner resources may include positive points of view about themselves, helping others, staying busy, and good problem-solving coping skills.

Some additional aspects of brief interventions suggested by Menninger (2002) include drinking agreements in the form of agreed-upon drinking limits that are signed by the patient and the practitioner, ongoing follow-up and support, and appropriate timing of the intervention with the patient's readiness to change. Completion rates for elder-specific alcohol treatment programs are modestly better than for mixed-age programs (Atkinson, 1995). Late-onset alcoholics are also more likely to complete treatment and have somewhat better outcomes (Liberto and Oslin, 1995). Alcoholics Anonymous may be helpful, particularly AA groups that are specifically oriented toward the elderly.

Babor and Higgins-Biddle (2000) discuss the use of brief interventions with people involved in "risky drinking" who are not as yet classified as alcohol dependent. Brief interventions are usually limited to three to five sessions of counseling and education. The intent of brief interventions is to prevent the onset of more serious alcohol-related problems. According to Babor and Higgins-Biddle (2000), "[m]ost programs are instructional and motivational, designed to address the specific behavior of drinking with information, feedback, health education, skill-building, and practical advice, rather than with psychotherapy or other specialized treatment techniques" (p. 676). Higgins-Biddle et al. (1997) analyzed 14 random studies of brief interventions that included more than 20,000 risky drinkers. They report a net reduction in drinking of 21% for males and 8% for females. To improve the effectiveness of short-term interventions, Babor and Higgins-Biddle (2000) encourage the use of early identification of problem drinking, life-health monitoring by health and mental health professionals, and risk counseling that includes screening and brief intervention to inform and motivate potential alcohol abusers of the risk of serious alcohol dependence and to help change their alcohol use. This approach requires a high degree of cooperation among health and education personnel who are often loathe to identify older adults as having "at risk" alcohol problems because they fear that doing so will exacerbate the problem through public identification and often believe, sometimes incorrectly, that more moderate drinking will take place as the older adult recognizes the problem and deals with it.

Fleming and Manwell (1998) report that people with alcohol-related problems often receive counseling from primary care physicians or nursing staff in five or fewer standard office visits. The counseling consists of objective information about the negative impact of alcohol use as well as practical advice regarding ways of reducing alcohol dependence and the availability of community resources. Gentilello et al. (1995) report that 25-40% of the trauma patients seen in emergency rooms may be alcohol dependent. The authors found that a single motivational interview, at or near the time of discharge, reduced drinking levels and re-admission for trauma during six months of follow up. Monti et al. (1999) conducted a similar study with 18- and 19-year-olds admitted to an emergency room with alcohol-related injuries. After six months, all participants had decreased their alcohol consumption; however, "the group receiving brief intervention had a significantly lower incidence of drinking and driving, traffic violations, alcohol-related injuries, and alcohol-related problems" (Monti et al., 1999, p. 3).

Cognitive-behavioral approaches are another form of short-term treatment where clients are taught to overcome addiction to alcohol. In cognitive-behavioral approaches, the client is taught to identify the situations that lead to drinking and to re-think those situations in more positive and rational ways. Perceptions of stressful events are important and clients are taught to logically rethink the situation and to reduce the stressful impact that may bring with it alcohol abuse. The Gerontology Alcohol Project (GAP) (Dupree et al., 1984) is an example of the cognitive-behavioral approach used to treat alcohol-related problems. GAP uses a day-treatment approach with older alcoholics and emphasizes self-management, skill acquisition, and social support. At a 12-month follow up, 75% of the participants in GAP maintained their drinking reduction goals and increased the size of their social support network. Rice et al. (1993) found that cognitive-behavioral therapy was significantly more effective for adults ages 50 and over than relationship enhancement and vocational-enhancement therapies in reducing alcohol dependence.

Lu and McGuire (2002) studied the effectiveness of out-patient treatment with substance abusing clients and came to the following conclusions:

1. the more severe the drug use problem before treatment was initi-ated, the less likely clients were to discontinue drug use during treatment when compared to other users;
2. clients reporting no substance abuse three months before admis-sion were more likely to maintain abstinence than those who reported abstinence only in the past one month;
3. heroin user were highly unlikely to sustain abstinence during treatment while marijuana users were less likely to sustain absti-nence during treatment than alcohol users;
4. clients with "psychiatric problems" were more likely to use drugs during treatment than clients without psychiatric problems;
5. clients with legal problems related to their substance abuse had reduced chances of improving during the treatment;
6. clients who had multiple prior treatments for substance abuse were less likely to remain abstinent during and after treatment;

7. more educated clients were more likely to sustain abstinence after treatment; and

8. clients treated in urban agencies were less likely to maintain abstinence than those treated in rural agencies.

12.3.2 Longer-term treatments

Connors et al. (2002) report that treatment attrition among substance abusers is such a pervasive problem in programs offering treatment services that it affects our ability to determine treatment effectiveness. Baekeland and Lundwall (1975) report dropout rates for inpatient treatment programs of 28% and that 75% of the outpatient alcoholic patients in their study dropped out of treatment before their fourth session. Leigh et al. (1984) report that of 172 alcoholic outpatients studied, 15% failed to attend their initial appointment, 28% attended only a session or two, and 19% attended only three to five times. In studying 117 alcoholism clinic admissions, Rees (1986) found that 35% of the clients failed to return after their initial visit and that another 18% terminated treatment within 30 days.

To try and reduce the amount of attrition in alcohol treatment programs, Connors et al. (2002) randomly assigned 126 clients entering an alcohol treatment program to one of three groups to prepare them for the treatment program: a role induction (RI) session, a motivational interview (MI) session, or a no-preparatory session control group (CG). They found that clients assigned to the motivational interview, "attended more treatment sessions and had fewer heavy drinking days during and 12 months after treatment relative to control group" (p. 1161). Clients assigned to the motivational interview also were abstinent more days during treatment and in the first three months following treatment than the control group but the difference, unfortunately, did not last for the remaining nine months of follow up. Clients assigned to the role induction group did no better than the control group in any of the variables studied.

In describing the motivational interview, Connors et al. (2002, p. 1164) indicate that it consists of the following:

(a) eliciting self-motivational statements;

(b) reflective, empathic listening;

(c) inquiring about the client's feelings, ideas, concerns, and plans;

(d) affirming the client in a way that acknowledges the client's serious consideration of and steps toward change;

(e) deflecting resistance in a manner that takes into account the link between therapist behavior and client resistance;
(f) reframing client statements as appropriate; and
(g) summarizing.

Kirchner et al. (2000) considered the factors related to entry into alcohol treatment programs following a diagnosis of alcoholism. They found that many patients who might benefit from treatment were not referred by their medical providers because of a belief that treatment wasn't effective, even though a number of "well-designed and methodologically sound studies have repeatedly shown that treatment for alcohol-related disorders can be effective not only for reducing the consumption of alcohol but also for improving the patient's overall level of functioning" (p. 339). The authors also report that improved detection of alcoholism, the first step in the provision of services, is negatively influenced by a number of factors, including older age, non-Caucasian ethnicity, the severity of the alcohol use, lower socioeconomic status, and male gender. Drug and alcohol use to self-medicate for psychiatric disorders is also a key predictor of detection as are alcohol-related medical problems such as liver disorders, high blood pressure and adult-onset diabetes. Herman (2000) reports that the reasons substance abusers enter treatment are usually external in nature and include legal problems with drug use (license suspension because of drunk driving), marital problems, work-related problems, medical complications caused by drug and alcohol abuse, problems with depression and anxiety that lead to self-medicating with alcohol and drugs, and referral by mental health professionals (a major reason women enter treatment programs).

12.3.3 Treatment strategies

Herman (2000) believes that the primary strategy in the treatment of substance abuse is to initially achieve abstinence. Once abstinence is achieved, the older adult substance abuser can begin to address relationship problems that might interfere with social and emotional functioning. Herman (2000) believes that the key to treatment is to match the client with the type of treatment most likely to help. He suggests that the following phases exist in the treatment of substance abuse:

Phase 1: Abstinence.
Phase 2: Teaching the client coping skills to help prevent a relapse through cognitive-behavioral techniques that help clients manage stressful situations likely to trigger substance abuse. These

techniques may include recognizing internal cues that lead to substance abuse (depression and feelings of low self-esteem); managing external cues (responses by others and inter-personal relationships); avoiding peers who are likely to continue to abuse substances and encourage the client to do the same; and, alternative behaviors that help the client avoid drug use (substituting substance abuse with exercise, or attending social events where alcohol isn't available).

Phase 3: Since the underlying problems that contribute to substance abuse are often deeply internalized feeling of low self-worth, depression, and self-loathing, therapy should help the client deal with internalized pathologies that are likely to lead to relapse. The therapies that seem most effective in doing this are cognitive-behavioral therapies, the strengths approach, and affective therapies including Gestalt therapy (Herman, 2000). Herman also suggests the use of psychodynamic therapy but research evidence of the effectiveness of this form of treatment with substance abuse is not overly positive.

In a review of 30 years of research, the National Institute on Drug Abuse (1999) reports that the following are necessary elements of effective treatment of substance abuse:

1. correctly matching the client with the appropriate treatment approach;
2. providing treatment that is readily available and may be useful in treating other psychosocial problems experienced by the client;
3. the treatment plan is comprehensive, the length of treatment is adequate, and the treatment plan is regularly reviewed;
4. medication is available if needed;
5. treatment is more than helpful with detoxification;
6. treatment is useful for involuntary clients;
7. there is frequent monitoring of the patient's substance use;
8. there is an assessment made of HIV/AIDS and other potential diseases; and
9. treatment is offered again even after multiple relapses. (Found in Lennox and Mansfield, 2001, p. 169)

Other factors found to provide best evidence of treatment effectiveness include the following: Dahlgren and Willander (1989) compared women-only and mixed-gender treatment groups. Clients in the women-only group remained in treatment longer, had higher completion rates, and had improved bio-psychosocial rates as compared to women who were in mixed-gender programs. Burtscheidt et al. (2002) studied the treatment effects of long-term treatment by comparing nonspecific supportive therapy with two different forms of behavioral therapy (coping skills training and cognitive behavioral therapy). One-hundred-and-twenty patients were randomly assigned to each of the three therapy approaches and were seen in treatment for 26 weeks with a follow-up period of two years. Patients receiving behavioral therapy showed consistently higher abstinence rates. Differences in treatment effectiveness between the two behavioral therapies could not be established. The study also established that cognitively impaired and severely personality disordered clients experienced less benefit from any of the therapies than other clients. The authors conclude that behavioral treatment had the best long-term effects and met high client acceptance, but that a great deal still needs to be done to develop even more effective behavioral therapies for clients who abuse substances.

12.3.4 Natural recovery

Granfield and Cloud (1996) estimate that as many as 90% of all problem drinkers never enter treatment and that many end their abuse of alcohol without any form of treatment (Hingson et al., 1980; Roizen et al., 1978; Stall and Biernacki 1989). Sobell et al. (1993) report that 82% of the alcoholics they studied who terminated their addiction did so by using natural recovery methods that excluded the use of professional treatment. As an example of natural recovery techniques, Granfield and Cloud (1996) report that most ex-smokers discontinue their tobacco use without treatment (Peele 1989) while many addicted substance abusers "mature-out" of a variety of addictions including heavy drinking and narcotics use (Snow 1973; Winick 1962). Biernacki (1986) reports that people who use natural methods to end their drug addictions utilize a range of strategies, including discontinuing their relationships with drug users, avoiding drug-using environments (Stall and Biernacki, 1986), having new goals and interest in their lives (Peele, 1989), and using friends and family to provide a support network (Biernacki, 1986). Trice and Roman (1970) indicate that self-help groups with substance abusing clients are particularly helpful because they develop and continue a support network that assists clients in maintaining abstinence and other changed behaviors.

Granfield and Cloud (1996) studied middle class alcoholics who used natural recovery alone without professional help or the use of self-help groups. Many of the participants in their study felt that some self-help groups were overly religious while others stressed a belief that alcohol abuse is a disease that suggested a lifetime struggle. The subjects in the study believed that some self-help groups encouraged dependence on the group and that associating with other alcoholics would probably complicate recovery. In summarizing their findings, Granfield and Cloud (1996) report that:

> Many [research subjects] expressed strong opposition to the suggestion that they were powerless over their addictions. Such an ideology, they explained, not only was counterproductive but was also extremely demeaning. These respondents saw themselves as efficacious people who often prided themselves on their past accomplishments. They viewed themselves as being individualists and strong-willed. One respondent, for instance, explained that "such programs encourage powerlessness" and that she would rather "trust her own instincts than the instincts of others." (p. 51)

Waldorf et al. (1991) found that many addicted people with jobs, strong family ties, and other close emotional supports were able to "walk away" from their very heavy use of cocaine. Granfield and Cloud (1996) indicate that many of the respondents in their study had a great deal to lose if they continued their substance abuse and that their sample consisted of people with stable lives, good jobs, supportive families and friends, college educations, and other social supports that gave them motivation to "alter" their drug-using behaviors.

12.3.5 Self-help groups

Humphreys (1998) studied the effectiveness of self-help groups with substance abusers by comparing two groups: one receiving in-patient care for substance abuse, and the other attending self-help groups for substance abuse. At the conclusion of the study, the average participant assigned to a self-help group (AA) had used $8,840 in alcohol-related health care resources as compared to $10,040 for the inpatient treatment participants. In a follow-up study, Humphreys (1998) compared outpatient services to self-help groups for the treatment of substance abuse. The clients in the self-help group had decreased alcohol consumption by 70% over three years and consumed 45% less health care services (about $1,800 less per person). Humphreys (1998) believes that "From a cost-conscious point of view, self-help groups should be the first option evaluated when an addicted individual makes initial contact with professional services (e.g., in a primary care appointment or a clinical assessment at a substance abuse agency or employee assistance program)" (p. 16). Additional data on the effectiveness of self-help groups may be found in Chapter 14.

CASE STUDY: EVIDENCE-BASED PRACTICE WITH AN OLDER ADULT SUBSTANCE ABUSER

Wanda Anderson is a 69-year-old single woman who lives in an upscale retirement community in Arizona. Wanda was a successful real estate agent in Kansas City for many years and decided to sell her home at the height of the real estate boom in 2005 and buy a nice home in a retirement community. Wanda moved to her new home in January, 2006, and was ecstatic to find 70-degree weather and many activities in which she could not participate in Kansas City during the winter. However, her first summer in Arizona was a shock with temperatures hovering in the 100–115-degree range for almost six months without stop. During the hot months, Wanda found that many people left for cooler climates and that her fantasy of many close friends to accompany her on "adventures" evaporated. She was alone and there were few people with whom she could socialize. The community had a bar with a happy hour where cheap drinks and food were available, and Wanda began going every afternoon around 4:00 p.m. and staying increasingly later.

Wanda had never been much of a drinker, but after going to happy hour almost every day for a year, she found that thinking about having a drink gave her great joy. She couldn't wait until 4:00 p.m. to begin. The bar was only a short distance from her home and she either walked or drove her electric golf cart. Driving home from the bar in her cart about 11:00 p.m. when most people were asleep, Wanda missed a turn and her cart went down a steep embankment. She and a friend were to go walking at 6:00 a.m. the next morning before the summer heat became unbearable. Not finding Wanda at home, the friend contacted security and, after a long search, they found Wanda unconscious at the bottom of the embankment with the cart lying partially on top of her.

Wanda was rushed to the hospital and, thankfully, her injuries were limited to a broken arm and a number of cuts and bruises. More serious was the fact that her blood pressure and blood sugars were extremely high. Wondering about the possibility of alcohol abuse, the attending physician checked her alcohol level and even after many hours without alcohol, found it high. He also found evidence of the onset of liver damage and possible heart problems.

When Wanda was awake, the doctor and a social worker interviewed her about her accident and her alcohol consumption. At first she was very defensive, but after a few minutes of avoiding their questions she admitted that she drank 10–15 drinks, usually Martinis, every day at the bar and had even begun having a few drinks before happy hour. A social worker and nurse met with Wanda three additional times over the course of a three-day stay in the hospital. They gave her information about the health impact of drinking and did a screening test to determine Wanda's level of abusive drinking. They concluded that she was at very high risk of becoming an alcoholic since her drinking impaired her judgment and was thought to be responsible for high blood pressure and high blood sugar readings consistent with adult-onset diabetes.

A psychosocial history taken by the social worker revealed that Wanda was painfully lonely and that the drinking seemed to be a response to early retirement without a plan for what she would do with herself after a lifetime of hard, successful work. The history also revealed that Wanda had come from a family of alcoholics, had vowed to keep her drinking limited, but now realized she was romanticizing about alcohol the way many members of her family had. Wanda had her driver's license revoked and her ability to drive her golf cart in the retirement community grounds was curtailed to daylight hours and only if someone was with her. She was told by the retirement community CEO that the bylaws of the community required her to go for counseling and that she had to maintain sobriety for six months before she could have full use of her cart privileges. She was also banned from any of the bars in the retirement community.

Wanda met with her substance abuse counselor and for the first few sessions was very angry and could only talk about the "hoity-toity" CEO and who did he think he was? She'd seen lots of men like him and she would just like to tell him a thing or two. But in the third session, Wanda broke down and cried, telling the counselor she made a mistake retiring and leaving her support network in Kansas City. Little did she know, she told the counselor, that she had an aversion to "old people" and hated it here in the community. She thought she'd meet a man but most of the men were either "jerks, and the same Casanovas she'd been meeting most of her life" or too old and sick to be any fun. She'd spent her first 18 years taking care of "drunks" and she never wanted to take care of anyone again. Still, she was lonely and loneliness was everything it was cracked up to be.

The first item on the agenda was to focus on resolving the alcohol problem and the issues that seemed to bring about the late-life drinking problem. After some discussion Wanda pointed out that she didn't like the words "alcoholic or drunk" since they were words used to describe members of her family. She did agree that she was drinking too much and that the drinking had health and mental health implications. The worker asked that Wanda do what she had done so often in her lifetime and that was to take control of her problem by assertively looking for more information that she could use in counseling. Wanda agreed and the worker gave her a list of articles on the Internet she might read for the next session and encouraged Wanda do her own reading about late life drinking problems, loneliness, and early retirement.

From the work of Kuperman et al. (2001), they agreed that Wanda had a number of problems that should be dealt with, including feelings of loneliness, lack of work to keep her occupied, little ability to handle leisure time, and alcohol abuse. They decided that a cognitive-behavioral approach would work best, with homework assignments and cognitive restructuring as additional aspects of the treatment. Wanda was intrigued with an article she found on the strengths approach and showed the therapist an article by Moxley and Olivia (2001) that they both found quite useful. Another article on self-help groups by Humphreys (1998) convinced them that a self-help group for older adult alcohol abusers might also be helpful. Finally, Wanda brought up the issue of understanding the impact her alcoholic family had on her current situation. Several articles on the dynamic approach to treatment were suggested which Wanda read and found relevant.

After months of treatment, during which time Wanda would often avoid answering questions directly or would go off on tangents, she began to talk about her feelings and admitted that she has continued drinking heavily. She also drives, although her license has been suspended. She feels strong when she drinks, and loves the peaceful feeling that comes over her as she gets drunk. Like her parents, she romanticizes her drinking and can hardly wait to have her first drink of the day. Sometimes she drinks when she wakes up and often drinks rather than eats. She is aware that this cycle of drinking to feel better about herself can only lead to serious life problems, but she doesn't think she's capable of stopping. A number of women in the community are secret drinkers, she tells the counselor, and like many of them, drinking is one of the few pleasures they have. Life has stopped having meaning and, faced with many years of living alone and doing nothing, she finds solace in alcohol.

Her counselor has seen the same pattern in older adult alcoholics and has allowed for the fact that the problem will take much longer to resolve because Wanda lacks a support group. The therapist thought that an older adult support group of problem drinkers would help Wanda but found out from Wanda that all the members have continued drinking and have even formed a club, of sorts, to drink together.

During one session several months into treatment, the counselor admitted to Wanda that the treatment wasn't helping Wanda with her drinking. While Wanda read articles and came prepared to discuss them, it was an intellectual exercise and it wasn't helping Wanda change her behavior. Wanda pleaded with the counselor not to give up on her. She was the only person in Wanda's life with whom Wanda could talk. She didn't know what she would do if the counselor gave up on her and had openly considered suicide as an option.

The session was electric, as Wanda spoke of her early life, her co-dependency, and how it had made relationships impossible. She had lied about her drinking and had a pattern of binge drinking from early adolescence, but had never done anything about it. She thought of herself as a tough-minded woman who had lapses, only this relapse wasn't going away. She promised to "hunker down" and get to work, and she did. On her 70th birthday, she passed six months of sobriety and had her cart privileges back. With the counselor's recommendation she also got her driver's license back. She has joined a real estate firm selling re-sales in the retirement community and is busier than ever. And she has found a man her age who she considers her best friend and companion. In the time she has available after work, they take advantage of the wonderful cultural events in the community. During the hottest months of the summer, they go to the mountains. Little happens during those months at work. If someone contacts the agency she can handle it on the Internet and by phone.

Wanda's counselor said, "I want to applaud the professionals Wanda worked with in the hospital. Even thought the treatment was brief, it made a lasting impact on her to hear that she was considered an alcoholic, and it did bring her into treatment along with the loss of her license and the recognition in the retirement community that she had a drinking problem. That's exactly what you hope for in serious alcoholics who are in denial. It took Wanda longer to turn the corner and get down to work than most younger adults. The reason, I've come to believe since I see the same thing in other older substance abusers, is that there is a sense of hopelessness in many older adults. They accept cultural stereotypes that older people have no useful function, and they tend to give up. They also think that retirement will be a magical time when they'll meet interesting people, have intimate relationships, and are active much of the time. That isn't always the case and many people retire before they are ready because they're burned out and angry about their jobs. They don't realize that work gives them a schedule and fills in free time that many older adults haven't learned to handle.

"I'm never surprised when people tell me that they have a history of drinking even though they deny it early in treatment. I wonder about late-onset alcoholism and, while I'm sure it exists, many older people with no actual history of drinking problems find alcohol aversive both in taste and in its effect. I think Wanda is one of many tough-minded successful women in our society who fill their lives so full that when they take a break and try and relax, many emotional issues come up they'd rather not deal with. So they work hard, have lots of acquaintances, and stay very busy. When they retire, many years of denial and ignoring problems begin to have an impact. The fact that Wanda read the articles I suggested and came prepared to discuss them gave her a large body of information. When she was ready to begin changing, the material she read came in very handy".

"I don't want to define Wanda as a success story. Alcohol isn't her only problem. When she becomes too tired to work or fill up her time with other activities, it wouldn't surprise me if she had a relapse. Right now, she's had a scare and she's very motivated. I've referred her for therapy that's more insight-oriented to help her understand the impact of her early life, but she's put it off. I suspect she's had some very bad traumas and maybe she can avoid discussing them but I think sooner or later they'll come back to haunt her."

12.4 RESEARCH PROBLEMS AND BEST EVIDENCE

A major problem with the treatment of substance abuse is the lack of best evidence because of compelling research problems. Clifford et al. (2000) suggest that many research studies on the effectiveness of treatment for substance abuse have numerous methodological problems and write, "It is recommended that treatment outcome studies be interpreted cautiously, particularly when the research protocols involved frequent and intensive follow-up interviews conducted across extended periods of time" (p. 741). As an example of the type of research errors made in substance abuse research, Ouimette et al. (1997) compared 12-step programs such as AA with cognitive-behavioral programs and programs that combined both approaches. One year after completion of treatment, all three types of programs had similar improvement rates when alcohol consumption was measured. Participants in the 12-step program had more "sustained abstinence" and better employment rates than the other two programs, but Ouimette et al. (1997) caution that readers should not make more of these findings than is warranted because of non-random assignment of patients to the different treatment types. Clifford et al. (2000) indicate that many substance abuse studies have methodological problems that affect their validity and include infrequent follow up, compounding effects that may suggest better results than are warranted, the lack of quality data, and research protocols that are influenced more by existing politics and social correctness than science.

12.5 SUMMARY

In this chapter on EBP and older adult substance abuse, research findings are reported that suggest disagreement regarding the effectiveness of certain types of treatment, particularly very brief treatment with high-risk abusers. However, promising research on natural recovery and self-help groups suggests that treatment effectiveness may be consistently positive with these two approaches. Research issues are discussed that make the development of best evidence on the efficacy of all forms of treatment of substance abuse questionable, and the suggestion is made that before we can develop best evidence, more effective studies must take place that include adequate research designs and controls. A case study is provided that demonstrates the use of EBP with substance-abusing older adult clients.

12.6 QUESTIONS FROM THE CHAPTER

1. In the case presented, the client admitted she had been a binge drinker since adolescence. The worker indicated that she was dubious about late-life onset of heavy drinking and wasn't surprised when Wanda finally admitted to binge drinking. Does this case make you wonder if the data indicating that 35% of all heavy drinking begins after age 60 is true?

2. Brief treatment of substance abuse flies in the face of what many people believe about the long-term addictive nature of alcohol and drug dependence. What's your view about the effectiveness of brief treatment?

3. Is it fair to criticize the lack of adequate research for self-help groups treating addictions? Shouldn't we take at face value the overwhelmingly positive feedback from participants that they work very well?

4. The idea that people will walk away from their addictions when they're ready is contraindicated in studies of weight loss.

In these studies, people cycle back and forth and fail to sustain weight loss. Might not the same thing be said about addictions to substances?

5. Focusing on positive behavior seems like a worthy way to treat substance abusers, but aren't there dangerous behaviors (unprotected sex, automobile accidents, negative effects on health) that need to be stopped immediately, and don't they require a type of "tough love?"

REFERENCES

Adams, W. L., Barry, K. L., & Fleming, M. F. (1996). Screening for problem drinking in older primary care patients. *Journal of the American Medical Association, 276*(24).

Atkinson, R. (1995). Treatment programs for aging alcoholics. In T. Beresford & E. Gomberg (Eds.), *Alcohol and Aging* (pp. 186–210). New York: Oxford University Press.

Babor, T. F., & Higgins-Biddle, J. C. (2000). Alcohol screening and brief intervention: Dissemination strategies for medical practice and public health. *Addiction, 95*(5), 677–687.

Backer, K. L., & Walton-Moss, B. (2001). Detecting and addressing alcohol abuse in women. *Nurse Practitioner, 26*(10), 13–22.

Baekeland, F., & Lundwall, L. (1975). Dropping out of treatment: A critical review. *Psychology Bulletin, 82*, 738–783.

Banta, J. E., & Montgomery, S. (2007). Substance abuse and dependence treatment in outpatient physician offices, 1997–2004. *The American Journal of Drug and Alcohol Abuse, 33*, 583–593.

Barrick, C., & Connors, G. J. (2002). Relapse prevention and maintaining abstinence in older adults with alcohol-use disorders. *Drugs and Aging, 19*, 583–594.

Bien, T. J., Miller, W. R., & Tonigan, J. S. (1993). Brief interventions for alcohol problems: A review. *Addictions, 88*(3), 315–335.

Biernacki, P. (1986). *Pathways from heroin addiction: Recover without treatment.* Philadelphia, PA: Temple University Press.

Bisson, J., Nadeau, L., & Demers, A. (1999). The validity of the CAGE scale to screen heavy drinking and drinking problems in a general population. *Addiction, 94*(5), 715–723.

Blow, F. C. (1991). *Short michigan alcoholism screening test-geriatric version (SMAST-G).* Ann Arbor, MI: University of Michigan Alcohol Research Center.

Blow, F.C. (2007). Substance abuse among older adults: Treatment improvement Protocol (TIP) series 26. *Substance Abuse and Mental Health Services Administration.* Retrieved 17.11.2007 from <http://ncadi.samhsa.gov/govpubs/BKD250/>

Blow, F. C., Brower, K. J., Schulenberg, J. E., Demo-Dananberg, L. M., Young, J. P., & Beresford, T. P. (1992). The michigan alcoholism screening test-geriatric version (MAST-G): A new elderly-specific screening instrument lill. *Alcoholism: Clinical and Experimental Research, 16*.

Burge, S. K., Amodei, N., Elkin, B., Catala, S., Andrew, S. R., Lane, P. A., & Seale, J. P. (1997). An evaluation of two primary care interventions for alcohol abuse among Mexican-American patients. *Addiction, 92*(12), 1705–1716.

Burtscheidt, W., Wolwer, W., Schwartz, R., et al. (2002). Alcoholism, rehabilitation and comorbidity. *Acta Psychiatrica Scandinavica, 106*(3), 227–233.

Chang, G., Wilkins-Haug, L., Berman, S., & Goetz, M. A. (1999). Brief intervention for alcohol use in pregnancy: A randomized trial. *Addiction, 94*(10), 1499–1508.

Clifford, P. R., Maisto, S. A., & Franzke, L. H. (2000). Alcohol treatment research follow-up and drinking behaviors. *Journal of Studies on Alcohol, 61*(5), 736–743.

Connors, G. J., Walitzer, K. S., & Dermen, K. H. (2002). Preparing clients for alcoholism treatment: Effects on treatment participation and outcomes. *Journal of Consulting and Clinical Psychology, 70*(5), 1161–1169.

Dahlgren, L., & Willander, A. (1989). Are special treatment facilities for female alcoholics needed? *Alcoholism, Clinical and Experimental Research, 13*, 499–504.

Dupree, L. W., Broskowski, H., & Schonfeld, L. (1984). The gerontology alcohol project: A behavioral treatment program for elderly alcohol abusers. *Gerontologist, 24*, 510–516.

Fleming, M., & Manwell, L. B. (1998). Brief intervention in primary care settings: A primary treatment method for at-risk, problem, and dependent drinkers. *Alcohol Research and Health, 23*(2), 128–137.

Fleming, M. F., Barry, K. L., Manwell, L. B., Johnson, K., & London, R. (1997). Brief physician advice for problem alcohol drinkers: A randomized controlled trial in community-based primary care practices. *JAMA, 277*(13), 1039–1045.

Gentilello, L. M., Donovan, D. M., Dunn, C. W., & Rivara, F. P. (1995). Alcohol interventions in trauma centers: Current practice and future directions. *JAMA, 274*(13), 1043–1048.

Granfield, R., & Cloud, W. (1996). The elephant that no one sees: Natural recovery among middle-class addicts. *Journal of Drug Issues, 26*, 45–61.

Grant, B. F., & Dawson, D. A. (1997). Age at onset of alcohol use and its association with DSM-IV alcohol abuse and dependence: Results from the national longitudinal alcohol epidemiologic survey. *Journal of Substance Abuse, 9*, 103–110.

Herman, M. (2000). Psychotherapy with substance abusers: Integration of psychodynamic and cognitive-behavioral approaches. *American Journal of Psychotherapy, 54*(4), 574–579.

Higgins-Biddle, J. C., Babor, T. F., Mullahy, J., Daniels, J., & Mcree, B. (1997). Alcohol screening and brief interventions: Where research meets practice. *Connecticut Medicine, 61*, 565–575.

Hingson, R., Scotch, N., Day, N., & Culbert, A. (1980). Recognizing and seeking help for drinking problems. *Journal of Studies on Alcohol, 41*, 1102–1117.

Humphreys, K. (1998). Can addiction-related self-help/mutual aid groups lower demand for professional substance abuse treatment? *Social Policy, 29*(2), 13–17.

Kirchner, J. E., Booth, B. M., Owen, R. R., et al. (2000). Predictors of patient entry into alcohol treatment after initial diagnosis. *Journal of Behavioral Health Services & Research, 27*(3), 339–347.

Kuperman, S., Schlosser, S. S., Kramer, J. R., Bucholz, K., Hesselbrock, V., Reich, T., & Reich, W. (2001). Risk domains associated with adolescent alcohol dependence diagnosis. *Addiction, 96*(4), 629–637.

Leigh, G., Ogborne, A. C., & Cleland, P. (1984). Factors associated with patient dropout from an outpatient alcoholism treatment service. *Journal of Studies on Alcohol, 45*, 359–362.

Lennox, R. D., & Mansfield, A. J. (2001). A latent variable model of evidence-based quality improvement for substance abuse treatment. *Journal of Behavioral Health Services & Research, 28*(2), 164–177.

Liberto, J. G., & Oslin, D. W. (1995). Early versus late onset of alcoholism in the elderly. *International Journal of Addiction, 30*(13–14), 1799–1818.

Lu, M., & McGuire, T. G. (2002). The productivity of outpatient treatment for substance abuse. *Journal of Human Resources, 37*(2), 309–335.

Menninger, J. A. (2002). Assessment and treatment of alcoholism and substance-related disorders in the elderly. *Bulletin of the Menninger Clinic, 66*(2), 166–184.

Miller, W. R., & Sanchez, V. C. (1994). Motivating young adults for treatment and lifestyle change. In G. S. Howard & P. E. Nathan (Eds.), *Alcohol use and misuse by young adults* (pp. 55–81). Notre Dame, IN: University of Notre Dame Press.

Miller, K. E. (2001). Can two questions screen for alcohol and substance abuse? *American Family Physician, 64*, 1247.

Miller, W. R., & Roilnick, S. (1991). *Motivational interviewing: Preparing people for change*. New York: Guilford Press.

Monti, P. M., Colby, S. M., Barnett, N. P., et al. (1999). Brief intervention for harm reduction with alcohol-positive older adolescents in a hospital emergency department. *Journal of Consulting and Clinical Psychology, 67*(6), 989–994.

Moxley, D. P., & Olivia, G. (2001). Strengths-based recovery practice in chemical dependency: A transperson perspective. *Families in Society, 82*(3), 251–262.

Mukamal, K. J., Mittleman, M. A., Longstreth, W. T., Newman, A. B., Eried, L. P., & Siscovick, D. S. (2004). Self-reports alcohol consumption and falls in older adults: Cross-sectional and longitudinal analyses of the cardiovascular health study. *Journal of the American Geriatrics Society, 52*, 1174–1179.

National Institute of Alcohol Abuse and Alcoholism (2000). *Alcohol alert* (Vol. 49). NIAAA.

National Institute for Alcohol Abuse and Alcoholism, Department of Health and Human Services, Alcohol and Health (1997). *Ninth special report to the United States on alcohol and health* (NIH Publication No. 97–4017). Washington, DC: US Government Printing Office.

National Institute on Drug Abuse (1999). *Principles of drug addiction treatment: A Research-Based Guide*. Rockville, MD: National Institute on Drug Abuse; 1999. DHHS publication (ADM), pp. 99–4180.

Nemes, S., Rao, P. A., Zeiler, C., Munly, K., Holtz, K. D., & Hoffman, J. (2004). Computerized screening of substance abuse in a primary care setting: Older vs. Younger adults. *The American Journal of Drug and Alcohol Abuse, 30*(3), 327–642.

Onder, G., Landi, E., Delia Vedova, C., Atkinson, H., Pedone, C., Cesari, M., et al. (2002). Moderate alcohol consumption and adverse drug reactions among older adults. *Pharmacoepidemiological Drug Safety, 11*, 385–392.

Oslin, D. W. (2004). Late-life alcoholism: Issues relevant to the geriatric psychiatrist. *American Journal of Geriatric Psychiatry, 12*, 571–583.

Ouimette, P. C., Finney, J. W., & Moos, R. H. (1997). Twelve-step and cognitive-behavioral treatment for substance abuse: A comparison of treatment effectiveness. *Journal of Consulting and Clinical Psychology, 65*(2), 230–240.

Peele, S. (1989). *The diseasing of America: Addiction treatment out of control*. Lexington, MA: Lexington Books.

Pennington, H., Butler, R., & Eagger, S. (2000). *The diseasing of America: Addiction treatment out of control*. Lexington, MA: Lexington Books.

Rees, D. S. (1986). Changing patients' health beliefs to improve compliance with alcohol treatment: A controlled trial. *Journal of Studies on Alcohol, 47*, 436–439.

Rice, C., Longabaugh, R., Beattie, M., & Noel, N. (1993). Age-group differences in response to treatment for problematic alcohol use. *Addiction, 88*, 1369–1375.

Roizen, R., Calahan, D., Lambert, E., Wiebel, W., & Shanks, P. (1978). Spontaneous remission among untreated problem drinkers. In D. Kandel (Ed.), *Longitudinal research on drug use*. Washington, DC: Hemisphere Publishing.

Seligman, M. E. P. (1995). The effectiveness of psychotherapy: The consumers report study. *American Psychologist, 50*(12), 965–974.

Snow, M. (1973). Maturing out of narcotic addiction in New York City. *International Journal of the Addictions, 8*(6), 932–938.

Sobell, L., Sobell, M., Toneatto, T., & Leo, G. (1993). What triggers the resolution of alcohol problems without treatment? *Alcoholism: Clinical and Experimental Research, 17*(2), 217–224.

Sorocco, K. H., & Ferrell, S. W. (2006). Alcohol use among older adults. *The Journal of General Psychology, 133*(4), 453–467.

Stall, R., & Biernacki, P. (1989). Spontaneous remission from the problematic use of substances. *International Journal of the Addictions, 21*, 1–23.

Stewart, K. B., & Richards, A. B. (2000). Recognizing and managing your patient's alcohol abuse. *Nursing, 30*(2), 56–60.

Substance Abuse and Mental Health Services Administration (SAMHSA) (1998). *Substance abuse among older adults: Treatment improvement protocol* (TIP; Series #26). Rockville, MD: US Department of Health and Human Services.

Substance Abuse and Mental Health Services Administration (SAMHSA) (2004). *National survey on drug use and health*. Rockville, MD: US Department of Health and Human Services.

Trice, H., & Roman, P. (1970). Delabeling, relabeling, and Alcoholics Anonymous. *Social Problems, 17*, 538–546.

US Department of Health and Human Services (2000a). *Healthy people 2010. Understanding and improving health and objectives for improving health* (2nd ed.). Washington, DC: US Government Printing Office 2 vols.

US Department of Health and Human Services. (2000b). *National Household Survey on Drug Abuse.* Retrieved 13.10.2002 from <http://www.samhsa.gov/oas/dependence/chapter2.htm/>

Waldorf, D., Reinarman, C., & Murphy, S. (1991). *Cocaine changes: The experience of using and quitting*. Philadelphia, PA: Temple University Press.

Winick, C. (1962). Maturing out of narcotic addiction. *Bulletin on Narcotics, 6*(1).

Part four

The Impact of Spirituality and Religion and the Significance of Self-Help Groups

Evidence-Based Practice and the Significance of Religion and Spirituality in the Lives of Older Adults

13.1 INTRODUCTION

A number of studies provided in this chapter suggest that spirituality and religious involvement may have a positive influence on health and mental health even though the helping professions have generally separated themselves from religious and spiritual ideologies. Despite this sense that spirituality and religious involvement somehow lie outside of the orthodox notions of what human service professionals should do with the two issues in their practice, researchers agree that it has been a neglected area (Canda, 1988).

This chapter will consider the evidence of the impact of religion and spirituality on health and mental health. It will also look at the role of the human services in dealing with issues of religious and spiritual belief. Several case studies are provided to help the reader better understand the relationship between religion and spirituality and practice.

A section at the end of the chapter considers the special research questions posed in an attempt to understand best evidence that spirituality and religion may serve a beneficial role in the lives of people.

13.2 DEFINITIONS OF SPIRITUALITY AND RELIGIOUS INVOLVEMENT

Confusion sometimes exists over the appropriate definitions of spirituality and religious belief. Glicken and Fraser (2004) define *spirituality* "as the means by which one finds wholeness, meaning, and purpose in life. It arises from an innate longing for fulfillment through the establishment of loving relationships with self and the community. Spirituality suggests harmony with self, others, and the world" (p. 65). Using a somewhat different definition, Manheimer (1994) writes that "Spirituality, while certainly overlapping with church or synagogue affiliation, refers to a psychological and personal inward experience that may be totally independent of institutional membership" (p. 72).

Derezotes (1995) defines *religious involvement* as "A system of beliefs, rituals, and behaviors, usually shared by individuals within an institutionalized structure. It is an external expression of faith" (p. 1). George et al. (2000, p. 105) report an attempt by the National Institute of Aging, in conjunction with the Fitzer Work Group (1997), to define spirituality and religious involvement. They found the following common elements in the definitions of both:

1. Religious/spiritual preference or affiliation: Membership in or affiliation with a specific religious or spiritual group.
2. Religious/spiritual history: Religious upbringing, duration of participation in religious or spiritual groups, life-changing religious or spiritual experiences, and "turning points" in religious or spiritual participation or belief.
3. Religious/spiritual participation: Amount of participation in formal religious or spiritual groups or activities.
4. Religious/spiritual private practices: Private behaviors or activities, including but not limited to prayer, meditation, reading sacred literature, and watching or listening to religious or spiritual radio or television programs.
5. Religious/spiritual support: Tangible and intangible forms of social support offered by the members of one's religious or spiritual group.

6. Religious/spiritual coping: The extent to which and ways in which religious or spiritual practices are used to cope with stressful experiences.

7. Religious/spiritual beliefs and values: Specific religious or spiritual beliefs and values.

8. Religious/spiritual commitment: The importance of religion/ spirituality relative to other areas of life and the extent to which religious or spiritual beliefs and practices serve to affect personal values and behavior.

9. Religious/spiritual motivation for regulating and reconciling relationships: Most measures in this domain focus on forgiveness, but other issues may be relevant as well (e.g., confession, atonement.

10. Religious/spiritual experiences: Personal experience with the divine or sacred, as reflected in emotions and sensations (p. 105).

13.3 THE IMPACT OF SPIRITUALITY AND RELIGIOUS INVOLVEMENT ON THE HEALTH AND MENTAL HEALTH OF OLDER ADULTS

Blazer (1991) found that 90% of all older adults surveyed describe spirituality and religion as one of their most frequently used coping and support mechanisms. Musick (1996) found that the use of religion and spirituality as coping mechanisms may be even more prevalent in racial and ethnic minority elderly than in white elderly. Religion and spirituality have been described as a "buffer against depression, a way to maintain meaning at the end of life, a mechanism for preparation for death and dying, increased happiness and life satisfaction and higher levels of adjustment for older adults" (Lewis, 2001, p. 232). Musick (1996) report that religious beliefs and spirituality have been linked to positive physical health and inversely related to physical illnesses. Koenig et al. (1996) report that religiously committed older adults are healthier, abuse alcohol less often, have lower blood pressure, experience fewer strokes, and have longer survival rates than those older adults not committed to religion. Lewis (2001) writes, "Therefore, it seems that utilizing religion and spirituality in counseling with religiously and spiritually committed older adults would be especially useful when discussing coping mechanisms for dealing with mental health concerns or developmental issues [concerns about aging]" (p. 231).

George et al. (2000) report a growing body of research showing the positive health benefits of religious involvement. According to the authors, religious involvement was found to reduce the likelihood of disease and disability in 78% of the studies attempting to determine the existence of a relationship between religion and health. The positive health benefits of religion were particularly noted with certain medical conditions, including coronary disease and heart attacks, emphysema, cirrhosis, and other varieties of liver disease (Comstock and Partridge, 1972; Medalie et al., 1973), hypertension (Larson et al., 1989), and disability (Idler and Kasl, 1992, 1997). In these studies, "the strongest predictor of the prevention of illness onset is attendance at religious services" (George et al., 2000, p. 108). The authors also point to a relationship between religious observance and longevity, noting that "multiple dimensions of religion are associated with longevity, but attendance at religious services is the most strongly related to longevity" (p. 108).

Ellison et al. (2001) studied the relationship between religious involvement and positive health and mental health outcomes. Among their key findings were the following:

1. there is a positive relationship between church attendance and well-being, and an inverse association with distress;
2. the frequency of prayer is inversely related to well-being and only slightly positively related to distress;
3. a belief in eternal life is positively related to well-being but unrelated to distress;
4. church-based support networks are unrelated to well-being; and
5. "[t]here is limited evidence of stress-buffering effects, but not stress-exacerbating effects, of religious involvement" (Ellison et al., 2001, p. 215)

Gartner et al. (1991) comprehensively reviewed over 200 psychiatric and psychological studies and concluded that religious involvement has a positive impact on both health and mental health. In another review of the literature, Ellison et al. (2001) concluded that, "there is at least some evidence of mental health benefits of religion among men and women, persons of different ages and racial and ethnic groups, and individuals from various socioeconomic classes and geographical locations. Further, these salutary effects often persist even with an array of social, demographic, and health-related statistical controls" (p. 215).

Manheimer (1994) reports that church membership plays a significant role in the health and mental health of ethnic and racial minorities. According to Manheimer (1994), church attendance is a strong predictor of happiness among older African Americans while social activities in church contribute to life satisfaction and personal adjustment. As Haight (1998) notes in her study of the spirituality of African American children:

> Available empirical evidence suggests a relationship between socialization experiences emanating from the African American church and a number of positive developmental outcomes. For example, Brown and Gary (1991) found that self-reports of church involvement were positively related to educational attainment among African American adults. In an interview study of African American urban male adolescents, Zimmerman and Maton (1992) found that youths who left high school before graduation and were not employed, but who attended church, had relatively low levels of alcohol and drug abuse. In a questionnaire administered to African American adults (Seaborn-Thompson and Ensminger, 1989), 74% responded "very often" or "often" to the statement, "The religious beliefs I learned when I was young still help me." On the basis of data from the 1979–80 National Survey of Black Americans, Ellison (1993) argued that participation in church communities is positively related to self-esteem in African American adults. (p. 215)

Baetz et al. (2002) studied the level of religious interest of psychiatric inpatients to determine whether religious commitment had an impact on selected outcome variables. In the study, 88 consecutive adult patients (50% men) admitted to an inpatient facility were interviewed about their religious beliefs and practices. Patients with a Beck Depression score of 12 or more were included for outcome analysis. The researchers report the following results: (1) frequent worship attendees had fewer symptoms of depression, shorter hospital stays, were more satisfied with their lives, and had much lower rates of current or lifetime use of alcohol when compared to subjects with less frequent or non-existent worship attendance; and (2) the authors believe that worship may protect clients against greater severity of symptoms, longer hospital stays, increased satisfaction with life, reduced severity of symptoms, and enhanced quality of life among psychiatric patients.

Kissman and Maurer (2002) report that "[p]eople with strong faith, regardless of religious persuasion, live longer, experience less anxiety, cope better with stressful life events, have lower blood pressures and stronger immune systems (Koening, 1998; Dossey, 1997)." Krucoff and Crater (1998) found that coronary surgery patients who were prayed for by congregations had a better recovery rate when compared with patients in a control group where prayer was not used. George et al. (2000) report that religious involvement and spirituality have been shown to reduce the onset of illness. Once the illness is present, recovery is faster and longevity is greater than in those who are not involved with religion or spirituality. The authors write that healthy religious involvement may positively affect the course of an illness and lead to longer survival after heart transplants (Harris et al., 1995); reduce risk of repeated heart attacks which might be fatal or non-fatal (Thoresen, 1990); reduce death rates among women with breast cancer (Spiegel et al., 1989); increased the ability to cope with pain (Kaczorowski, 1989; Landis, 1996; O'Brien, 1982); and may prove to be the most significant reason for better medical recoveries and outcomes (George et al., 2000).

Religious involvement appears to be associated with faster and more complete recovery from mental illnesses, substance abuse/dependence, and depression (George, 1992; Koenig, in press; Koenig et al., 1998). Compared to patients who report no or low levels of religious involvement, those who report stronger religious involvement are more likely to recover and to do so more quickly. Evidence indicating a relationship between religious or spiritual involvement with recovery from substance abuse is based upon studies of Alcoholics Anonymous (AA) and other 12-step programs (Emrick, 1987; Montgomery et al., 1995; Project Match Research Group, 1997). According to George et al. (2000), "A central component of these programs is the belief that one has no personal control over the addiction, but that there is a higher power who can help the individual to conduct it" (p. 109). The authors indicate that all of the studies cited are multivariate studies that control for a variety of intervening variables and that longitudinal studies following subjects over a long period of time confirm the existence of a relationship between spirituality and religious involvement and better recovery for mental illness, depression, and substance abuse.

One of the criticisms of studies involving the impact of religious and spiritual involvement is that methodologies are problematic. However, George et al. (2000) indicate that the studies cited above were multivariate (other factors that might affect improved health results were controlled for), and that longitudinal studies showing the long-term impact on health of religious/spiritual involvement continue to show a strong relationship. The authors also indicate that the evidence for the impact of religious/spiritual involvement on mental health is even stronger than it is for physical health.

13.4 DISSENTING VIEWS ABOUT THE BENEFIT OF RELIGIOUS INVOLVEMENT AND PRAYER

Although the evidence presented thus far suggests a positive relationship between church attendance and positive health and mental health benefits, Rauch (2003) reports that the proportion of people who say they never go to religious services has increased 33% from 1973 to 2000. To further confuse the relationship between religious attendance and health and mental health benefits, Rauch quotes Theology Professor John G. Stackhouse, Jr. as saying: "Beginning in the 1990s, a series of sociological studies has shown that many more Americans tell pollsters they attend church regularly than can be found in church when teams actually count. In fact, actual church-going may be half the professed rate" (Rauch, 2003, p. 34). This suggests that the validity of research on church attendance and positive health and mental health benefits may be in doubt.

Furthermore, there is some evidence that certain religious beliefs may cause harm. Simpson (1989) found that a sample of Christian Scientists died at younger ages than their peers while Asser and Swan (1998) studied child deaths in families refusing medical care in favor of faith healing and found much higher rates of death. Both sets of authors believe that there are healthy and unhealthy uses of spirituality and religious involvement but have thus far been unable to determine precisely what they are and how health and mental health are affected.

Dembner (2005) reports that researchers studied 748 patients who were undergoing heart procedures such as angioplasty or cardiac catheterization. Congregations of various religions at locations outside the hospital were randomly assigned to pray for half of the patients, without the patients or their doctors knowing into which group they fell. The patients weren't told because the researchers wanted to separate any impact of prayer from possible placebo effects. The prayers followed the traditions of the congregation involved, and continued for five to 30 days. The congregations were told the name, age, and illness of the patient. Over a six-month period, the study found no difference in serious side effects, death rate, or readmissions between the patients who had received prayers and those who had not. In a further review of the benefits of prayer, Dembner (2005) reports that a review of 17 past studies of "distant healing," published in 2003 by a British researcher, found no significant effect for prayer or other healing methods.

The largest studies have focused on cardiac care. In one study of 990 cardiac patients conducted at Saint Luke's Hospital in Kansas City, Mo., and published in 1999, researchers found prayer did not affect hospital length of stay, but did improve health based on a composite score of measures that the researchers created for the study. A study of 799 patients at the Mayo Clinic in Rochester, Minn., published in 2001, found prayer made no difference in the outcomes of patients after discharge from the cardiac care unit. The study looked at the number of deaths, cardiac arrests, and repeat hospitalizations, among other outcomes.

13.5 WHY DOES RELIGIOUS AND SPIRITUAL INVOLVEMENT IMPACT HEALTH AND MENTAL HEALTH?

Ellison and Levin (1998) suggest three reasons for the beneficial impact of religious involvement and spirituality.

1. **Controlling health-related risks**. Some religions have specific prohibitions against at-risk health behaviors. These prohibitions may include the use of tobacco and alcohol, premarital sexual experiences and other risky sexual activity, use of foods that may contribute to high cholesterol and heart problems, and strong prohibitions against the use of illegal drugs. Many religions encourage good health practices. The Mormons, Seventh Day Adventists, and other religious adherents with strict prohibitions concerning health-related behaviors are healthier and live longer, on average, than members of other faiths and those who are uninvolved in religion (Enstrom, 1978, 1989; Gardner and Lyon, 1982; Lyon et al., 1976; Phillips et al., 1980). However, George et al. (2000) indicate that strict prohibitions on health-related behaviors only explain 10% of the reasons that religious and spiritual beliefs have a positive impact on health and mental health.

2. **Social support**. A second possible reason that religion may affect health and mental health is the fellowship, support, and social bonds developed among people who are religiously affiliated. When compared to their nonreligious peers, people who regularly attend religious services report: (a) larger social networks; (b)

more contact with those social networks; (c) receipt of more help from others; and (d) more satisfaction with their social support network (Zuckerman et al., 1984). Despite this, social support provides only a 5–10% explanation of the relationship between religion and health (Idler, 1987; Zuckerman et al., 1984).

3. **Life meaning or the coherence hypothesis**. A third explanation for the health benefits of religion is that people who are religious understand "their role in the universe, the purpose of life, and develop the courage to endure suffering" (George et al., 2000, p. 110). The authors call this the "coherence hypothesis" and note that the connection between a sense of coherence about the meaning of life and one's role in the universe affects 20–30% of a client's health and mental health, largely because it buffers clients from stress (Antonovsky, 1980; Idler, 1987; Zuckerman et al., 1980).

Other writers have noted the positive impact of spirituality and religious belief when serious illness is present. Kubler-Ross (1969, 1997) suggested that coping with the possibility of death and disability often leads to life-changing growth and new and more complex behaviors that focus on the meaning of life. Greenstein and Breitbart (2000) write, "Existentialist thinkers, such as Frankl, view suffering as a potential springboard, both for having a need for meaning and for finding it" (p. 486). Frankl (1978) believed that life meaning could be found in our actions, our values, and in our suffering. Commenting on the meaning of suffering, Frankl (1978) wrote that even while facing imminent death, there is still the opportunity to find meaning in the experience. "What matters, then, is the stand he takes in his predicament, the attitude we choose in suffering" (Frankl, 1978, p. 24). However, Balk (1999) believes that three issues must be present for a health or mental health crisis to create coherence: "The situation must create a psychological imbalance or disequilibrium that resists readily being stabilized; there must be time for reflection; and the person's life must forever afterwards be colored by the crisis" (p. 485).

One further study of the coherence hypothesis is a recent longitudinal study of a Catholic order of women in the Midwest by Danner et al. (2001). The study found that a person's positive view of life and life meaning can have a significant impact on physical and emotional health. The authors found that positive and affirming personal statements written by very young women entering the religious order correlated with a life span as long as 10 years beyond the mean length of life for women in the religious order and as much as 20 years or longer than the general population. Many women in a sample of 650 lived well into their nineties, while six women in the order were over 100 years of age. The authors believe that the reasons for longer life could be explained by good nutritional and health practices and a communal environment that focused on spirituality and helping others.

Emery and Pargament (2004) believe that there are five reasons religion and spirituality are so important to older adults:

1. Religion offers personal stability – as part of a sacred tradition religion, may provide older adults with a sense of continuity in the midst of rapidly unfolding changes of late life.
2. Religion offers intimacy and belonging to a large social network that may provide friendships and the opportunity for intimate relationships.
3. Feeling close to God offers many older adults a sense of intimate support and understanding.
4. "In spite of social, physical, and psychological change and loss, confronted with transitions that may be difficult to comprehend, religion offers individuals a larger framework of meaning and a benevolent and hopeful vision of past, present, and future" (Emery and Pargament, 2004, p. 6).
5. "Through a relationship with God, people can experience a greater sense of efficacy and control. Congregational involvement can also empower the elderly by building on their experience, wisdom, and talents" (Emery and Pargament, 2004, p. 7).

13.6 SHOULD ISSUES OF RELIGION AND SPIRITUALITY BE INCLUDED IN THE WORK OF HUMAN SERVICE PROFESSIONALS WITH OLDER ADULTS?

Although the prior research discussed in this chapter indicates that religious involvement and spirituality may have a positive impact on health and mental health, there is a lack of agreement about whether helping professionals should learn about both issues in their training or even include either in their work with clients. In a study of 53 social work faculty members, Dudley and Helfgott (1990) found that those opposed to a course on spirituality were concerned about conflict with the mission of social work, problems stemming from the separation of church and state, and concerns that religious and spiritual material in the curriculum would conflict with the personal beliefs of faculty members and students. Sheridan and Wilmer (1994) asked educators from 25 schools of social work questions regarding the inclusion of religious and spiritual content in social work programs. The majority (82.5%) supported inclusion in a specialized elective course. In another study, Sheridan et al. (1992) surveyed 328 social work practitioners and found that 83% received little training in religion and spirituality during their graduate studies, although a third of their clients discussed religious or spiritual concerns during treatment.

Sheridan (2000) found that 73% of the social workers surveyed had generally positive attitudes about the appropriateness of discussing religion and spirituality in practice. Forty-three percent of the respondents said that religion played a positive role in the lives of their clients, while 62% said that spirituality played a positive role in the lives of their clients. Spirituality was reported to play a harmful role in their clients' lives only 12% of the time, while religion was reported detrimental to client functioning 21% of the time (Sheridan, 2000). A majority of the social workers responding said that they had used spiritually and religiously based interventions with clients even though most (84%) reported little or no prior instruction. However, over half of the respondents had attended workshops and conferences on religion and spirituality after their professional training was completed.

Amato-von Hemert (1994) believes we should include material on religious involvement and spirituality in graduate training and writes, "Just as we train and evaluate how workers address issues of class, gender, and race, we must maintain our professionalism by training workers to deal with religious issues" (p. 16). Tobias et al. (1995) say that, "Today's multiethnic America encompasses a wide-ranging spiritual orientation that is, if anything, diverse" (p. 1), while Dudley and Helfgott (1990) suggest that, "Understanding spirituality is essential to understanding the culture of numerous ethnic groups that social workers help" (p. 288).

In trying to find a definition of practice that includes religious and spiritual content, Boorstein (2000) reports that a study by Lajoie and Shapiro (1992) came up with more than 200 definitions of transpersonal (spiritual) psychology. However, the authors summarized those definitions by writing that, "Transpersonal psychology is concerned with the study of humanity's highest potential, and with the recognition, understanding, and realization of intuitive, spiritual, and transcendent states of consciousness" (p. 91). Boorsten (2000) notes the following difference between traditional psychotherapy and spiritually based psychotherapy: (1) Traditional psychotherapy is pessimistic. For example, Freud said that psychoanalysis attempts to convert "neurotic misery to ordinary misery" (Boorstein, 2000, p. 413); (2) spiritually-based psychotherapy tries to help clients gain awareness of the existence of joy, love and happiness in their lives; and (3) spiritually-based therapy is concerned with life meaning and not just symptom removal.

Older adults tend to underutilize mental health services. Tobias et al. (1995) suggests that one reason is that older adults believe counselors will ignore or ridicule spiritual concerns and that it will not be useful for end-of-life issues. To deal with the need to discuss spiritual concerns, Lewis (2001) suggests the use of the Life Review Technique (LRT). Lewis describes LRT as follows:

> In general, the life review is one type of reminiscence therapy (Haight et al., 1998), but is different from reminiscence in that it is an active, rather than passive process. Specifically, memories are recalled, evaluated, and then reintegrated into the individual's self-concept during synthesis (Webster and Young, 1988). Developmentally, the life review facilitates integrity as "a recalled and evaluated past may lead to a new organization and acceptance of self both past and present" (Webster and Young, 1988, p. 320). In summary, the technique consists of asking the therapy client existential questions such as "who are you?" and "how have you lived your life?" for the purpose of taking stock of the past and integrating life experiences into the individual's present identity (see Butler, 1963, for a fuller description of the life review process). (pp. 234–235)

Research on LRT with older adults has shown that it helped in preventing despair, as measured by depression and hopelessness scales (Haight et al., 1998) and that it promoted integrity, as measured by psychological well-being, with the effect lasting for a year (Haight et al., 1998). Lewis (2001) says that advantages of using LRT "include its flexibility to accommodate many topics, applicability to older adults of diverse backgrounds, and use in either individual, family, or group counseling settings" (p. 234).

Finally, Bracki and Thibault (1990) write, "For *older adults*, religion is a significant part of everyday life. To ignore this aspect of the whole person is to miss both a strength for coping with adversity and loss and a support system important enough to enhance quality of life" (p. 55). The authors believe that many clinicians are uncomfortable with discussions of religion and spirituality because professional training may have "fostered the idea that the topic was not valuable and even to be avoided. This is a professional and personal issue with which the counselor must come to terms" (p. 58). The authors continue by noting that while no counselor can fully understand all religions and their nuances and beliefs, it is important to be "attuned to the languages of the various religions that are most likely to be influencing clients, to understand the traditions of the religions and to understand what the expectations of a specific religion might be for a given client" (p. 58) so that we can determine if the client is using religion in a way that aids or detracts from good health and mental health.

13.7 DISSENTING VIEW

In a dissenting view of the inclusion of religious and spiritual issues in practice, Sloan and Bagiella (2001) conclude that while interest in the impact of religious involvement and spirituality on health is great,

> The empiric support required to convert this interest into recommendations for health practice is weak and inconclusive at best, with most studies having numerous methodological shortcomings. Even if there were methodologically solid findings demonstrating associations between religious and spiritual activities and health outcomes, problems would still exist. (p. 33)

The authors point out the following methodological problems in trying to demonstrate a positive relationship between religious and spiritual involvement and improved health benefits: First of all, "We have no idea, for example, whether recommending that patients attend religious services will lead to increased attendance and, if so, whether attendance under these conditions will lead to better health outcomes" (Sloan and Bagiella, 2001, p. 34). Many factors influencing health are beyond the scope of practice. While marital status is strongly associated with health effects, most practitioners would "recoil" at recommending marriage because of its positive relationship to health. Furthermore, "Recommending religion to patients in this context may be coercive" (Sloan and Bagiella, 2001, p. 34) since it creates two classes of people: those who comply and those who don't. This may lead to the implication that poor health may be linked to insufficient spiritual or religious involvement. The authors conclude that, "the absence of compelling empiric evidence and the substantial ethical concerns raised suggest that, at the very least, it is premature to recommend making religious and spiritual activities adjunctive treatments" (Sloan and Bagiella, 2001, p. 34).

13.8 CONCLUSIONS

In summary, there is compelling evidence that many older adult clients have strong religious and spiritual beliefs that play an important role in the way they cope with social, emotional, and physical difficulties. While many practitioners understand and value the importance of religious and spiritual beliefs, few feel prepared to work with either issue and most feel that professional education should include content related to understanding and applying knowledge related to spirituality and religious beliefs. However, concerns are raised when faculties are asked how material will be taught given the diverse nature of faculties and student bodies in the helping profession.

CASE STUDY: RELIGIOUS ISSUES DISCUSSED IN TREATMENT

Isaac Grossman is a 67-year-old man seen in treatment for problems of depression, anxiety and substance abuse. In the course of gathering information for a psychosocial history, Isaac told the therapist that he had been sexually molested outside his synagogue in Poland when he was 10 years old and has been unable to attend religious services since. He used to find great meaning in his religion and realizes that a terrible event has shaken his willingness to take part in something that he thinks is important for his well-being. Isaac asked the therapist if they could talk about the molestation and his subsequent absence from religious participation. The therapist agreed but told Isaac that the actual reentry into the functions of the religion would be a decision that he alone could make.

Isaac said that because of the intense anti-Semitism in Poland when he was molested by a non-Jewish army officer in the Polish Army, it was impossible to file charges against the man. Although he realizes that it's irrational to blame his religion or God, still, he had just attended services when the molestation happened and because of official anti-Semitism in Poland, being Jewish made him powerless to do anything about the molestation. Had God cared, he reasoned, this would not have happened to him.

Isaac spent the last two years of the Second World War in a concentration camp. He was then repatriated and spent the final years of his adolescence in Israel, where he joined the Israeli Army and became proficient in the art of assassination. He along with other former concentration camp inmates then living in Israel formed a death squad in which Nazis and SS members and collaborators were killed. Isaac tracked down the army officer who molested him and tortured and killed him. He felt that this act of revenge would wipe the slate clean but instead his personal life slowly deteriorated. He worked at a menial job in Israel, one well below his ability, and began to drink heavily and experience depression. Out of desperation to turn his life around, he recently moved to the USA to be close to his children. The experience has not been a good one and the children openly resent him. They think he's a sad old drunk and they much prefer their mother, who left Isaac when the children were still small. Isaac now feels hopeless and has toyed with the idea of suicide but can't quite get himself to follow through.

Using a cognitive approach to treatment, Isaac's progress in treatment has been very limited and, believing that it could be a key to his problems and that he might progress at a faster pace, the therapist began discussing Isaac's religious beliefs. In the midst of an early discussion, Isaac burst out crying and said that the thoughts he was having were too painful for him to manage and asked that they not talk about religion anymore. The next week he came for treatment prepared to discuss the issue that had upset him so. It wasn't only the molestation that had troubled Isaac, he told the therapist, it was the reason Isaac's parents had used with him for not reporting his molester to the police. Perhaps, they explained, Isaac was partly responsible and had led the man on. He should ask God's forgiveness for his sinful behavior. And, they said, Poland being what it was, did Isaac want to cause problems for other Jews? Isaac told the therapist that he had never stopped believing that he was a sinful and flawed human being, and because no one in the synagogue pushed his parents to report the molestation, he now saw his fellow Jews as unkind and selfish. The religion had not led to acts of kindness toward him and, after the molestation, he was ostracized by the congregants. He didn't think he could ever believe in any religion again, but he had nothing to take its place and felt spiritually adrift.

"You have to believe in something," he told the therapist, "or how can you survive? When I was in the camps I believed in retribution and it didn't get me anywhere. Maybe if I could find something to believe in the problems I'm having will go away."

The therapist referred Isaac to a community group that discussed spirituality. Many of the people in the group had feelings about religion that were similar to his. Perhaps the group could serve as a substitute for his religious needs. Isaac reluctantly attended the group meetings but came back with ambivalent feelings. "I don't know what to say," he told his therapist. "It's like being in synagogue without the sermons and the ceremonies. People in the group believe in something, but I can't be certain what it is. They say negative things about religion, but they have no substitute that makes any sense to me. And most of them are very angry at religion. They think that whatever they believe now is a substitute, but I can't see that it is. I think we should talk about my other problems. Religion is a dead issue to me now."

Discussion

Should the therapist have discussed religion with Isaac? Certainly Isaac asked her to. Why the feeling of dead-endedness then? Perhaps the issues that Isaac wanted to talk about had more to do with his reasons for leaving his religion. That seems like a safer and more productive avenue of discussion. And rather than offering the spirituality group as a substitute, perhaps the therapist might have asked Isaac to define his religious and spiritual beliefs and to use them as a guide for finding a like-minded group of people. Finally, the need to understand his parent's behavior and a religious philosophy of human behavior that makes victims into perpetrators seems more in keeping with the therapist's area of expertise. Perhaps focusing on Isaac's reaction to his parents and his relationship with them may have also proven more beneficial. Finally, Isaac's lack of progress in treatment may be completely unrelated to his religious experiences. Perhaps the issue of religion is a smokescreen to prevent discussion of other more compelling issues, such as his feelings of failure as a parent and a man. The fact that he killed his molester, but that it resulted in no real improvement in Isaac's functioning, is a good indication that what Isaac needs to discuss only marginally has to do with religion and probably relates more to the impact of the molestation and his adaptation to it. Issues of religious and spiritual belief are important matters in people's lives, but in therapy they may be secondary to other more pressing problems that if resolved, may ultimately lead to the resolution of religious and spiritual conflict. And finally, perhaps the therapist might have consulted the literature to find similar cases or spoken to a rabbi who might have been able to offer advice and direction. When in doubt, seeking information and advice seems the professional thing to do.

13.9 PROBLEMATIC RESEARCH ISSUES

Many unresolved research issues still remain as we consider the relevance of religious involvement and spirituality in overall health and mental health. Those issues are as follows:

1. Is there clear evidence that religion plays an important role in health and mental health? This is still a fairly new field, and

do we have sufficient evidence to suggest a link? Not all of the research to date has been positive, nor has it found a relationship between positive health and religious involvement. In a review of the available correlational studies that attempt to link religion with positive mental health, Batson and Ventis (1982) write:

> Being more religious is not associated with greater mental health or happiness or with greater social compassion and concern. Quite the contrary, there is strong evidence that being more religious is associated with poorer mental health, with greater intolerance of people who are different from ourselves, and with no greater concern for those in need. The evidence suggests that religion is a negative force in human life, one we would be better off without. (p. 306)

2. We need clear definitions about the distinctions between religious belief and spirituality. Most of us consider ourselves to be spiritual people. If that's the case, we should all be healthier than we really are. This raises a fundamental research problem. If you ask people whether they are healthy, most people will say yes. When you ask them if they are spiritual or religious, most people will also say yes. If this is the case, how can we determine a link between religious involvement, spirituality, and well-being? Most research studies use self-reports to do this, but one wonders about their accuracy. If we're trying to show connections with mental health, we have to prove that people are spiritual and/or religious and we need behavioral measures of well-being. How might we do this, since most measures of well-being are based on self-reports or on instruments that lack reliability and validity? These several research issues suggest great difficulty in showing links between well-being and spiritual or religious convictions, beliefs and involvement. The wise consumer will pay great attention to a study's methodology before using the findings.

3. Do all religious groups have an equally positive impact on health and mental health? We know that some religious groups are antagonistic toward gays and lesbians. Some groups are exclusionary and believe that non-members are inferior. Some religious groups have moral codes that demand such high commitment that most people break those codes with resulting feelings of guilt. Can these groups have a positive impact on the health and mental health of participants? In responding to these issues, George et al. (2000) note that, "[g]roups of people who feel that their

religion has harmed them should be studied in depth. It also would be helpful to study people who profess no religious or spiritual involvement. These patterns may have different implications for health" (p. 112).

4. Do religious affiliation and spirituality actually answer questions about life meaning considered so important to good health and mental health? Many people see religious attendance as primarily a social experience and not as an existential one. Rauch (2003) finds that many people have only a vague notion of the theology of their religion and then are tolerant of other people's belief to such a degree that Rauch has coined the term, "apatheist" to describe someone "Who cares little about one's own religion and has an even stronger disinclination to care about other people's" (p. 34).

5. Is it religious attendance that impacts health? That appears to be a rather vague concept. We all know people who attend religious services and are not ethical, healthy, or spiritual. And how do we resolve the dilemma of people saying they attend religious services when they don't? These concerns have major significance for attempts to relate religious attendance to better health and mental health.

6. Does becoming spiritual or religious late in life have any relevance for overall health? For religious affiliation and spirituality to be significant, shouldn't it occur early in life when the positive effects of either would have their most compelling impact? George et al. (2000) believe that we need to know more about a person's religious or spiritual history. Most current research focuses on a person's current religious or spiritual involvement, but to really see a connection between religious involvement and well-being, designs must be longitudinal in nature and should consider a person's life course. George et al. (2000) write, "Does a lifetime of religious involvement have greater health benefits than a shorter, more recent history of spirituality? What about dramatic changes in one's involvement (e.g., conversion experiences, switching denominations, losses of faith)? Any or all of these might have differential effects on health" (p. 112).

7. Are men, women, and diverse ethnic and racial groups equally affected by religious/spiritual involvement? Was the composition of religious groups studied in the research offered in this chapter

mostly mainstream? And if so, how would marginal groups fare whose practices are sometimes thought to be cultish, disturbing, and even unlawful?

8. Is SES a better explanation for good health and mental health than religious and spiritual involvement? Are healthy communities more important to health and mental health than religious and/or spiritual involvement? A good study should factor in all the probable variables to explain well-being and test them against one another to determine which of the variables has the most positive or negative impact. Religious and spiritual involvement may be influenced by where one lives, the safety of a community, friendships, support networks, and finances, to name only a few potential reasons for good physical and emotional health. Some congregations require very high membership dues or tithing of a certain amount of income, requirements that may actually drive people away from religion. Might the greater the amount one pays for dues be a stronger influence than positive associations with the religious experience? Might tithing represent a sort of spiritual investment in the future that is more superstitious than real? If one tithes or pays higher dues, might this encourage people to believe that their experiences in life and in the afterlife will be more positive? In other words, is the amount of money paid a more powerful influence on well-being than the actual religious experience?

9. Does membership in groups that give people a sense of purpose (self-help groups, therapy groups, community action groups, political groups, charitable involvement) have an equally positive impact on health and mental health when compared to religious involvement and spirituality?

10. While some of the writers in this chapter suggest that helping professionals should discuss issues of religion and spirituality with clients, is that a good idea and might the practitioner lose objectivity in the process? Clinicians working with clients who have a fundamentalist approach to religion may have a difficult time containing their bias. Religious discussions may also lead to proselytizing by the practitioner. These issues certainly need to be explored more fully before clinicians are encouraged to become involved in issues pertaining to religious and spiritual beliefs.

11. Are people who are inclined to become spiritually or religiously involved more likely to be physically and emotionally healthy to begin with? The study of the religious order of women in the Midwest seems to suggest this.

12. Is there a hierarchy in power between religious involvement and spirituality? Is one more significant to well-being than the other? How do we deal with people who are deeply ambivalent about religion, have no real philosophy regarding life meaning, and don't think of themselves as spiritual but are, nonetheless, very good people who are also physically and emotionally healthy?

13. And a fundamental final question: Is it even possible to study the impact of religious and spiritual involvement because of the methodological problems inherent in such research? Going to church, saying you believe in God, and finding meaning in religious observances are not easily quantifiable issues. Just saying that a relationship exists between attendance and better health may be entirely spurious. Can methodologies be constructed that avoid spurious arguments and provide meaningful answers? This is a fundamental question we need to ask when we continue research efforts to find the relationship between religious involvement, spirituality, and well-being.

EVIDENCE-BASED PRACTICE WITH A FUNDAMENTALIST CLIENT: A CASE STUDY

Joan Byers is a 69-year-old woman whose anxiety and panic attacks brought her to a mental health clinic in rural Arkansas. She is being seen for the first time by a clinical social worker. Joan believes she is being punished by God for the sins she committed as a young women when she had an abortion after an affair with a married man. Joan has felt increasing guilt about the abortion since her daughter lost a child when Joan's son-in-law accidentally ran the child over in the driveway of their home. Joan belongs to a fundamentalist church that is generally antagonistic toward mental health services and therapy, believing that the church and God can cure everything and that therapists are basically sinful people who are Godless in their beliefs. Joan is assigned to a social worker without strong religious beliefs.

The worker allowed Joan to talk about her fears that the worker would try and change her beliefs, and that in the process Joan would alienate God even more so than she's alienated him now. The worker told Joan that these were good concerns to have and if she ever felt she was discouraging Joan from her religious beliefs that she should confront the worker in no uncertain terms. Joan wants some suggestions from the worker about how to lessen her anxiety and panic attacks. She refuses to take medication, saying that it's something the Devil would give her to make her lose her belief in God. After taking a psychosocial history and setting some goals for treatment, the worker made an appointment for the next day.

The worker immediately went to the literature to find treatment approaches that might reduce Joan's anxiety without alienating her, and found a description of the Life Review Technique (LRT). Lewis (2001) says that LRT can be useful in resolving past conflicts. Webster and Young (1988) believe that the life review can "help clients reach a sense of acceptance or integrity" (Tobias et al. (1995), p. 218). Lewis (2001) notes that "discussing spirituality as part of a life review may erode the misperception that a psychologist would ignore spiritual concerns in counseling, build trust, and facilitate the development of the therapeutic relationship" (p. 235).

The next day the worker asked Joan to tell her about Joan's journey toward her religious beliefs. Joan was able to do this and provided the worker with a fairly concise personal history in the process. Her abortion had prompted a search for meaning that had included many different churches and religions. "When I found The Gospel of the Church of Jesus Christ it seemed right for me. It's strict and there's no compromising, but when I let Jesus into my life it made a lot of pain go away and I felt content until this awful tragedy with my grandson. Then all the bad feelings I had about myself, they just came back. I asked the preacher about it and we prayed together and read scripture, but God had left me then and it didn't do no good. Seeing how much I was hurting, the preacher said I should see a doctor, which I did, and he said I should come here for help. I told the preacher, and the people in the church had a meeting. They decided that if I could find someone who would respect my beliefs that it would be fine so long as I asked Jesus to be with me and to comfort me."

The worker asked Joan if she wanted to talk about the abortion in more detail. "Well, it hurts, you know, but I was in love with the man. I knew he was married, but my young heart had gone wild and I hadn't accepted Jesus yet, so I didn't have no support in my life to be strong. It was a sin to get pregnant and a worse sin to kill my baby. No other way to see it. I should suffer for my sins and God is right to make me so upset. Still, I got to work, old as I am, and if this worrying gets any worse, I can't be at my job. At my age, I'll never get another one."

The worker wondered if her pastor had given her any advice that she could use to help with the anxiety. "Yup, he said God was testing me and if I came through this as good as I came through the abortion and finding my way to Jesus, then I'd be a cinch to be in heaven with my Savior and my baby. He said my baby was alive in heaven and just waiting for me." Joan said she had tried everything in her to capture the strength she'd had earlier in life but the anxiety only got worse. The worker wondered if Joan had any ideas why. Joan thought for a minute or two and said, "I'm old, and sad, and I don't have the strength I had when I was young. And maybe I wonder if my beliefs are really strong enough. I mean lots of times I think I go to church for the social events and I know that my beliefs aren't so strong; not as strong as some. Maybe God is testing me."

They spoke more about Joan's life. The worker asked if Joan could think of a reason why God was testing her. Joan thought for a long time and then began to cry. Between her tears she said, "I never liked that son-in-law of mine. He's mean to my daughter and he drinks. I wanted to take my daughter away from him before this ever happened and I couldn't do it. When my grandson got killed, my son-in-law was drunk. He just run over the baby and kept driving, and no one has seen him since. And I feel that the whole thing was my fault, I truly do."

Joan came back several days later and told the worker that her anxiety had improved. "I don't know why but I never admitted to anyone that I felt responsible for my grandson's death. You let me think about that and to set myself right with Jesus. I went home and I prayed, and you know what? I could feel a big weight off my shoulders. After I prayed, I opened the Bible and this is the first thing I came to: 'For everything there is a season and a time for every matter under heaven. A time to be born, and a time to die; a time to kill, and a time to heal' (Ecclesiastics 3.1). I saw it as a sign, and when I woke up the next morning, I felt better. Maybe not as good as gold, but much better, and I thank you. My faith is stronger than ever and I feel better. Maybe it's a miracle that you was the one I worked with."

Joan left therapy after three sessions. Several days after Joan's last appointment the pastor of the church called the worker and asked if they could chat a bit about how the clinic could work with some of the folks in the church who once in a while had problems that were beyond his ability to help. If Joan could get so much better and have her faith restored, other people might benefit. The worker met with the pastor who invited her to a service and to talk after the service about what she did and how she worked. The visit went well and periodically members of the church would call and ask to only see her. She, of course, always agreed but thinks it's ironic that someone who has very weak feelings about religion would find themselves identified as the "religious counselor."

Discussion

In discussing her work with Joan, the worker said that she felt very uncomfortable talking to Joan about religious issues. She still does but "people with fundamentalist beliefs sometimes have serious emotional problems. You can't turn them away, and you certainly don't want to challenge their beliefs or you'll very likely drive them away. So you listen and if you can be neutral about religion and understand that it's an important factor in some people's lives, then you get your cues from the client. Clients let you know what they want, and what they usually want is not to hurt so much emotionally. That's my job – to lessen pain. I think I can do that while respecting people's beliefs and not creating needless conflict by challenging those beliefs. And I think there is a growing literature to guide our work with religious issues that can be very useful. If you work in a part of the country where people take their beliefs very seriously you know that to be condescending or superior about religion is going to alienate clients and then, who have you helped and whose needs have you met?"

13.10 SUMMARY

This chapter reports a number of positive studies showing a relationship between religious and spiritual involvement and better health and mental health. Concerns are raised about methodological problems and whether positive findings suggest a role for mental health practitioners. The chapter notes the attempts to change curricula in programs training helping professionals to include content on religious and spiritual beliefs and the difficult nature of the process. Even so, many professionals believe that these issues are fundamental to client well-being and that the effective practitioner should know about religious and spiritual belief and use them, in some fashion, in their work with clients. Two case studies of clients with religious concerns are provided along with the approach to treatment used by each worker.

13.11 QUESTIONS FROM THE CHAPTER

1. Do you think religious and spiritual issues should be acknowledged and even discussed in our work with older adult clients? Give compelling reasons why you do or don't feel this way.

2. Much of the chapter deals with the religious experience. Research on spirituality seems much less in evidence and was only mentioned in passing. Why do you think this is the case?
3. How would you explain people who regularly attend religious services, are observant, but are not "good" people (they're unethical, unhelpful to others, bigoted, self-centered, do illegal things, etc.)?
4. How can religions that have unhealthy beliefs about other people have a healthy impact on participants, particularly older adults facing end-of-life issues?
5. Would you become involved in discussions of religious and spiritual practices with clients? If so, would there be limits to the discussion? What might they be?

REFERENCES

Amato-von Hemert, K. (1994). Point/counterpoint. Should social work education address religious issues? Yes! *Journal of Social Work Education, 30*, 7–11.

Antonovsky, A. (1980). *Health, stress, and coping*. San Francisco: Jossey-Bass.

Asser, S. M., & Swan, K. (1998). Child fatalities from religion-motivated medical neglect. *Pediatrics, 101*, 625–629.

Baetz, M., Larson, D. B., Marcoux, G., Bowen, R., & Griffin, R. (2002). Canadian Psychiatric Inpatient Religious Commitment: An Association with Mental Health. *Canadian Journal of Psychiatry, 47*(2), 159–167.

Balk, D. E. (1999). Bereavement and spiritual change. *Death Studies, 23*(6), 485–493.

Batson, C. D., & Ventis, W. L. (1982). *The religious experience. A social-psychological perspective*. New York: Oxford University Press.

Blazer, D. (1991). Spirituality and aging well. *Generations, 15*(1), 61–65.

Boorstein, S. (2000). Transpersonal psychotherapy. *American Journal of Psychotherapy, 54*(3), 408–423.

Bracki, M. A., & Thibault, J. M. (1990). *Generations, 14*(4), 55–59.

Brown, D. R., & Gary, L. E. (1991). Religious socialization and educational attainment among African Americans: An empirical assessment. *Journal of Negro Education, 3*, 411–426.

Butler, R. N. (1963). The life review: An interpretation of reminiscence in the aged. *Psychiatry, 26*, 65–76.

Canda, E. R. (1988). Spirituality, religious diversity, and social work practice. *Social Casework, 69*, 238–247.

Comstock, G. W., & Partridge, K. B. (1972). Church attendance and health. *Journal of Chronic Diseases, 25*, 665–672.

Danner, D. D., Snowdon, D. A., & Friesen, W. V. (2001). Positive emotions in early life and longevity: Findings from the nun study. *Journal of Personality and Social Psychology, 80*(5), 804–813.

Dembner, A. (2005). *Scientists attempt to measure what religions accept on faith.* The Boston *Globe* (July). Retrieved from the Internet 7.06.2007 <http://www. boston.com/news/globe/health_science/articles/2005/07/25/a_prayer_for_ health?mode = PF/>

Derezotes, D. S. (1995). Spirituality and religiosity: Neglected factors in social work practice. *Arête, 20*(1), 1–15.

Dossey, L. (1997). *Prayer is good medicine: How to reap the healing benefits of prayer.* San Francisco, CA: Harper Publisher.

Dudley, J. R., & Helfgott, C. (1990). Exploring a place for spirituality in the social work curriculum. *Journal of Social Work Education, 26*(3), 287–294.

Ellison, C. G., & Levin, J. S. (1998). The religion-health connection: Evidence theory and future directions. *Health Education and Behavior, 25*, 700–720.

Ellison, G., Boardman, J. D., Williams, D. R., & Isaacson, J. S. (2001). Religious involvement, stress and mental health: Findings from the 1995 Detroit area study. *Social Forces, 80*(1), 215–235.

Emery, E. E., & Pargament, K. I. (2004). The many faces of religious coping in late life: Conceptualization, measurement, and links to well-being. *Aging International, 29*(1), 3–27.

Emrick, C. D. (1987). Alcoholics Anonymous: Affiliative processes and effectiveness as treatment. *Alcoholism: Clinical and Experimental Research, 12*, 416–423.

Enstrom, J. E. (1978). Cancer and total mortality among active Mormons. *Cancer, 42*(19), 13–1951.

Enstrom, J. E. (1989). Health practices and cancer mortality among active California Mormons. *Journal of the National Cancer Institute, 81*, 807–1814.

Frankl, V. E. (1978). *Psychotherapy and existentialism: Selected papers on logotherapy.* New York: Touchstone Books.

Gardner, J., & Lyon, J. L. (1982). Cancer in Utah Mormon men by lay priesthood level. *American Journal of Epidemiology, 116*, 243–257.

Gartner, J., Larson, D. B., & Allen, G. D. (1991). Religious commitment and mental health: A review of the empirical literature. *Journal of Psychology and Theology, 19*, 625.

George, L. K. (1992). Social factors and the onset and outcome of depression. In K. W. Schaie, J. S. House, & D. G. Blazer (Eds.), *Aging, health behaviors, and health outcomes* (pp. 137–159). Hillsdale, NJ: Erlbaum.

George, L. K., Larsson, D. B., Koenig, H. G., & McCullough, M. E. (2000). Spirituality and health: What we know, what we need to know. *Journal of Social and Clinical Psychology, 19*(1), 102–116.

Glicken, M. D., & Fraser, L. (2004). Spiritual and religious belief. In M. D. Glicken, *Using the strengths perspective in social work practice* (pp. 65–76). Boston, MA: Allyn and Bacon/Longman.

Greenstein, M., & Breitbart, W. (2000). Cancer and the experience of meaning: A group psychotherapy program for people with cancer. *American Journal of Psychotherapy, 54*(4), 486–500.

Haight, W. L. (1998, May). "Gathering the spirit" at First Baptist Church: Spirituality as a protective factor in the lives of African American children. *Social Work, 43*(3).

Haight, B. K., Michel, Y., & Hendrix, S. (1998). Life review: Preventing despair in newly relocated nursing home residents – short- and long-term effects. *International Journal of Aging and Human Development, 47,* 142–199.

Harris, R. C., Dew, MA., & Lee, A. (1995). The association of social relationships and activities with mortality: Prospective evidence from the Tecumseh Community Health Study. *American Journal of Epidemiology, 116,* 123–140.

Idler, E. L. (1987). Religious involvement and the health of the elderly: Some hypotheses and an initial test. *Social Forces, 66,* 226–238.

Idler, E. L., & Kasl, S. V. (1992). Religion; disability, depression, and the timing of death. *American Journal of Sociology, 97,* 1052–1079.

Idler, E. L., & Kasl, S. V. (1997). Religion among disabled elderly persons II: Attendance at religious services as a predictor of the course of disability. *Journal of Gerontology: Social Sciences*, S306–S316.

Kaczorowski, J. M. (1989). Spiritual well-being and anxiety in adults diagnosed with cancer. *Hospice Journal, 5,* 105–126.

Koening, H. G. (1998). *The healing power of faith.* New York: Simon & Schuster.

Koenig, H.G. (in press). Does religiosity contribute to the remission of depression? *Harvard Mental Health Letter.*

Koenig, H. G., Larson, D. B., & Matthews, D. A. (1996). Religion and psychotherapy with older adults. *Journal of Geriatric Psychiatry, 29,* 155–184.

Koenig, H. G., George, L. K., Cohen, H. J., Hays, J. C., Larson, D. B., & Blazer, D. G. (1998). The relationship between religious activities and smoking in older adults. *Journal of Gerontology: Medical Science, 53A,* M426–M434.

Kissman, K., & Maurer, L. (2002). East meets west: Therapeutic aspects of spirituality in health, mental health and addiction recovery. *International Social Work, 45*(1), 35–44.

Krucoff, M. and Crater, S. (1998). *Paper presented at the american heart association national meeting*, Dallas, Texas.

Kubler-Ross, E. (1969, 1997). *On death and dying.* New York: Touchstone.

Lajoie, D. H., & Shapiro, S. Y. (1992). Definitions of transpersonal psychology: the first twenty-three years. *Journal of Transpersonal Psychology, 24*(1), 79–98.

Landis, B. J. (1996). Uncertainty, spiritual well-being, and psychosocial adjustment to chronic illness. *Issues in Mental Health Nursing, 27,* 217–231.

Larson, D. B., Koenig, H. G., Kaplan, B. H., & Levin, J. S. (1989). The impact of religion on men's blood pressure. *Journal of Religion and Health, 28,* 265–278.

Lewis, M. M. (2001). Spirituality, counseling, and elderly: An introduction to the spiritual life review. *Journal of Adult Development, 8*(4), 231–240.

Lyon, L., Klauber, M. R., & Gardner, J. Y. (1976). Cancer incidence in Mormons and non-Mormons in Laah, 1966–1970. *New England Journal of Medicine, 294,* 129–133.

Manheimer, R. J. (Ed.). (1994). *Older Americans Almanac*. Detroit: Gale Research.

Medalie, J. H., Kahn, H. A., Neufeld, H. N., Riss, E., & Goldbourt, U. (1973). Five-year myocardial infarction incidence II: Association of single variables to age and birthplace. *Journal of Chronic Disease, 26*, 329–349.

Montgomery, H. A., Miller, W. R., & Tonigan, J. S. (1995). Does Alcoholics Anonymous involvement predict treatment outcome? *Journal of Substance Abuse Treatment, 22*, 241–246.

Musick, M. A. (1996). Religion and subjective health among black and white elders. *Journal of Health and Social Behavior, 37*, 221–237.

National Institute on Aging/Fetzer Institute Working Group (1997). *Measurement scale on religion, spirituality, health, and aging*. Bethesda, MD: National Institute an Aging.

O'Brien, M. E. (1982). Religious faith and long-term adjustment to hemodialysis. *Journal of Religion and Health, 21*, 68–80.

Phillips, R. L., Kuzma, J., & Beeson, W. L. (1980). Influence of selection versus lifestyle on risk of fatal cancer and cardiovascular disease among Seventh Day Adventists. *American Journal of Epidemiology, 112*, 296–314.

Project MATCH Research Group. (1997). Matching alcoholism treatments to client heterogeneity: Project MATCH posttreatment drinking outcomes). *Journal of Studies on Alcohol, 58*, 7–29.

Rauch, J. (2003). Let it be. *Atlantic Monthly, 291*(4), 34.

Seaborn-Thompson, M., & Ensminger, M. E. (1989). Psychological well-being among mothers with school age children: Evolving family structures. *Social Forces, 67*, 715–730.

Sheridan, M.J. (2000). The use of spiritually-derived interventions in social work practice. *46th Annual Program Meeting of the Council on Social Work Education, 1*, 22.

Sheridan, M. J., Bullis, R. K., Adcock, C. R., Berlin, S. D., & Miller, P. C. (1992). Practitioners' personal and professional attitudes and behaviors toward religion and spirituality: Issues for social work education and practice. *Journal of Social Work Education, 28*, 190–203.

Sheridan, M. J., Wilmer, C. M., & Atcheson, L. (1994). Inclusion of content on religion and spirituality in the social work curriculum. *Journal of Social Work Education, 30*(3), 363–377.

Simpson, W. F. (1989). Comparative longevity in a college cohort of Christian Scientists. *Journal of the American Medical Association, 262*, 1657–1658.

Sloan, R. P., & Bagiella, E. (2001). Spirituality and medical practice: A look at the evidence. *American Family Physician, 63*(1), 33–34.

Spiegel, D., Bloom, J. R., & Kraemer, H. C. (1989). Effect of psychosocial treatment on survival of patients with metastatic breast cancer. *Lancet, 142*, 888–897.

Thoresen, C. E. (1990). *Long-term 8-year follow-up of recurrent coronary prevention (monograph)*. Uppsola, Sweden: International Society of Behavioral Medicine.

Tobias, M., Morrison, J., & Gray, B. (Eds.), (1995). *A parliament of souls.* San Francisco: KQED Books.

Webster, J. D., & Young, R. A. (1988). Process variables of the life review: Counseling implications. *International Journal of Aging and Human Development, 26*(4), 315–323.

Zimmerman, M. A., & Maton, K. I. (1992). Life-style and substance use among male African American urban adolescents: A cluster analytic approach. *American Journal of Community Psychology, 20,* 121–138.

Zuckerman, D. M., Kasl, S. V., & Ostfeld, A. M. (1984). Psychosocial predictors of mortality among the elderly poor: The role of religion, well-being, and social contacts. *American Journal of Epidemiology, 179,* 410–423

Chapter | fourteen

Evidence-Based Practice and the Effectiveness of Self-Help Groups with Older Adults

14.1 INTRODUCTION

This chapter discusses the benefits of self-help groups in the treatment of health and mental health problems for older adults. Because there is such passion for self-help groups in the absence of supportive data, the chapter considers the available research information on the treatment effectiveness of self-help groups and the reasons self-help groups have become so popular in the USA. In suggesting the need for cooperation among human service professionals and self-help groups, Humphreys and Ribisl (1999) note that "self-help groups can provide benefits that the best health care often does not: identification with other sufferers, long-term support and companionship, and a sense of competence and empowerment" (p. 326). However, Kessler et al. (1997a) caution that self-help groups will "never be a substitute for professional care. Such groups should not be looked to as a cheap and quick fix to the health care crisis" (p. 27).

14.2 DEFINING SELF-HELP GROUPS

Wituk et al. (2000) write that "self-help groups consist of individuals who share the same problem or concern. Members provide emotional support to one another, learn ways to cope, discover strategies for improving their condition, and help others while helping themselves" (p. 157). The authors indicate that an estimated 25 million Americans have been involved in self-help groups at some point during their lives (Kessler et al., 1997a). Positive outcomes have been found in groups treating substance abuse (Humphreys and Moos, 1996), bereavement (Caserta and Lund, 1993), care giving (McCallion and Toseland, 1995), diabetes (Gilden et al., 1992), and depression (Kurtz, 1990, 1997). Riessman (2000) reports that, "More Americans try to change their health behaviors through self-help than through all other forms of professional programs combined" (p. 47).

Kessler et al. (1997b) indicate that 40% of all therapeutic sessions for psychiatric problems reported by respondents in a national survey were in the self-help sector, as compared to 35.2% receiving specialized mental health services, 8.1% receiving help from the general physicians medical sector, and 16.5% receiving help from social service agencies. Wuthnow (1994) found that self-help groups are the most prevalent organized support groups in the USA today. The author estimated that eight to ten million Americans are members of self-help groups and that there are at least 500,000 self-help groups in the USA.

Fetto (2000) notes a study done by the University of Texas at Austin that found that approximately 25 million people will participate in self-help groups at some point in their lives, and that eight to 11 million people participate in self-help groups each year. Men are somewhat more likely to attend groups than women and Caucasians are three times as likely to attend self-help groups as African-Americans. This number is expected to be much higher with the full use of the Internet as a tool for self-help. Participants most likely to attend self-help groups are those diagnosed with alcoholism, cancer (all types), diabetes, AIDS, depression, and chronic fatigue syndrome. Those least likely to attend suffer from ulcers, emphysema, chronic pain and migraines, in that order (Fetto, 2000).

Riessman (1997) identifies the following principles defining the function and purpose of self-help groups:

1. members share a similar condition and understand each other;
2. members determine activities and policies that make self-help groups very democratic and self-determining;

3. helping others is therapeutic;
4. self-help groups build on the strengths of the individual members, the group, and the community, charge no fees, and are not commercialized;
5. self-help groups function as a social support system that helps participants cope with traumas through supportive relationships between members;
6. values are projected that define the intrinsic meaning of the group to its members;
7. self-help groups use the expertise of members to help one another;
8. seeking assistance from a self-help group is not as stigmatizing as it may be when seeking help from a health or mental health provider; and
9. self-help groups focus on the use of self-determination, inner strength, self-healing, and resilience.

Wituk et al. (2000), studied the characteristics of self-help groups and report the following:

1. groups had been in existence an average of eight years and 30% met weekly with an average attendance of 13 participants;
2. 20 new members joined the group in the prior year;
3. 68% of the participants were female, and minority participation was proportionally in keeping with the minority population of the regions studied;
4. group outreach was usually done by word of mouth, but some groups used newspaper ads and radio and television spot ads;
5. 34% of the groups were peer led with some professional involvement, 28% were led by professionals, and 27% had no professional involvement, while 86% of the groups had two or more members acting in leadership capacities;
6. the primary function of the groups was to provide emotional and social support to members (98% of the groups reporting), while 32% provided information and education, and 58% provided advocacy services for members and their families;
7. 77% of the groups felt that networking with the larger community was important and did this through guest speakers, buddy systems, training seminars open to the public, and social events open to the community;
8. a large majority of the groups held meetings in very easily accessible places. Many offered childcare during meetings,

transportation, and bi-lingual meetings for non-English-speaking participants;

9. over half the groups had national affiliations and reported a great deal of help from these organizations through brochures, newsletters, conferences and workshops, but very little helped with finances or information about advances in research;

10. 75% of the groups had local affiliations with hospitals, churches, and social service agencies; and

11. the self-help groups were very well connected to the professional community.

14.3 THE INDIGENOUS LEADERS OF SELF-HELP GROUPS

Patterson and Marsiglia (2000) note remarkable similarities in the characteristics of two cohorts of natural helpers coming from two distinct geographic locations in the USA. Those similarities include offering assistance to family and friends before it was asked for, an attempt to reduce stress in those helped and a desire to help strengthen coping skills. Lewis and Suarez (1995) have identified the primary functions of indigenous helpers as buffers between individuals and sources of stress, providers of social support, and information and referral sources and lay consultants. Waller and Patterson (2002) believe that indigenous helpers strengthen the social bond that holds communities together through a sense of civic responsibility that increases the well-being of individuals and communities.

Patterson et al. (1972) found that natural helpers used one of three helping styles: (1) active listening and encouragement, emphasizing positives about the client, and suggesting alternative solutions to problems; (2) direct intervention by doing something for the client that has an immediate impact; and (3) a combination of numbers one and two in a way that fits the client's needs. Memmott (1993), however, found little difference between natural helpers and professionals, although natural helpers were more inclined to advocate and intervene on behalf of the client than professionals, tended to think much less about causal reasons for a client's problems than professionals, and used direct methods of help that were atheoretical but often sound.

Robert Bly (1985) suggests that we seek out others in the community, our close family, or people in our work environment for advice and support. He calls these natural helpers "People of Wisdom," because they listen well, are empathic and sensitive, and are known for their expertise in solving certain types of problems. We gravitate to these people because they help us in unobtrusive and informal ways, which are often profoundly subtle since the lack of formal training by natural helpers is offset by their kindness, patience, common sense, and good judgment.

When older adults were used as volunteers, the evaluation of the Family Friends program found that volunteer home visitors age 55 and older significantly reduced hospitalization rates among chronically ill and disabled children and improved the overall well-being of parents and families (Rinck and Naragon, 1995). When adolescents with behavioral problems or struggles in school were linked with older mentors in the Across Ages program, they showed improved class attendance, more positive attitudes toward school, and reductions in substance use (Rogers and Taylor 1997). More generally, Wheeler et al. (1998) reviewed 37 studies across a variety of program models and found that 85% of the individuals served by older adults showed significantly improved results. Nonprofits increasingly rely on volunteers, a significant portion of whom are older adults.

Over 6 in 10 nonprofits report working with volunteers between the ages of 65 and 74 (VolunteerMatch, 2007). Volunteers who manage or deliver social services allow nonprofits to save money and get more done, extending the reach of their staff and stabilizing their resources (Rabiner et al., 2003). Finally, both paid work and formal volunteer activities benefit the economy. Johnson and Schaner (2006) value formal volunteering activities among older adults at $44.3 billion in 2002. Paid work also increases the retirement security of older adults. Even a few additional years can significantly boost retirement income, especially among lower-paid workers (Butrica et al., 2006).

CASE STUDY: AN OLDER ADULT INDIGENOUS LEADER STARTS A SELF-HELP GROUP FOR DEPRESSED OLDER ADULTS

Thanks to Sage Publications for permission to use this case, which first appeared in Glicken (2005, pp. 269–271).

Jack Holden is a 71 year-old leader of a support group for older adults with chronic depression. Jack has been depressed much of his life and has come to believe that it's a condition he has to live with, much as he would if he had diabetes or heart problems. Jack is a kind and empathic person, and after reading about a support group for depressed people in another community, Jack volunteered his time to organize a similar group in his community. In preparing for this commitment, Jack met with a number of other leaders of various types of support groups in the community and attended meetings of a local volunteer organization in town to get additional ideas. He wrote to a national organization for depressed people asking for assistance in setting up a group. They sent him a kit that explained how one might go about developing a group that included many practical ideas about advertising, screening people, where to hold meetings, and how to plan an agenda. Jack was able to use free ads in local newspapers and some spot ads on radio and television. Even so, the response was slow and Jack almost gave up. After four months, he had 10 names of people over 60 who wanted to be part of the group and who were willing to help in its organization.

The group met over a two-month period and, much to Jack's delight, they were willing to work hard, entered into some very useful discussions about the mission and focus of the group, and asked Jack to be their leader under the supervision of a professional from the community who had agreed to help. The professional gave Jack some books to read on group leadership, and the national association Jack had contacted held a one-week leadership workshop for new leaders. Jack found the experience invaluable. During the first several meetings of the new self-help group, the professional observed the group, but after that she assured Jack that what he was doing was just fine. She agreed to meet with him periodically to discuss the group and to enter into a loose supervisory arrangement. She assured Jack that if there was a crisis, he could always call and that they would immediately meet to discuss it. They also decided that if any member was unwilling to promise not to commit suicide, if this came up in discussion or if group members were concerned about the possibility that the professional would be contacted, a further assessment would be done by the professional. Thankfully, this has never happened in the three years the group has been actively meeting.

Gradually, the group has settled in with about 15 regular members, most of whom are dealing with issues related to failing health, retirement and the illness of a significant other. That's about all Jack thinks he can handle at one time. A few people have left the group because it hasn't worked for them, but others have taken their place. There are 20 people on the waiting list and Jack is trying to organize another group to be led by one of the current members with very strong leadership skills. The group meets once a week for two hours in the evening. All of the members have suffered from chronic depression for more than two years, and all of the members actively see professionals in therapy or are being seen medically to monitor medication. The mission of the group is to offer support, encouragement, help with problem solving, to plan social events to help group members stay socially active, and to disseminate and discuss research information about depression. All the members are responsible for sending one another new articles or research reports via the Internet at least once or twice a month. The group has become so adept at finding new literature that many have brought information to their therapists or psychiatrists that were new even to them. The professionals have found that group members who take a very active role in their treatment are also people who do much better in their lives, even though they continue to feel depressed some of the time. Depression, for many of the participants, is a struggle, but one they have learned to live with as a result of a combination of professional care and the self-help group.

The group believes that it should evaluate whether its work is helpful and has developed a testing instrument that measures life functioning in several key areas, including excessive sleep, exercise, weight, blood pressure, attendance at social events, reports from spouses, mates, or friends providing a weekly social functioning measure, and a 20-question depression inventory with good reliability and validity called the CES-D (Radloff, 1977). A copy of the CES-D can be found in the Appendix to this chapter. Over time, the use of an evaluation mechanism has shown a gradual improvement in social functioning. People exercise more, maintain normal weight, sleep less than before joining the group, and have less depression through reports from others and on scores from the depression instrument. Depression hasn't gone away completely for most participants, but they have learned to live with it and to get on with their lives more successfully than before.

This author observed the group. It is a kind, supportive, and warm group and many people have benefited from Jack's unobtrusive and affirming leadership approach. One group member said:

> Jack is so warm and kind, it filters down to the group. People come here and they're pessimistic and hopeless about their depression, but after a few weeks, Jack's optimism is contagious. We all suffer together and depression is an awful thing, but we love one another, we love Jack, and we all live with the hope that we will get better. If Jack left, we'd fall apart. Maybe that's not a good thing to admit but Jack is the glue that holds us together. I don't mind saying that. He's a wonderful person, and that he suffers from depression like the rest of us makes us love him that much more. There are days when he's too depressed to lead the group and others fill in. We have a buddy system that gives us

people to talk to when things get too tough. We go out together for dinner and socialize some. It's like the extended family many of us don't have anymore. We're lonely and isolated people and having this group is the best thing that's ever happened to me. And I'm glad that we have to maintain our contacts with professionals. It's a safety valve, in my opinion. Depressed people run a high risk of committing suicide. Were it not for the group and the professionals we work with, I couldn't promise not to do it if the feeling came over me really strongly. But the support network we've developed and the professional help keep us from going to extremes, and they give us hope. And for people who feel down most of the time, that's saying a lot.

14.4 BEST EVIDENCE OF THE EFFECTIVENESS OF SELF-HELP GROUPS

The Surgeon General's Report on Mental Health and Older Adults (Satcher, 1999) indicates that:

> Despite the scant body of research, there is reason to believe that support and self-help group participation is as beneficial, if not more beneficial, for older people with mental disorders. Older people tend to live alone and to be more socially isolated than are other people. They also are less comfortable with formal mental health services. Therefore, social networks established through support and self-help groups are thought to be especially vital in preventing isolation and promoting health. Support programs also can help reduce the stigma associated with mental illness, to foster early detection of illnesses, and to improve compliance with formal interventions. (p. 1)

Kessler et al. (1997a) report that while the research is somewhat limited on the subject of the effectiveness of self-help groups, "the little available data suggest that self-help groups are sometimes able to promote emotional recovery from life crises (Emrick et al., 1993; Galanter, 1984, 1988; Lieberman and Borman, 1991; Videcka-Sherman and Lieberman, 1985), [although] methodological limitations make it impossible to draw firm conclusions (Levy, 1984; Humphreys and Rappaport, 1994)" (p. 30). Recognizing the methodological limitations of the research reports summarized next is important for the reader to understand, because self-help groups are not under the same obligation to test for effectiveness as their professional counterparts. For that reason alone, there are a number of explanations for methodological limitations in determining best evidence of the effectiveness of non-professionally led self-help groups. They include the following:

1. Self-help groups pride themselves on confidentiality and sometimes discourage research because it can be intrusive;
2. most self-help groups don't think of themselves as competing with professional helpers and trying to prove their effectiveness isn't seen as part of their mission;
3. there is no real way to force people to accept research responsibilities when services are led by volunteers, free to the public, and make no claims to be alternatives to professional help;
4. the research process sets up barriers to the functioning of self-help groups that may subtly or overtly change the way a group operates;
5. many people attend self-help groups to avoid the way professional treatment sometimes compromises individuality. Adding a research component may make people feel as if they have lost their uniqueness;
6. self-help groups are loosely organized and run. People come and go as they please. It's difficult to make research effective in an atmosphere where the experimental group has only a very loose attendance pattern; and
7. as Kessler et al. (1997a) report, more than half of the people attending self-help groups also receive professional help, making it difficult to determine whether self-help, the professional help, or a combination of both causes improvement. With these caveats in mind, let's consider the data to date on the effectiveness of self-help groups.

14.4.1 Substance abuse

In an evaluation of a large study by *Consumers Reports* on the effectiveness of psychotherapy, Seligman (1995) concluded that, "Alcoholics Anonymous (AA) did especially well … significantly bettering mental health professionals [in the treatment of alcohol and drug related problems]"(p.10). Humphreys and Moos (1996) found that during three years period of study, alcoholics who initially chose Alcoholics Anonymous over professional help had a 45% ($1,826) lower average per-person treatment cost than those receiving professional treatment. Even with the lower costs, A.A. participants had reduced alcohol consumption, fewer number of days intoxicated, and lower rates of depression when compared to alcoholic clients receiving professional help. In follow-up studies, these findings were consistent at one year and three years after the start of the study. Humphreys et al. (1994) report that African-American participants ($N = 253$) in Narcotics Anonymous and Alcoholics Anonymous showed improvements over twelve months in six problem areas (employment, alcohol and drug use, and legal, psychological, and family problems). African- American group members had much more improvement in their medical, alcohol, and drug problems than did African-American patients not involved in self-help groups.

In a meta-analysis of more than 50 studies, Emrick et al. (1993) report that AA members who were also professionally treated were somewhat more likely to reduce drinking than are those who did not attend AA meetings. Membership in AA was also found to reduce physical symptoms and to improve psychological adjustment. Alemi et al. (1996) assigned two groups of pregnant women with substance abuse histories to either a self-help group meeting bi-weekly or to self-help groups operated over a bulletin board accessed by telephone. Bulletin board participants made significantly fewer telephone calls and visits to health care clinics than did the group assigned to participate in the face-to-face group. Both groups had similar health status and drug use at the end of the study.

Christo and Sutton (1994) report that members of Narcotics Anonymous who stayed off drugs for three years or more as a result of their involvement in the group had the same level of anxiety and self-esteem as a random sample of people who had never been drug addicted. McKay et al. (1994) report on African-American participants in self-help groups for substance abuse after a seven-month follow-up. Participants with high rates of attendance at group meetings reduced their use of alcohol and drugs by half as much as those who were poor attenders of meetings. Both groups were similar in their use of substances prior to the start of their group involvement. Tattersall and Hallstrom (1992) report on a self-help group offering telephone counseling and a support group formed to help members reduce their reliance on tranquilizers. Members had been addicted to tranquilizers for more than 12 years on average. Most members of the group reported that the symptoms for which tranquilizers had initially been prescribed had lessened and that 65% were at least moderately satisfied with their withdrawal from tranquilizers as self-evaluated by their quality of life.

14.4.2 Medical problems

Riessman (2000) reports on a project to use self-help groups with older patients suffering from heart disease. Initially the project used patient-led groups to help keep patients on their diet and exercise regimens, but Reissman says that it soon became apparent that, "participation in the groups themselves was one of the most powerful interventions" (p. 48). Spiegelet al. (1989) studied 86 older women receiving treatment for metastatic breast cancer. Fifty of the 86 women were randomly chosen to supplement their ontological care with a weekly support group. The support groups were lead by a psychotherapist with breast cancer in remission and a psychiatrist or social worker. The sessions offered an opportunity to talk about living life fully, improving communication with significant others, coping with death, discussing grief, and controlling pain through self-hypnosis. Support group members lived twice as long as controls, for an average of 18 months longer. Nash and Kramer (1993) studied 57 African-Americans who were involved in self-help groups for sickle-cell anemia. Those involved the longest had the fewest psychological symptoms and the fewest problems from the disease, particularly in work and relationships. Hinrichsen and Revenson (1985) compared older scoliosis patients in a self-help group who had undergone bracing or surgery with patients having the same treatment who were not in a self-help group. Participants in the self-help group had a more positive outlook on life, better satisfaction with their medical care, fewer psychosomatic symptoms, better self-esteem, and fewer feelings of "shame and estrangement."

14.4.3 Caregiver groups

Toseland et al. (1989) divided 103 adult women caring for frail older relatives into three conditions: participation in a peer-led self-help group, participation in a professionally led support group, and no participation in either group. Groups met for eight weekly two-hour sessions. Both groups focused on enhancing coping skills. Compared to non-participants, women who participated in either type of group experienced significantly greater (1) increases in the size of their support network; (2) increases in their knowledge of community resources;

(3) improvement in their interpersonal skills and ability to deal with the problems of caregiving; (4) improvement in their relationships with their care receivers; and (5) decreases in pressing psychological problems.

14.4.4 Groups for older adults

Lieberman and Bliwise (1985) compared participants (86 women and 22 men) in peer-led and professionally-led SAGE (Senior Actualization and Growth Explorations) self-help groups for the elderly to those who were on a waiting list to join the groups. Members of both types of SAGE groups felt they achieved their desired goals to a greater extent than those in the waiting-list group. Participation in either SAGE group also reduced psychological problems, such as nervousness and depression. Caserta and Lund (1993) found that widows and widowers over age 50 who participated in bereavement self-help groups ($n = 197$) experienced less depression and grief than non-participants ($n = 98$) if their initial levels of interpersonal and coping skills were low. Those with initially high interpersonal skill levels also benefited from participation if they participated in the groups for longer than eight weeks. Lieberman and Videka-Sherman (1986) followed 36 widowers and 466 widows, 376 of whom were members of the bereavement self-help group THEOS. Over a period of one year, THEOS members who formed social relationships with other group members outside group time experienced less psychological distress (depression, anxiety, somatic symptoms) and improved more in psychological functioning (well-being, mastery, self-esteem) than did non-members and members who did not form such relationships.

Marmar et al. (1988) studied bereaved older women who sought treatment for grief after the death of their husbands. The participants were randomly assigned to either professional psychotherapy ($n = 31$) or self-help groups ($n = 30$). Self-help groups worked just as well as the therapy. Participants and non-participants in the self-help groups reduced stress-specific and general psychiatric symptoms such as depression equally. They also experienced similar improvements in social adjustment and work functioning. Vachon et al. (1980) studied women over a two-year period ($N = 162$) whose husbands had died within the past month. Half of these women were assigned to participate in a "widow-to-widow" program. After six months in the program, participants were more likely than non-participants to feel more healthy and to feel "better," and less likely to anticipate a difficult adjustment to widowhood. After 12 months, participants were more likely than non-participants to feel "much better," to have made new friends, and to have begun new activities, and were less likely to feel constantly anxious or to feel the need to hide their true emotions. Participation facilitated adjustment both inside the person (in their relationship with themselves) and outside the person (in their relationships with others).

14.5 Q AND A WITH THE AUTHOR ABOUT THE MEANING OF THESE STUDIES

The following mock question-and-answer exercise is offered to help the reader better understand the limitations, meaning, and practical use of reported findings on the efficacy of self-help groups. Thanks to Sage Publications for permitting the use of this material which first appeared in somewhat modified form in Glicken (2005, pp. 277–280).

Question (Q): Do these studies prove anything?

Answer (A): Probably not. What they *do* show is that people in self-help and support groups report better functioning and a higher level of life satisfaction. Whether that's the case remains to be seen. Self-reports are notoriously susceptible to social desirability. People say positive things about self-help groups even though there may be no empirical evidence that change in social functioning has actually taken place. The halo effect is also likely to influence responses. People in any type of treatment often report better results than may be the case because, in the short run, they may actually feel better and because, in the case of self-help groups, they may feel a sense of loyalty to the group that encourages them to report better social functioning than may be the case. Whether better functioning has actually occurred in the studies cited in this chapter requires evidence that only an empirical study can provide. *Saying* that you feel better is not the same as actually *being* better when social functioning is considered.

Methodological problems are considerable in the measurement of self-help group effectiveness. Ouimette et al. (1997) compared 12-step programs such as AA with cognitive-behavioral programs and programs that combined both approaches. One year after completion of treatment, all three types of programs had similar improvement rates related to alcohol consumption. Participants in 12-step had more "sustained abstinence" and better employment rates than the other two programs, but Ouimette et al. (1997) caution the reader not to make more of these findings than are warranted because of non-random assignment of patients to the different types of treatment. A careful look at many other substance abuse treatment studies suggests similar methodological concerns in a field where empirically based studies are essential if we are to believe and then use the results in treatment. Clifford et al. (2000) reinforce concerns about research methodologies used to study sub-stance abuse programs when they point out that "[i]t is recommended that treatment outcome studies be interpreted cautiously, particularly when the research protocols involve frequent and intensive follow-up interviews conducted across extended periods of time" (p. 741) because many external variables can confound the results and suggest improved functioning as a result of treatment when other factors are more suggestive of the reasons the client has improved.

Q: Shouldn't we feel elated by studies that people live longer or use substances less as a result of self-help groups?

A: Not until the evidence is substantiated by empirical studies using random selection and very scientific methodology. Certainly one should not say that self-help groups are more effective than professional help given the weakness of self-help research to date. Statements such as the following are not warranted: "The emergence of self-help groups may reflect a societal response to failures within the mental health commu-nity. Self-help groups have developed where society has fallen short in meeting the needs of its members." (Felix-Ortiz et al., 2000, p. 339).

Q: But aren't we being too harsh? Isn't it likely that self-help groups, through support and affiliation, help people feel more accepted, appreciated, and cared for, and isn't that important for positive mental health?

A: Certainly, but self-help groups may have short-term benefits that, in the long run, aren't likely to continue, or may actually cause harm. T-Groups and the encounter movement come to mind as examples.

Q: But what's wrong with short-term results if they're positive? Can't we say the same thing about professional treatment?

A: There's nothing wrong with short-term results and professional treatment may have the same limited results as self-help groups. But the studies cited don't permit us to make long-term predictions because they don't show cause–effect relationships between self-help groups and long-term improvement rates. A belief that self-help groups can replace pro-fessional help, without appropriate data, is troubling since it gives people confidence in a treatment that may not actually help and may, in some cases, do harm. During the current health care crisis, suggesting that self-help groups may replace professional help because it works better may leave a large number of clients who desperately need professional help without that option because managed care might increasingly rely on self-help groups to treat a number of serious social, emotional, and medical problems.

Q: So what's the answer?

A: Much more research but, in the meantime, a sense of optimism that perhaps self-help groups are an alternative or at least an adjunct to professional help.

Q: Why feel optimistic in view of the weak research data to support the benefits of self-help groups?

A: A preponderance of positive results tends to suggest that something works. It may not prove that something works, but the weight of the evidence suggests that many self-help groups do help. This should make us optimistic without making us true believers. EBP is a conservative and cautious paradigm. It doesn't accept best evidence until it's been proven. At the same time, the evidence thus far would suggest that we cautiously use the findings. A case study is presented in this chapter that might be instructive about how best to use self-help groups when professional services are also being provided.

Q: Would the author refer a client to self-help group?

A: Yes, but only after meeting with the group leader and evaluating the group objectives to make certain they were consistent with the needs of the client. And even then, I would suggest that the client use high standards and caution before joining the group. I would also want to be involved in a discussion with the client about what was taking place in the group and the client's feelings about the worth of the group. Perhaps contacting current and former group members would also help. If the group is legitimate, I wouldn't mind this happening unless, of course, confidentiality issues are involved.

Q: Aren't you being overly cautious?

A: Yes, but self-help groups, just as professional help, have the potential for doing harm.

Q: Really? What harm could they do?

A: Some self-help groups have been likened to cults. The tendency to make people accept a philosophy through group pressure that may be contrary to their own belief systems or to a process that might not be right for them, and may actually cause harm. Similarly, groups that are badly run may inhibit client progress. Relationships develop among group members that may be harmful, as in the case of substance abusers developing romantic or sexual attachments to one another that lead to more substance abuse. Granfield and Cloud (1996) studied middle class alcoholics who used self-healing approaches alone with neither professional help nor self-help group intervention. Many of the participants felt that the "ideological" base of some self-help groups were in conflict with their own philosophies of life. Concerns were raised that some groups were overly religious, or that alcoholism was seen by the group as a lifelong struggle. The subjects in the study by Granfield and Cloud also felt that some self-help groups encouraged dependence and that associating with other alcoholics would probably make recovery more difficult. In summarizing their findings, the authors concluded:

> Many [research subjects] expressed strong opposition to the suggestion that they were powerless over their addictions. Such an ideology, they explained, not only was counterproductive but was also extremely demeaning. These respondents saw themselves as efficacious people who often prided themselves on their past accomplishments. They viewed themselves as being individualists and strong-willed. One respondent, for instance, explained that "such programs encourage powerlessness" and that she would rather "trust her own instincts than the instincts of others." (Granfield and Cloud, 1996, p. 51)

Q: But couldn't the same thing happen in a professionally led group?

A: Yes, but all professionals are bound by codes of ethics and, in a number of states, licensure laws provide certain protections for clients against extreme behavior by professionals. Non-professional leaders may be less sensitive to inappropriate relationships among group members, or they may not see the harm in developing their own relationship with a group member. Professionals are also guided by a belief that they should respect the rights of clients. That would hopefully eliminate religious proselytizing or other behaviors in conflict with a client's belief system that might be found in some self-help groups.

Q: Doesn't the fact that self-help groups are usually free of cost and are non-discriminating suggest that, at the very least, they may provide a helping intervention that is an alternative to professional help?

A: Yes, but is this a financial argument or an argument about best evidence of effectiveness? Shouldn't clients in need be offered the best help available rather than the help that's cheapest?

Q: Yes, of course, but you can't argue that professional help is always excellent help or that it works, can you?

A: No, I certainly can't, and that's what makes this entire discussion so troubling. When professional help isn't effective, it means that something is fundamentally wrong with our system of treatment. An analogy would be finding that folk healers are more effective than medical doctors. If *that's* the case, we really would need to reexamine what we believe and whether it's worth maintaining that belief.

Q: Don't a lot of people get better on their own? Is it always necessary to compare self-help groups against professional services?

A: Good point. Waldorf et al. (1991) found that many addicted people with supportive elements in their lives (a job, family, and other close emotional supports) were able to "walk away" from their very heavy use of cocaine. The authors suggest that the "social context" of a drug user's life may positively influence their ability to discontinue drug use. Granfield and Cloud (1996) add to the social context notion of recovery by noting that many of the respondents in their sample had a great deal to lose if they continued their substance abuse, and write,

> The respondents in our sample had relatively stable lives: they had jobs, supportive families, high school and college credentials, and other social supports that gave them reasons to alter their drug-taking behavior. Having much to lose gave our respondents incentives to transform their lives. However, when there is little to lose from heavy alcohol or drug use, there may be little to gain by quitting. (p. 55)

Q: So do you feel positively or negatively about self-help groups? You sound awfully negative.

A: Actually, I feel very positively about self-help and I think the research makes a compelling argument that self-help groups may be very effective with a number of health and mental health problems. And, I confess that my heart is in the notion of people helping one another, but in a book on best evidence, I think the jury is still out until we have a substantial body of knowledge to show a relationship between self-help and its level of effectiveness with a range of problems experienced by a cross section of people across gender, age, ethnicity, and socio-economic class. In other words, I would hope self-help groups would develop the same body of research data to show effectiveness that I expect, but often don't find, for services provided by professionals. When that happens, we'll have a basis for comparison. Until then, I'm hopeful and optimistic while still being cautious. I don't believe, however, that self-help is a substitute for professional help and I worry that a health care system in crisis will turn to self-help as a last resort before needed services are withdrawn completely.

CASE STUDY: REFERRAL OF AN OLDER ADULT CLIENT TO A SELF-HELP GROUP FOR SEVERE DEPRESSION

Leonard is a 67-year-old client suffering from chronic depression that has lasted almost five years and began when his wife of 30 years passed away. Leonard is being seen by a psychiatrist to monitor his anti-depression medication and has been in therapy with a clinical psychologist for almost five years. The medication and therapy have a negligible impact and he still suffers from very severe depression that interferes with his retirement plans to start a second career and to travel. Leonard is too depressed to exercise and has become a compulsive eater with almost 100 pounds gained over the past five years. His therapist suggested a self-help group for people with chronic depression as an adjunct to therapy and medication, but Leonard has been unwilling to attend meetings, believing that the group will be as unsuccessful as his current treatments. The therapist arranged for Leonard to meet with the group leader, someone whom, like Leonard, fights chronic depression but has successfully learned to cope with it.

The leader invited Leonard to attend a meeting and asked participants to stay after so they could honestly discuss their feelings about the group and to answer questions Leonard might have about the group's effectiveness. The group leader also shared effectiveness research, which the national chapter of the group had accumulated on the effectiveness of the self-help group across the country that, while subjective and not terribly sound methodologically, still suggested positive results. Over 2,000 former participants of group chapters around the country returned questionnaires. Five thousand questionnaires representing a 10% sample of the 50,000 former national participants in the organization were sent out. Over 70% of the participants who stayed in the group more than two years reported fewer missed days at work, fewer doctor visits, less use of anti-depressants, and fewer days of depression. The average length of depression before the respondents began their group partici-pation was more than five years. Participants who stayed with the group two years or longer had better results than those who discontinued participation before completing a full year of group participation. Those who dropped out of the group early cited personality clashes with the group leader and differences of opinion about the purpose of the group as the major reasons for attrition.

Since Leonard was unwilling to attend the meeting alone, the therapist met him at the group meeting place and sat with him. After group, people spoke about what the group had done to help them. Following the meeting, Leonard shared his positive sense of the group with the therapist and his surprise at how strongly the members felt the experience had helped them. He decided to give it a try and began attending sessions on a regular basis while also seeing his therapist weekly and continuing with his anti-depression medication. After six months as a participant, Leonard told the therapist about the experience: "It's very supportive. Everyone there is like me. They're all older people struggling with depression. The difference is that they get on with their lives. That's what I've begun doing. I've been assigned a woman about my age as a mentor who I call when I feel so down I can't function. We've begun walking together and it's helped me lose weight. I feel a lot of positive acceptance from the other people, and that helps a lot. We have speakers who talk about depression and who keep us informed about the latest research. I've been assigned as a mentor to a new member and surprisingly, he seems to find a lot of solace from our contacts. I still feel really depressed, but while it used to be everyday, now I have good and bad days. Overall, I think I'm less depressed than I was before I started the group. Mainly, I think the support, the camaraderie, the loving environment, and the sense that we're all experts on depression and have something to say worth listening to about how to handle depression are what helps the most. I've made a couple of good friends from the group and instead of staying home and being lonely and blue, I go out to movies or have dinner with my friends. It helps from feeling lonely, which is one of the things depressed people often experience. Do I feel better than I did six months ago? Yes. Is it because of the group? I think some of it is but I have to admit that because of the group, I'm using therapy better. So overall, yes, I give it high marks. I'll stay with it and maybe, in time, I'll be able to get by without any help at all. That's my goal, for sure."

14.6 A PERSONAL SUPPORT GROUP STORY: COPING WITH THE DEATH OF LOVED ONES

"I was 60 years old – it was my birthday – when I got the news. When the phone rang, I assumed it was one of my children calling to wish me well. Instead, it was the call no mother ever wants to get. My son and grandson had been killed in a car accident. They had been returning home from a basketball game, and were hit by a drunk driver. The car flipped over, and both were apparently killed instantly.

"I still have no words to explain what that was like. I have repeated that story thousands of times, and it still has an unreal quality to it. It was the beginning of a very dark time in my life. To be able to talk about it now is nothing short of a miracle.

"The days and weeks after the accident are a blur. I know we had a funeral, but I can't tell you anything about it, except that there were so many people there. I just wanted it to end. My daughter-in-law and I went our separate ways for a long time – I couldn't look at her or talk to her or even say her name without cascading back into a kind of grief I never imagined. Everyone expressed their concern, but I was sitting on the floor of my closet at night, crying and asking why. I could not imagine a reason for living or how to go on with my life after the loss of my son.

"I know now that others were hurting, too. My husband grieved very differently, and neither of us knew what to say. We spent many nights just holding on to one another, never speaking a word.

"After some months had passed, a friend told me about a support group she had read about, and gave me a phone number. "It might help you start to feel better," she said. There was a part of me that was angry about this, too – because no one understood that I did not want to feel better – that would be a betrayal of David, my son, and Jonathan, my grandson.

"Three weeks later, I looked at myself in the mirror. I didn't recognize who I saw. I was 60, but I looked terrible. The lines in my face, the weight loss, the dark circles – I was a mess. And I was so tired of feeling that way – miserable, really. I called the number on the card my friend had given me, and spoke to a woman who was, thankfully, not too chipper. 'This is the grief center. My name is Loni. Would you like to talk to someone about a death or a loss?' Finally, I thought – someone who doesn't avoid the topic. Yes, I wanted to talk to someone. Yes, I was available tomorrow morning. And yes, I could find the place on my own.

"I can fast forward to what happened next. I entered the office of a young woman, and that meeting was a turning point for me. I think she only asked me one question: 'Can you tell me about your family?' I don't remember what I said, really, but the floodgates opened, and I found myself talking about David and Jonathan and my life before and after their death. I was hungry to say their names, and I did so often – to my surprise, she talked about them as if she knew them. Loni asked if I was ready to talk to others who had experienced the death of their children – they incorporated many ages, many ways of dying, and varying lengths of time since the death. She said, 'I think you may find something in our group that you have not found anywhere else. Why not join us, just for a visit?'

"It happened that the group was meeting the following evening, and so I went. Alone, since my husband said, 'I don't think that kind of thing is for me, but I'm glad you are going.' This group was my life raft, as it turned out. Others who had been treading water shared their stories, showed pictures of the children who had died, and cried and laughed and were honest about who they were. That's what I think I appreciated the most – no pretending. It was a place, this support group, where I didn't have to pretend to be all right. They weren't afraid of the intensity of my feelings, and they did not try to make it go away. They listened, and they understood. I could see among this group of mostly mothers (and a few fathers) parents who had struggled but were at peace, parents who were still struggling, like me, and even a few who appreciated what I said to them. Slowly, I began to see David and Jonathan's deaths as a gift – likely no one will understand that – but it truly became an opportunity for me to honor their lives by helping others. I stayed in the support group for 8 months, when Loni asked me if I would be interested in attending a training for support group facilitators. It seems they needed people to help with some new groups. When I look back now, I can see how the support group helped with my transformation – from incapacitated grief to being ready to help others navigate the treacherous road of grief. My husband and I grew closer – and we are the perfect examples of how people deal with their losses differently." – SB.

14.7 SUMMARY

This chapter on self-help groups offers some hopeful evidence that self-help may provide assistance to a variety of clients experiencing problems with addictions, health, mental health, and other social and emotional problems. A large number of Americans use self-help, but questions remain about the validity of findings indicating that self-help may be an effective alternative to professional assistance. Most of these questions relate to research issues that may be difficult to resolve given the fact that self-help groups do not have the same expectations as professional help to prove effectiveness. Self-help is generally supportive in nature and usually provides an affirming and positive approach to problem-solving. Some concern is raised that self-help groups may not be effective for everyone because they often have an unacceptable religious ideology and sometimes encourage people to believe that recovery is a life-long struggle. Still, the weight of findings provides a reason for optimism until empirically based research, with strong methodologies provide more compelling evidence of effectiveness.

14.8 QUESTIONS FROM THE CHAPTER

1. Do you agree that treatment provided in self-help groups can harm people? If so, under what circumstances might that be the case?
2. What possible harm is there in a group of people with the same problem getting together and offering support and encouragement? Why must we think of this as treatment and why should we even consider researching the effectiveness of this type of benign helping process?

3. If self-help groups turn out to be more effective than professional help, how would professionals justify their existence? What might they do to improve the effectiveness of their services?

4. Leaders of self-help groups can sometimes be officious or power hungry. Do you think either, in pursuit of honest help to people in need, would be an inhibitor to good treatment? If so, why might this be the case?

5. The research seems to suggest that the most effective self-help groups are the ones in which people attend regularly and stay in the group for two or more years. Couldn't people get better as a result of other factors during that time? What might some of the reasons be for improvement other than the self-help received by the client?

REFERENCES

Alemi, F., Mosavel, M., Stephens, R., et al. (1996). Electronic self-help and support groups. *Medical Care, 34*(Suppl.), OS32–OS44.

Bly, R. (1986, April–May). Men of wisdom. *Utne Reader*.

Butrica, B. A., Smith, K. E., & Steurle, C. E. (2006). *Working for a good retirement*. Washington, DC: The Urban Institute Older Americans' Economic Security, Brief 9.

Caserta, M. S., & Lund, D. A. (1993). Intrapersonal resources and the effectiveness of self-help groups for bereaved older adults. *Gerontologist, 33*(5), 619–629.

Christo, G., & Sutton, S. (1994). Anxiety and self-esteem as a function of abstinence time among recovering addicts attending Narcotics Anonymous. *British Journal of Clinical Psychology, 33*, 198–200.

Clifford, P. R., Maisto, S. A., & Franzke, L. H. (2000). Alcohol treatment research follow-up and drinking behaviors. *Journal of Studies on Alcohol, 61*(5), 736–743.

Emrick, C. D., Tonigan, J. S., et al. (1993). Alcoholics anonymous: What is currently known? In B. S. McCrady & W. R. Miller (Eds.), *Research on alcoholics anonymous: Opportunities and alternatives* (pp. 41–75). New Brunswick, NJ: Rutgers Center of Alcohol Studies.

Felix-Ortiz, M., Salazar, M. R., Gonzalez, J. R., Sorensen, J. L., & Plock, D. (2000). Addictions services: A qualitative evaluation of an assisted self-help group for drug-addicted clients in a structured outpatient treatment setting. *Community Mental Health Journal, 36*(4), 339–350.

Fetto, J. (2000). Lean on me. *American Demographics, 22*(12), 16.

Galanter, M. (1988). Zealous self-help groups as adjuncts to psychiatric treatment: A study of recovery, inc. *American Journal of Psychiatry, 145*(10), 1248–1253.

Gilden, J. L., Hendryx, M. S., Clar, S., Casia, C., & Singh, S. P. (1992). Diabetes support groups improve health care of older diabetic patients. *Journal of the American Geriatrics Society, 40*, 147–150.

Granfield, R., & Cloud, W. (1996). The elephant that no one sees: Natural recovery among middle-class addicts. *Journal of Drug Issues, 26*, 45–61.

Hinrichsen, G. A., & Revenson, T. A. (1985). Does self-help help? An empirical investigation of scoliosis peer support groups. *Journal of Social Issues, 41*(1), 65–87.

Humphreys, K., & Moos, R. H. (1996). Reduced substance-abuse-related health care costs among voluntary participants in alcoholics anonymous. *Psychiatric Services, 47*, 709–713.

Humphreys, K., & Rappaport, J. (1994). Researching self-help/mutual aid groups and organizations: Many roads, one journey. *Applied & Preventive Psychology, 3*, 217–231.

Humphreys, K., & Ribisl, K. M. (1999). The case for partnership with self-help groups. *Public Health Reports, 114*(4), 322–329.

Humphreys, K., Mavis, B. E., & Stoffelmayr, B. E. (1994). Are twelve step programs appropriate for disenfranchised groups? Evidence from a study of post-treatment mutual help involvement. *Prevention in Human Services, 11*(1), 165–179.

Johnson, R. W., & Schaner, S. A. (2006). *Value of unpaid activities by older Americans Tops $160 billion per year*. Washington, DC: The Urban Institute.

Kessler, R. C., Mickelson, K. D., & Zhao, S. (1997a). Patterns and correlates of self-help group membership in the United States. *Social Policy, 27*, 27–46.

Kessler, R. C., Frank, R. G., Edlund, M., Katz, S. J., Lin, S. J., & Leaf, P. (1997b). Differences in the use of psychiatric outpatient services between the United States and Ontario. *New England Journal of Medicine, 336*, 551–557.

Kurtz, L. F. (1990). The self-help movement: Review of the past decade of research. *Social Work with Groups, 13*(3), 101–115.

Kurtz, L. F. (1997). *Self-help and support groups: A handbook for practitioners*. Thousand Oaks, CA: Sage Publications.

Levy, L. H. (1984). Issues in research and evaluation. In A. Gartner & F. Riessman (Eds.), *The self-help revolution* (pp. 155–172). NY: Human Sciences Press.

Lewis, E. A., & Suarez, Z. E. (1995). Natural helping networks. In: *Encyclopedia of social work* (19th ed.) Silver Spring, MD: National Association of Social Workers (pp. 1765–1772). (19th ed.).

Lieberman, M. A., & Bliwise, N. G. (1985). Comparisons among peer and professionally directed groups for the elderly: Implications for the development Caserta of self-help groups. *International Journal of Group Psychotherapy, 35*(2), 155–175.

Lieberman, M. A., & Borman, L. D. (1991). The impact of self-help groups on widows' mental health. *National Reporter, 4*, 2–6.

Lieberman, M. A., & Videka-Sherman, L. (1986). The impact of self-help groups on the mental health of widows and widowers. *American Journal of Orthopsychiatry, 56*, 435–449.

Marmar, C. R., Horowitz, M. J., et al. (1988). A controlled trial of brief psychotherapy and mutual-help group treatment of conjugal bereavement. *American Journal of Psychiatry, 145*(2), 203–209.

McCallion, P., & Toseland, R. W. (1995). Supportive group interventions with caregivers of frail older adults. *Social Work with Groups, 18*(1), 11–25.

McKay, J. R., Alterman, A. I., et al. (1994). Treatment goals, continuity of care, and outcome in a day hospital substance abuse rehabilitation program. *American Journal of Psychiatry, 151*(2), 254–259.

Memmott, J. L. (1993). Models of helping and coping: A field experiment with natural and professional helpers. *Social Work Research and Abstracts, 29*, 11–22.

Nash, K. B., & Kramer, K. D. (1993). Self-help for sickle cell disease in African American communities. *Journal of Applied Behavioral Science, 29*(2), 202–215.

Ouimette, P. C., Finney, J. W., & Moos, R. H. (1997). Twelve-step and cognitive-behavioral treatment for substance abuse: A comparison of treatment effectiveness. *Journal of Consulting and Clinical Psychology, 65*(2), 230–240.

Patterson, S.L., Holzhuter, J.L., Struble, V.E., & Quadagno, J. S. (1972). *Final report, utilization of human resources for mental health* (Grant No. MH 16618). Unpublished report. Washington, DC: National Institute of Mental Health.

Patterson, S. L., & Marsiglia, F. F. (2000). Mi casa es su casa: Beginning exploration of Mexican Americans' natural helping. *Families in Society, 81*(1), 22–31.

Rabiner, D. J., Koetse, E. C., Nemo, B., & Helfer, C. R. (2003). An overview and critique of the experience corps for independent living initiative. *Journal of Aging and Social Policy, 15*(1), 55–78.

Radloff, L. S. (1977). The CES-D scale: A self-report depression scale for research in the general population. *Applied Psychological Measurements, 1*, 385–407.

Riessman, F. (2000). Self-help comes of age. *Social Policy, 30*(4), 47–49.

Rinck, C., & Naragon, P. (1995). *Family Friends Evaluation*. Kansas City, MO: UNKC Institute for Human Development.

Rogers, A. M., & Taylor, A. S. (1997). Intergenerational mentoring: A viable strategy for meeting the needs of vulnerable youth. *Journal of Gerontological Social Work, 28*(1 and 2), 125–140.

Satcher (1999). *Surgeon General's Report: Chapter 5: Older adults and mental health*. Retrievd 12.12.2007 form <http://www.surgeongeneral.gov/library/mentalhealth/chapter5/sec1.html/>

Seligman, M. E. P. (1995). The effectiveness of psychotherapy: The consumers report study. *American Psychologist, 50*(12), 965–974.

Spiegel, D., Bloom, J. R., Kraemer, H. C., & Gottheil, E. (1989). Effect of psychosocial treatment on survival of patients with metastatic breast cancer. *Lancet, 8668*, 888–891.

Tattersall, M. L., & Hallstrom, C. (1992). Self-help and benzodiazepine withdrawal. *Journal of Affective Disorders, 24*(3), 193–198.

Toseland, R. W., Rossiter, C. M., & Labrecque, M. S. (1989, September). The effectiveness of two kinds of support groups for caregivers. *Social Service Review*, 415–432.

Vachon, M. L. S., Lyall, W. A. L., et al. (1980). A controlled study of self-help intervention for widows. *American Journal of Psychiatry, 137*(11), 1380–1384.

Videcka-Sherman, L., & Lieberman, M. A. (1985). The effects of self-help and psychotherapy intervention on child loss: The limits of recovery. *American Journal of Orthopsychiatry, 55*, 70–82.

VolunteerMatch (2007). *Great expectations: Boomers and the future of volunteering. VolunteerMatch user study*. San Francisco: MetLife Foundation.

Waldorf, D., Reinarman, C., & Murphy, S. (1991). Cocaine changes: The experience of using and quitting. Philadelphia: Temple University Press.

Waller, M. A., & Patterson, S. (2002). Natural helping and resilience in a Dine (Navajo) community. *Society, 81*(1), 73–84.

Wheeler, J. A., Gorey, K. M., & Greenblatt, B. (1998). The beneficial effects of volunteering for older volunteers and the people they serve: A meta-analysis. *International Journal of Aging and Human Development, 47*(1), 69–79.

Wituk, S., Shepherd, M. D., Slavich, S., Warren, M. L., & Meissen, G. (2000). A topography of self-help groups: An empirical analysis. *Social Work, 45*(2), 157–165.

Wuthnow, R. (1994). Sharing the journey: Support groups and America's quest for community. New York: Free Press.

APPENDIX: THE CES-D: A MEASURE OF DEPRESSION

The CES-D is a widely used and simple instrument to measure depression with good reliability and validity. Scores of 16 to 30 indicate the presence of depression requiring intervention. Scores over 30 would suggest concern for suicide and would require very serious interventions. For further information on scoring, the article by Radloff (1977) might be an initial first source to consider.

Directions: I am going to read you some statements about the ways people act and feel. On how many of the last seven days did the following statements apply to you?

		None or 1 day	2 or 3 days	4 days	5 or more days
1.	I was bothered by things that usually don't bother me.	0	1	2	3
2.	I did not feel like eating. My appetite was poor.	0	1	2	3
3.	I felt that I could not shake off the blues even with help from my friends and family.	0	1	2	3
4.	I felt I was just not as good as others.	0	1	2	3
5.	I had trouble keeping my mind on what I was doing.	0	1	2	3
6.	I felt depressed.	0	1	2	3
7.	I felt that everything I did was an effort.	0	1	2	3
8.	I felt hopeful about the future.	0	1	2	3
9.	I thought my life was a failure.	0	1	2	3
10.	I felt fearful.	0	1	2	3
11.	My sleep was restless.	0	1	2	3

12.	I was happy.	0	1	2	3
13.	I talked less than usual.	0	1	2	3
14.	I felt lonely.	0	1	2	3
15.	People were unfriendly.	0	1	2	3
16.	I enjoyed life.	0	1	2	3
17.	I had crying spells.	0	1	2	3
18.	I felt sad.	0	1	2	3
19.	I felt people disliked me.	0	1	2	3
20.	I could not get going.	0	1	2	3

Part five

Evidence-Based Practice and Health Issues of Older Adults

Chapter fifteen

Evidence-Based Practice with Alzheimer's Disease and Dementia

15.1 INTRODUCTION

The author wishes to thank Dr. Suzanne Bushfield for her contributions to this chapter on Alzheimer's disease and dementia.

The National Institute for Aging (2006) estimates that as many as 4.5 million Americans suffer from Alzheimer's disease (AD). The disease usually begins after age 60, and risk goes up with age. While younger people may also get AD, it is much less common. About 5% of men and women ages 65 to 74 have AD, and nearly half of those over the age of 85 may have the disease, with the number of people suffering from the disease doubling every five years beyond age 65. Grady (2007) reports that caring for patients with AD costs 100 billion dollars a year. With estimates of the rates of AD as high as 11–15 million people by 2050, the disease could well swamp the health care system. Of the over four million Americans estimated to have an intellectual decline because of AD, one-third have severe dementia and are so impaired that they can no longer manage without assistance in the simplest daily activities, including eating, dressing, grooming and toileting.

15.2 DEFINITIONS OF ALZHEIMER'S DISEASE AND DEMENTIA

The term dementia is not a specific disorder or disease, but a group of symptoms associated with a progressive loss of memory and other intellectual functions. Dementia can be serious enough to interfere with the performance of daily life tasks. Dementia, although associated with aging, can occur to anyone at any age and is the leading cause of older adult institutionalization (Psychiatry Online, 2007). Symptoms of dementia include loss of memory, extreme mood changes, and communication problems, which include a decline in the ability talk, write, and read. While AD is the most common disease in which dementia is a symptom, people with dementia may suffer from the effects of strokes and heart problems causing brain damage due to oxygen deprivation. Dementia can also result, to a lesser extent, from the conditions of multiple sclerosis, motor neurone disease, Parkinson's disease and Huntington's disease.

15.3 DIAGNOSIS

There are several distinct types of memory: sensory, short-term, working, and long-term. Sensory memory is fleeting unless we pay attention to it. Short-term memory serves as a temporary holding tank for things that we do pay some attention to, but it has limited storage capacity. Interference frequently disrupts short-term memory. Working memory is also a limited area, but it allows us to hold and store information while we are processing or reasoning various steps. Long-term memory, which endures for more than 30 seconds, is either declarative (involving facts and events available through conscious recall), semantic (independent of context), or episodic (highly contextual). No one area of the brain is entirely responsible for memory, since this complex process involves various parts of the brain, depending on the type of memory, the emotional content, and the perceiving, processing, and analyzing necessary for the memory. The brain's nerve cells (neurons) communicate with each other, providing important transmission of signals which are responsible for complex tasks and processing (www.alz.org). The firing of synapses (neurons being transmitted) is a part of the brain's memory process. Different synapses work differently for short- and long-term memory (National Institute on Aging, 2008.)

In AD, the neurons are unable to connect signals due to a build up of plaque between brain cells and tangles within brain cells. This development of plaque and tangles is the hallmark of AD, but diagnosis has been difficult, as the tangles are not readily evident. Early stage and early onset AD manifests itself as problems with memory, thinking, and concentration. People with AD may also exhibit physical and verbal outbursts, emotional distress, pacing, restlessness, hallucinations, and delusions. AD is usually diagnosed after ruling out other physical and medical causes, assessing cognitive functioning through such tests as the Mini Mental Status Examination (MMSE), and various brain scans. However, the MMSE is not always accurate, making the definitive diagnoses of AD more difficult (Shiroky et al., 2007).

The diagnosis of AD is disturbing for its terminal prognosis (albeit slow) and for the multiple losses that ensue. Early onset AD has certain genetic features, and recent developments in DNA testing (using genotype tests) may be useful in determining the existence of AD and the presence of apolipoprotein E (APOE), which is a marker for AD (Nee et al., 2004).

Children of AD patients have a higher-than-average risk of developing dementia, suggesting a genetic predisposition (Grady, 2007). Grady also notes that studies of IQ early in life indicate that people who develop AD have lower scores on early tests than healthy people, and that therefore AD may develop early in life and progress slowly until symptoms become more obvious, sometimes in early mid-life. The good news is that early detection of AD and understanding risk factors may lead to therapies that slow and even stop brain deterioration.

15.4 STAGES OF ALZHEIMER'S DISEASE

Although people with AD die an average of four to six years after diagnosis, the duration of the disease can vary from three to 20 years (Alzheimer's Association, 2007). This is the reason stages in the development of the disease may be important to clinicians so they understand how rapidly the disease is progressing and they can provide some concrete information about the future to loved ones. It should be noted that not everyone advances through the stages in a similar manner. Clients can sometimes seem to be in two or more stages at once, and the rate at which people advance through the stages is different for everyone. Still, the stages help us understand the probable symptoms and their challenges for caregivers and professionals. The stages of AD are as follows (Alzheimer's Association, 2007):

Stage 1: No impairment noted during an assessment.
Stage 2: Very mild cognitive decline that may be age-related or may suggest the early stages of AD. Individuals may feel as if they have some memory lapses such as forgetting familiar words or names or the location of keys, eyeglasses or other everyday

objects. These problems are usually not evident during an assessment or apparent to friends, family, or co-workers.

Stage 3: Mild cognitive decline in which the early stages of AD might be indicated. Others begin to notice problems with memory and performance at work and in many otherwise normal activities. The client may be unable to organize time and activities and social situations may become problematic because of memory lapses or the inability to remember what the event is about or the people attending the event.

Stage 4: Moderate cognitive decline indicating early-stage AD. At this stage clinicians will note a decreased knowledge of current events, an impaired ability to do simple mathematical tasks, an inability to pay bills or managing finances, and a change in affect with the client appearing more withdrawn or subdued.

Stage 5: Moderately severe cognitive decline indicating moderate or mid-stage AD. In this stage major memory gaps are apparent and some assistance with everyday activities becomes necessary, although assistance with eating or using the toilet are not necessary. At stage 5 one can expect confusion about the date, time of day, the week or the season, but people at stage 5 usually know their names and the names of loved one.

Stage 6: Severe cognitive decline indicating moderately severe or mid-stage AD. At stage 6, memory continues to deteriorate and clients need extensive help with daily living. Clients may lose awareness of their surroundings and may frequently become lost. They also have increasing problems with incontinence and begin experiencing delusions, paranoia, and compulsive repetitive behaviors such as shredding newspapers or washing hands.

Stage 7: Very serious cognitive decline indicating severe or late-stage AD. At stage 7, clients lose their ability to speak, to respond to others, to walk without assistance, to smile, or to hold their heads up. Reflexes become abnormal and muscles grow rigid. Swallowing is impaired. Clients may also groan, scream, mumble, speak gibberish and cry out. Clients in stage 7 need round-the-clock care.

15.5 EVIDENCE-BASED PRACTICE WITH AD CLIENTS AND CARETAKERS

Past research on senior centers and other community facilities serving elders has identified specific social supports and leisure activities related to the maintenance of physical and mental health among older adults (Fitzpatrick et al., 2005); however, few studies have examined brain fitness activities and their relationship to mental and physical health and cognitive abilities. Certain social, physical, and intellectual activities, such as learning new languages, computer programs and labs, aerobic exercises, listening to speakers and participating in strength-based exercises, and sports are thought to protect against cognitive decline (Colcombe et al., 2006).

Controlling the environment may be helpful, as people with AD are often distressed by moving to a new environment, changes in caregivers, perceived threats, hospital admission, bathing and dressing, fear and fatigue (alz.org, 2007). Remaining calm, avoiding confrontation, simplifying living surroundings, and providing safety and security may all assist in managing symptoms of clients with AD.

Certain social, physical and intellectual activities are thought to protect against cognitive decline and may lead to memory enhancement and better physical functioning. To date, little research has addressed the influence of brain fitness activities and their relationship to mental and physical health and cognition among older adults living in the community. Brain fitness activities can include aerobics, strength exercises, career decisions, working for pay, participating in a computer lab, learning new languages, group work on projects, and listening to speakers.

The concept of leisure activity participation and its relationship to health and cognitive functioning among older adults can also be understood from an activity theory perspective (Fitzpatrick, 1995; Maddox, 1988; Zarit, 1980) in which good adjustment and well-being in later life is positively associated with a high level of activities. Brain fitness activities represent a specific type of community activity in which older individuals may find additional intellectual and fitness challenges to promote and maintain physical and cognitive well-being. For example, these activities challenge the brain yet differ from activities that primarily involve reading, arts and crafts and bingo. Maintenance of brain fitness activities, especially physical activity and aerobic exercise, are said to protect cognition and benefit memory in midlife (Colcombe et al., 2006).

Other studies have also found that a specific and revolutionary computer-based program can potentially "revitalize the brain" (George, 2007) and improvements were found in areas of short-term memory and attention among the participants. Carle (2007) discusses several brain-training games such as "Nana" Technology, Posit Science, Mindfit and MyBrainTrainer.com, in which he describes programs that are "more than just a game" to maintain cognitive strength among residents in nursing homes and other long-term care facilities (p. 24). Therefore, brain fitness activities and various forms of physical fitness activities appear to serve as important mechanisms of support that have a strong relationship to health and cognitive well-being. The strength and quality of the activities may prove beneficial in warding off the negative effects of cognitive and memory decline associated with the aging process. Senior centers, retirement centers, and assisted living facilities are ideal locations for various forms of activities for social and physical participation. However, not all of these facilities offer brain fitness activities and certainly not everyone will wish to engage in these activities. George (2007) states that there is a "life-long ability to adapt, called brain plasticity and the ability to generate new brain cells." General health and nutrition through the adult years are also thought to serve a purpose in prevention of debilitating disease in late life. For those diagnosed with AD, exercise has been shown to have a positive effect on mood and in maintaining overall health (Williams and Tappen, 2007).

A promising but preliminary study suggests that elderly people who view themselves as self-disciplined, organized achievers may have a lower risk for developing AD than people who are less conscientious (Wilson et al., 2007). According to the researchers, a strong self-directed personality may somehow protect the brain, perhaps by increasing neural connections that can act as a reserve against mental decline. Surprisingly, when the brains of some of the strongly self-directed people in the study were autopsied after their deaths, they were found to have lesions that would meet accepted criteria for AD – even though these people had shown no signs of dementia. The authors point out that prior studies have linked social connections and stimulating activities like working puzzles with a lower risk of AD, while people who experience more distress and worry about their lives are at a higher risk.

At the start of the study, none of the participants ($n = 997$ older Catholic priests, nuns and brothers who participated in the Religious Orders Study) showed signs of dementia. The average age was 75. The subjects were given IQ tests and tests to measure self-direction (conscientiousness) and then were tracked for 12 years. Everyone took tests, including a standard personality test, and then the researchers tracked them for 12 years, with testing done yearly to determine if there were signs of cognitive decline and dementia. Brain autopsies were performed on most of those who died.

Over the 12 years, 176 people developed AD, but those with the highest scores for "conscientiousness" at the start of the study had an 89% lower risk of developing AD, compared to people with the lowest scores for that personality trait. The conscientiousness scores were based on how people rated themselves, on a scale of 0 to 4, on how much they agreed with statements such as: "I work hard to accomplish my goals," "I strive for excellence in everything I do," "I keep my belongings clean and neat" and "I'm pretty good about pacing myself so as to get things done on time."

When the researchers took into account a combination of risk factors, including smoking, inactivity, and limited social connections, they still found that the conscientious people had a 54% lower risk of AD compared to people with the lowest scores for conscientiousness. While these results are very promising because they seem to indicate that people with high expectations of themselves suffer far less chance of developing AD, it should be noted that the social and physical environments of the subjects (all members of religious communities) contain protective factors that may inhibit or delay the development of AD. Still, this is an exciting study because it suggests that strong personality traits related to conscientiousness should be encouraged and supported in children at early stages of development.

A study published in the *Annals of Neurology* in June 2006 (Scarmeas, 2006) suggests that people who eat a "Mediterranean" diet – rich in fruits, vegetables, olive oil, legumes, cereals and fish – have a lower risk of developing AD. Researchers examined the health and diet of more than 2,000 people over a four-year period. The average age of study participants was 76. None of the participants had AD at the start of the study. By the end of the study, 260 participants had been diagnosed with AD. Over the course of the study, researchers evaluated how closely participants followed a published definition of the Mediterranean diet. Participants who stuck most closely to the diet were less likely to develop AD than were participants who didn't follow the diet.

Researchers at the University of North Dakota (Pedraza, 2008, p. 2) have been studying the link between diets that are high in fat and the onset of AD. They found that one cup of coffee a day can neutralize the impact of fat on brain functioning and while the relationship between coffee and AD isn't conclusive, the researchers are optimistic that coffee reduces high levels of iron and cholesterol in the brain that have been associated with AD.

15.6 CARING FOR LOVED ONES WITH DEMENTIA

Persons with AD and related disorders (ADRD) generally live at home or in a community setting until the end stage of the disease, with family and friends meeting 75% of these care demands. The combination of an aging society and the correlation of age with ADRD will create exponential growth in the number of families undertaking the informal caregiving role and the need for in-home formal care services. Moreover, cultural differences can create additional critical challenges for service providers in their efforts to offer culturally competent services that meet the needs of our diverse aging society.

As growing numbers of older adults receive care in the community rather than in institutional settings, it is also critical to develop culturally competent strategies to ensure the safety of care recipients and prevent elder abuse, neglect and exploitation. A growing amount of research has uncovered racial and ethnic differences in caregiver characteristics, which impact caregiver perceptions of informal care-giving as well as the availability, accessibility and acceptability of formal care services (e.g., Aranda et al. (1997), Coon et al., 2004; Haley et al., 2004; Hinton, 2002). Decades of caregiver and caregiver intervention research document the burden and physical, psychological and social stressors associated with dementia caregiving in particular. (e.g., Ory et al., 1999; Schulz et al., 1995; Vitaliano et al., 2004).

Spousal caregivers have been called the "hidden victims" of AD. They are at high risk for isolation, stress, depression, and mortality. Older female caregivers show positive response to telephone support. (Winter and Gitlin, 2007). Persons who have dementia and other cognitive impairments live in the community and typically rely on formal caregivers, but as the disease progresses, they need additional community-based care. Higher levels of service used over long duration have been identified, suggesting that the average caregiver makes use of 6.9 community services (3.7 human services and 3.2 health services) in providing care for persons with dementia (Toseland et. al, 1999). Even when there is considerable use of services, caregivers report an increased burden of care-giving for persons with dementia, in part due to the greater need for services across longer periods of time. This suggests a need for better ways to organize, deliver, and shape services to the persons who need them.

Counseling and support have a positive effect on caregivers of community-dwelling patients with AD (six sessions of counseling, support group participation, and continuous availability of telephone counseling). This has also been shown to have a positive impact on self-reported health and the amount of illness in caregivers (Mittelman et al., 2007). The effects of focused intervention can be long lasting for caregivers (Selwood et al., 2007). Depressive symptoms among dementia caregivers, and distress from patient problem behaviors, were significant predictors of the length of time for developmentment of cardiovascular disease (Mausbach et al., 2007).

Caregivers and care receivers have different views of what constitutes quality of life with regard to dementia. Family caregivers rated quality of life (QOL) higher when the dementia patient had fewer depressive symptoms, less irritability, less apathy, less impairment in daily living, and lived at home. For the patient, self-rated QOL was associated with fewer depressive symptoms and living at home and are important to the dementia patient's feelings of a better quality of life (Hoe et al., 2007).

Activities of daily living for persons with dementia can be sources of considerable stress. Bathing is usually relaxing and pleasurable; for the elderly with dementia, it is often traumatic. Agitated behaviors are manifested most often during bathing than other times. This is influenced by the needs of the patient, the needs of the caregiver, environment, and institutional factors (Cohen-Mansfield and Parpura-Gill, 2007). Caring for a person with dementia requires increasing responsibilities for the caregiver and can be stressful and disruptive. Caregivers often feel angry, worried, guilty, distressed and isolated; they experience grief, particularly as the loved one begins to deteriorate beyond any reasonable chance of improvement and death seems clearly in view.

Caregiving may also be influenced by cultural norms. A longitudinal study by Mausbach (2004) compared rates of institutionalization of dementia patients cared for by Latina and Caucasian female caregivers, which concluded that Latina dementia caregivers delayed institutionalization much longer than female Caucasian caregivers. The researchers also found that Latino cultural values and positive views of the care-giving role were important factors that influenced their decision to delay placing loved ones with dementia in nursing homes.

Positive attitudes toward care-taking of loved ones with dementia are often reinforced by the inclusion of hospice services. Hunt-Raleigh et al. (2006) studied the impact of hospice and whether it influenced the family's decision to provide care at home or place the family member with AD in a nursing home. Hospice workers were frequently identified in the study as providing significant emotional support in making the caregiver feel cared for, respected and supported, and increased the caregiver's ability to cope with loved ones with AD at home. Family members receiving hospice service suffered fewer symptoms of bereavement than those not receiving services or those who decided to place loved ones in nursing homes at an earlier stage in the progression of AD.

The National Institute on Aging (2006) gives some helpful hints for caretakers of AD clients which may also help clinicians working with the family as well as the client with AD. Those suggestions include the following:

1. **Dealing with the diagnosis:** Caregivers should be encouraged to ask the doctor any questions they have about AD, including which treatments might work best to alleviate symptoms or address behavior problems. They might also contact organizations such as the Alzheimer's Association and the Alzheimer's Disease Education and Referral (ADEAR) Center for more information about the disease, treatment options, and caregiving resources. Some community groups may offer classes which teach caregiving, problem-solving, and management skills. Support groups where caregivers can share feelings and concerns can help. Online support groups make it possible for caregivers to receive support without having to leave home. If there are times of day when the person with AD is less confused or more cooperative, caregivers might plan their routine to make the most of those moments, keeping in mind that the way the person functions may change from day to day, and flexibility is needed. Adult day care or respite services which ease the day-to-day demands of caregiving allow caregivers to have a break, while knowing that the person with AD is being well cared for. It's a good idea to help caregivers get financial and legal documents in order, investigate long-term care options, and determine what services are covered by health insurance and Medicare.

2. **Communication:** Because communicating with a person who has AD can be a challenge, caregivers should choose simple words and short sentences and use a gentle, calm tone of voice. It helps to minimize distractions and noise – such as the television or radio – to help the person focus on what you are saying. Caregivers might find it helpful to call the person by name, make

sure they have his or her attention before speaking and allow enough time for a response. If the person with AD is struggling to find a word or communicate a thought, it helps to gently try to provide the word he or she is looking for and to frame questions and instructions in a positive way.

3. **Bathing:** For some people with AD, bathing can be a frightening and confusing experience. It helps to plan the bath or shower for the time of day when the person is most calm and agreeable. Caregivers might find it helpful to tell the person what they are going to do, step by step, and allow the client with AD to do as much as possible. Caretakers should make certain they have everything they need ready and in the bathroom before beginning. Safety risks can be minimized by using a handheld showerhead, shower bench, grab bars, and nonskid bath mats. Accidents are likely to happen and the person should never be left alone in the bath or shower. Bathing may not be necessary every day. A sponge bath can be effective between showers or baths.

4. **Dressing:** It helps to have the person get dressed at the same time each day so he or she will come to expect it as part of the daily routine. Caregivers should encourage the person to dress himself or herself to whatever degree possible and allow extra time so there is no pressure or rush. If he or she has a favorite outfit, caregivers might consider buying several identical sets. It helps to arrange the clothes in the order they are to be put on in order to help the person move through the process and provide clear, step-by-step instructions if the person needs prompting. Clothing that is comfortable, easy to get on and off, and easy to care for with elastic waists and Velcro enclosures minimize struggles with buttons and zippers.

5. **Eating:** Some people with AD want to eat all the time, while others have to be encouraged to maintain a good diet. Caregivers might want to view mealtimes as opportunities for social interaction and success for the person with AD. It helps to have a quiet, calm, reassuring mealtime atmosphere by limiting noise and other distractions. Maintain familiar mealtime routines, but adapt to the person's changing needs. Give the person food choices, but limit the number of choices. Serve small portions or several small meals throughout the day. In the earlier stages of dementia, caregivers should be aware of the possibility of overeating. If the person has trouble managing utensils, use a bowl instead of

a plate, offer utensils with large or built-up handles, use straws or cups with lids to make drinking easier, and encourage the person to drink plenty of fluids throughout the day to avoid dehydration. As the disease progresses, the caregiver should be aware of the increased risk of choking due to chewing and swallowing problems.

6. **Activities:** Don't expect too much. Simple activities often are best, especially when they use current abilities. Help the person get started on an activity. The caregiver might try breaking the activity down into small steps and praising the person for each step he or she completes. Watch for signs of agitation or frustration with an activity and try to include the person with AD in the entire activity process. Preparing a meal, setting the table, pulling out chairs, or putting away the dishes are good ways to keep the person with AD engaged. Caregivers should certainly take advantage of adult day services, which provide various activities for the person with AD, as well as an opportunity for caregivers to gain temporary relief from tasks associated with care-giving. Transportation and meals often are provided.

7. **Exercise:** Incorporating exercise into the daily routine has benefits for both the person with AD and the caregiver. The author knows a couple who play tennis together with the wife giving subtle prompts to her husband with AD about the score, who is serving, and when to change sides. He is a good tennis player and both spouses seem to enjoy the activity because those who play tennis with them are aware of the husband's AD and the benefits of doing something together they both enjoy. Senior centers may have group programs for people who enjoy exercising with others. Local malls often have walking clubs and provide a place to exercise when the weather is bad. Remember that exercise will help the AD client sleep better.

8. **Incontinence:** As the disease progresses, many people with AD begin to experience the inability to control their bladder and/or bowels. Caregivers might find it helpful to have a routine for taking the person to the bathroom every three hours or so during the day. They should watch for signs that the person may have to go to the bathroom, such as restlessness or pulling at clothes. Respond quickly. It helps to keep track of when accidents happen in order to help plan ways to avoid them. Limiting fluids with caffeine in the evening might limit night-time accidents.

9. **Sleep problems:** Many people with AD become restless, agitated, and irritable around dinnertime. Caregivers should encourage exercise during the day and limit daytime napping, but make sure that the person gets adequate rest during the day because fatigue can increase the likelihood of late afternoon restlessness. Physically demanding activities should be scheduled earlier in the day. Keeping lights dim in the evening, eliminating loud noises, and playing soothing music if the person seems to enjoy it are also helpful. Use nightlights in the bedroom, hall and bathroom if the darkness is frightening or disorienting.

10. **Hallucinations and delusions:** As the disease progresses, a person with AD may experience hallucinations and/or delusions. The caretaker should avoid arguing with the person about what he or she sees or hears and provide reassurance and comfort. Distracting the person to another topic or activity, moving to another room or going outside for a walk may help. Violent or disturbing programs should be avoided because the person with AD may not be able to distinguish television programming from reality.

11. **Wandering:** Some people with AD have a tendency to wander away from their homes or their caregivers. Caregivers should be informed that the person should carry some kind of identification or wear a medical bracelet. They may also want to enroll the person in the Alzheimer's Association Safe Return program. If the person becomes lost and is unable to communicate adequately, identification will alert others to the person's medical condition. Caregivers should notify their neighbors and local authorities in advance that the person has a tendency to wander. Keeping a recent photograph or videotape of the person with AD to assist police if the person becomes lost is helpful. Caregivers should be urged to keep doors locked and consider a keyed deadbolt or an additional lock up high or down low on the door. If the person can open a lock because it is familiar, a new latch or lock may help. Be sure that the caregiver secures anything that could cause danger, both inside and outside the house.

12. **Driving:** Caregivers should look for clues that safe driving is no longer possible, including the person becoming lost in familiar places, driving too fast or too slow, disregarding traffic signs, or becoming angry or confused. Using the doctor to stop the person with AD from driving may help, since clients with AD may view the doctor as an "authority" and may be willing to stop driving

if the doctor says he or she should. The doctor also can contact the Department of Motor Vehicles and request that the person be reevaluated. If necessary, caregivers may want to take the car keys. If all else fails, caregivers may need to disable the car or move it to a location where the person cannot see it or gain access to it.

13. **Choosing a nursing home:** There comes a point when many caregivers can no longer care for their loved one at home. Choosing a nursing home or an assisted living facility can be a difficult decision. It is helpful for caregivers to gather information about services and options before the need actually arises and to make a list of questions to ask the staff. Caregivers should be urged to observe the way the facility runs, how residents are treated and to drop by again unannounced to see if first impressions are the same. Caregivers should be encouraged to ask about staff training in dementia care, specialized programs and policies about family participation in planning patient care. Room availability, cost, method of payment, and participation in Medicare or Medicaid should also be determined. It is often wise to have caregivers place their loved ones on a waiting list even if they are not ready yet to make a decision about long-term care. Once they have made a decision, they should understand the terms of the contract and financial agreement. Having an attorney review the documents before signing is also a good idea. A human service professional may be able to help caregivers plan for and adjust to the move.

The Johns Hopkins Health Alert (2007) reports that people with AD often become agitated or have a deterioration in their symptoms in the late afternoon or early evening (often called sundowning). Some possible reasons for sundowning include end-of-the day fatigue, being overwhelmed by too much sensory input, a lack of activities or attention, and becoming confused in dim light. Sleep problems, such as sleep apnea and disturbances in the sleep/wake cycle (circadian rhythm), may also play a role. The publication suggests the following ways of dealing with sundowning:

1. Because people with AD have a disproportionately high degree of sleep disturbances, including sleep apnea, helping the person get a good night's sleep can reduce daytime sleepiness and may reduce disruption of the circadian rhythm, a common problem in elderly people.

2. Because Aricept and other cholinesterase inhibitors sometimes act as stimulants, it may be best to give the medication in the morning if the person is not sleeping well.
3. Because patients with AD become confused when light is too dim, encouraging the person to go outdoors during the day, placing the person's chair next to a sunny window and having sufficient light at night can remedy the problem of insufficient light.
4. Inactivity is a strong catalyst for sundowning. Scheduling activities the person has always enjoyed for most afternoons can reduce sundowning.
5. When sundowning occurs, distracting the person or engaging them in topics they have interests in can help reduce the symptoms of sundowning.

15.7 A PERSONAL STORY: TAKING THE CAR KEYS AWAY FROM A PARENT

"The toughest thing I've ever done was to tell my dad he had to stop driving. He was 82 at the time. His memory was fading. His reflexes were slowed. It was a conversation we should have had long before he became a hazard to himself and others on Cleveland's highways. But it was a conversation no one in the family wanted to have. So we put it off until we could no longer ignore the obvious. Dad, like some of the nearly 19 million drivers age 70 and older in the USA, was a hazard on the highways."

"We confronted him on a Sunday afternoon in 1997. My mom was in the hospital with two broken arms. The hospital's social worker had approached my brother Jim and me."

" 'We're concerned about your dad's driving,' she told us. 'Several people here at the hospital are worried about how he pulls into and out of the hospital parking lot. He's going to kill someone, including himself. It's simply a matter of time. Today, tomorrow, but soon, ' " she said.

"So, we devised a foolproof plan. First we'd talk to Mom. And she agreed. 'Your father should not be driving,' "she told us.

"We decided to meet in Mom's hospital room to talk to dad. According to our plan, the social worker would open the conversation in a non-threatening way. We'd second her concerns. Mom would agree with us. And dad would hand over the keys. Simple. Do-able. Right? We rehearsed the meeting several times. Mom was fabulous. Jim, a psychologist, was excellent, too."

"Dad arrived at noon. While he chatted with Mom, Jim and I went over the plan with the social worker. And then we walked into Mom's room."

" 'Saul,' the social worker began, 'we're worried about your driving. We care about you. We don't want you to hurt yourself or anyone else.' "

"Jim and I jumped in at that point, echoing her words.

"Dad looked like a kid who'd been cornered by bullies on the playground. His back literally against the wall, he looked from me to Jim, at the social worker and then at Mom, who'd said nothing so far."

" 'What are you talking about?' he whispered. 'I'd be the first to know if I had a problem driving. I've been driving for more than 60 years. I'm a good driver.' There were tears in his eyes. In mine, too."

"That's when Mom jumped in. 'Your father's a wonderful driver,' she said. 'The best. I should know, I've driven with him for more than 50 years.' "

"And that was it."

"Dad drove for another year or so until dementia made it impossible for him. At some point, he couldn't even remember how to start the car. We were lucky he didn't hurt himself or anyone else. But it was just dumb luck."

"The fact is, people over 70 have a disproportionate number of accidents per miles driven, according to the National Highway Traffic Safety Administration. Indeed, their statistics show that not only do older drivers have more accidents; they are more likely than any other age group to kill themselves or others in an accident."

"We knew Dad should have stopped driving long before he did. My guess is most family members know. But there's a long way from knowing to doing something about it. We need tough new laws to require annual driving tests, eye exams and other physical tests for older people. It's in their best interests and ours."

"What did we learn from our experience? Dad died in February 2000. Mom was still driving then, at 84. But we talked to her about our concerns and she agreed to sell the car. She's not happy about it, but today, at 87, she's alive and doing quite well." – RA.

15.8 SUMMARY

The diagnosis of AD or dementia is understandably distressing. The multiple losses associated with AD and the long-term burden of caregiving present challenges to individuals, families, and communities. As the population ages, the numbers of persons with AD is expected to reach epidemic proportions. Costs associated with care and the need for medical resources to manage this disease will likely become a major social problem. Finding ways to accurately diagnose AD, and effective strategies for prevention and treatment of this terminal illness, will require significant research efforts.

AD is characterized by problems with memory, associated personality changes, and a gradual loss of brain functioning due to build up of plaque and tangles within the brain. Persons with AD may initially notice short-term memory problems and other cognitive changes, progressing to an inability to recognize family or friends. The multiple losses associated with AD are challenging to caregivers.

15.9 QUESTIONS FROM THE CHAPTER

1. The diagnosis of AD seems to be as rampant as the diagnosis of ADHD in children. Do you think there's a possibility that what we call AD is actually depression brought on by loneliness and isolation?

2. Don't you think we ask too much of people caring for loved one's with AD? Shouldn't the state assume responsibilities to save caretakers stress and strain that might negatively affect their family life?

3. Research cited in the chapter found that self-directed people often have the biological signs of AD but not the symptoms. Isn't it possible that as people feel unwanted and ignored as they age that much of what we call AD is actually a type of learned helplessness?

4. AD seems to be associated with cognitive problems that can be (or will be) diagnosed early in life. Do you think an early diagnosis of AD will stigmatize people with AD and negatively affect their ability to lead productive lives?

REFERENCES

Alzheimer's Disease Education & Referral Center (ADEAR) (2007). http://www. niapublications.org/adear/

Aranda, M. P., & Knight, B. G. (1997). The influence of ethnicity and culture on the caregiver stress and coping process: A sociocultural review and analysis. *Gerontologist, 37*, 342–354.

Carle, A. (2007, February). More than a game: Brain training against dementia. Feature article in *Nursing Home Magazine*, 22–24.

Cohen-Mansfied, J., & Parpura-Gill, A. (2007). Bathing: A framework for intervention focusing on psychosocial, architectural, and human factors considerations. *Archives of Geronotlogy and Geriatrics, 45*(2), 121–135.

Colcombe, S., Erickson, K., Scalf, P., Kim, J., Prakash, R., McAuley, E., Elavsky, S., Marquez, D., Hu, L., & Kramer, A. (2006). Aerobic exercise training increases brain volume in aging humans. *Journal of Gerontology: Medical Sciences, 61A,* 1166–1170.

Coon, D. W., Rubert, M., Solano, N., et al. (2004). Well-being, appraisal, and coping in Latina and Caucasian dementia caregivers: Findings from the REACH study. *Aging & Mental Health, 8,* 330–345.

Creswell, J. W. (2007, April 9). *Qualitative inquiry & research design: Choosing among five approaches.* Thousand Oaks, CA: Sage.

Fitzpatrick, T. R. (1995). Stress and well-being among the elderly: The effect of recreational services. *The Journal of Applied Social Sciences, 19,* 95–105.

Fitzpatrick, T. R., Gitelson, R., Andereck, K., & Mesbur, E. S. (2005). Social support factors among a senior center population in southern Ontario, Canada. *Social Work in Health Care, 40,* 15–37.

George, L. (2007, April 9). The secret to not losing your marbles. *Macleans,* 36–39.

Grady, D. (2007). *Six killers: Alzheimer's disease, finding Alzheimer's before a mind fails.* NYTIMES.COM (Dec. 26). <http://www.nytimes.com/2007/12/26/health/26alzheimers.html?_r=1&th=&oref=slogin&emc=th&pagewanted=all/>

Haley, W. E., Gitlin, L. N., Wisniewski, S. R., Mahoney, D. F., Coon, D. W., Winter, L., Corcoran, M., Schinfeld, S., & Ory, M. (2004). Well-being, appraisal, and coping in African-American and Caucasian dementia caregivers: Findings from the REACH study. *Aging & Mental Health, 8,* 316–329.

Hinton, L. (2002). Improving care for ethnic minority elderly and their family caregivers across the spectrum of dementia severity. *Alzheimer Disease and Associated Disorders, 16*(Suppl. 2), 50–55.

Hoe, J., Katona, C., Orrell, M., & Livingston, G. (2007). Quality of life in dementia: Care recipient and caregiver perceptions of QOL in dementia. *International Journal of Geriatric Psychiatry, 22*(10), 1031–1036.

Hunt-Raleigh, E. D., Robinson, J. H., Marold, K., & Jamison, M. T. (2006). Family caregiver perception of hospice support. *Journal of Hospice & Palliative Nursing, 8*(1), 25–33.

Johns Hopkins Health Alert. (2007). *Coping Strategies for Alzheimer's Disease Behavioral Problems* (Jan. 6). <http://www.johnshopkinshealthalerts.com/alerts/memory/JohnsHopkinsHealthAlertsMemory_569-1.html?CMP = OTC-RSS/>

Maddox, G. L. (1988). *Aging and well-being.* The 1987 Boettner Lecture. Bryn Mawr, PA: Boettner Research Institute.

Mausbach, B., Coon, D. W., Depp, C., et al. (2004). Ethnicity and time to institutionalization: A comparison of Latina and Caucasian dementia caregivers. *Journal of the American Geriatrics Society, 52,* 1077–1084.

Mittelman, M., Roth, D., Clay, O., & Haley, W. (2007). Preserving health of Alzheimer's caregivers: Impact of a spouse caregiver intervention. *American Journal of Geriatric Psychiatry, 15*(9), 780–789.

National Institute on Aging (NIA) (2008). Alzheimer's Disease Education and Referral Center http://www.nia.nih.gov/Alzheimers/ResearchInformation/Newsletter/CurrentIssue.htm. *Referral Connections, 15*(4).

Nee, L., Tierney, M., & Lippa, C. (2004). Genetic features of early onset Alzheimer's Disease. *American Journal of Alzheimer's Disease and Other Dementias, 19*(4), 219–225.

Ory, M., Hoffman, R., Lee, J., Tennstedt, S., & Schulz, R. (1999). Prevalence and impact of Care-giving: A detailed comparison between dementia and nondementia caregivers. *The Gerontologist, 39*, 177–185.

Pedraza, J.M. (2008). *Dimensions: The University of North Dakota*, June, p. 2.

Psychiatry Online. (2007). *Alzheimer's disease*. <http://www.psychiatryonline.com/searchResult.aspx?searchStr=alzheimer%27s+disease&searchType=1&rootTerm=alzheimer%27s+disease&rootID=9680&bCount=44&pracCount=16&jCount=288&additional=0&tabID= 2/>

Scarmeas, N., Stern, Y., Tang, M-X., Mayeux, R., Luchsinger, J. (2006). Mediterranean Diet and risk of Alzheimer's disease. *Annals of Neurology*; Published online 18.04.2006 <http://www.eurekalert.org/pub_releases/2006-04/jws-mdl041106.php/>

Schulz, R., O'Brien, A. T., Bookwala, J., & Fleissner, K. (1995). Psychiatric and physical morbidity effects of dementia care-giving: Prevalence, correlates, and causes. *The Gerontologist, 35*, 771–791.

Selwood, A., Johnston, K. I., Katona, C., Lyketsos, C., & Livingston, G. (2007). Systematic review of the effect of psychological interventions on family caregivers of people with dementia. *Journal of Affective Disorders, 101*(1–3), 75–89.

Shiroky, J., Schipper, H., Bergman, H., & Chertkow, H. (2007). Diagnosis of Alzheimer's Disease. *Journal of Alzheimer's Disease and Other Dementias, 22*(5), 406–415.

Vitaliano, P., Young, H., & Zhang, J. (2004). Is care-giving a risk factor for illness? *Current Directions in Psychological Science, 13*, 13–16.

Williams, C., & Tappen, R. (2007). Effects of exercise on Alzheimer's disease. *Journal of Alzheimer's Disease and Other Dementias, 22*(5), 389–397.

Wilson, R. S., Schneider, J. A., Arnold, S. E., Bienias, J. L., & Bennett, D. A. (2007, October 20). Conscientiousness and the incidence of Alzheimer disease and congnitive impairment. *Arch Gen Psychiatry, 64*(1204), 1212.

Winter, L., & Gitlin, L. (2007). Evaluation of a telephone based support group intervention for female caregivers of community dwelling individuals with dementia. *American Journal of Alzheimer's Disease and Other Dementias, 21*(6), 391–397.

Zarit, S. H. (1980). Aging and mental disorders. New York: The Free Press.

Chapter sixteen

Evidence-Based Practice with Disabilities, Terminal Illness, and Assisted Living

16.1 INTRODUCTION

In self-reports of satisfaction with their health, the Older Americans Update 2006: Key indicators of well being (2007) reports a difference in health satisfaction by race/ethnicity. Caucasians aged 65–75 report an 81% health satisfaction level, while Blacks and Hispanics report a 64% level of health satisfaction. Between ages 75 and 85, 73% of Caucasians were satisfied with their health as opposed to 57% for Hispanics and Blacks. In older adults aged 85 and older, 67% of the Caucasian and 52% of the Black and Hispanic populations were satisfied with their health. While the report does not indicate why there is such disparity in health satisfaction by race/ethnicity, one has to be concerned about the quality of health care for ethnic minorities and the fact that income is a predictor of health care throughout the life span. If one receives poor health care growing up, the chances are good that general health will suffer as a person ages.

When considering these data it's important to recognize that health care in America doesn't measure up for many populations of older

343

Americans, particularly low income and minority Americans. An editorial in the New York Times (August 12, 2007) notes that in an evaluation of health care systems in 191 countries, the USA ranked 37th. In the area of fairness, the USA ranked dead last in the disparity of quality care between richer and poorer Americans. Americans with below-average incomes are much less likely than their counterparts in other industrialized nations to see a doctor when sick, to fill prescriptions or to get needed tests and follow-up care. In an eight-country comparison including England, Australia and Canada, the USA ranked last in years of potential life lost to circulatory diseases, respiratory diseases, and diabetes, and had the second-highest death rate from bronchitis, asthma and emphysema.

To support these findings the Rand Corporation (2004) reports that although more than 40 cents of every health care dollar is spent on people who are 65 or older there are problems in quality care that negate the large amount of money spent. In a study of quality of care delivered to a group of community dwelling older adults who were members of a managed care plan, a Rand Corporation research team concluded that:

1. Vulnerable elders in the study received about half of the recommended care, and the quality of care varies widely from one condition and type of care to another.
2. Preventive care suffers the most, while indicated diagnostic and treatment procedures are provided most frequently.
3. Care for geriatric conditions, such as incontinence and falls, is poorer than care for general medical conditions such as hypertension that affect adults of all ages.
4. Physicians often fail to prescribe recommended medications for older adults (Rand Corporation, 2004, p. 1).

16.2 DISABILITIES IN OLDER ADULTS

Cigolle et al. (2007) report that 18% of American men over 65 had at least one of the following disabilities: Inability to walk two blocks, difficulty writing, inability to stoop, kneel, reach over their heads, or lift 10 pounds. Thirty-two percent of American women in the same age range were unable to do one or more of the preceding physical activities. The report does not indicate why women have such a higher disability rate but life span is certainly a major reason. Women live longer than men and experience more disabilities because of longer life span. Cigolle et al. (2007) found that the definition of disability fails to include common geriatric problems of the elderly, including cognitive impairment, falls, incontinence, low body mass index, dizziness, vision impairment, hearing impairment, and dependency in activities of daily living, including bathing, dressing, eating, transferring, and toileting. When these common geriatric conditions were included, the researchers found high rates of disability in men and women over 65. For example, incontinence affects 12% of all women 60–64. At age 85 and older, the level is over 20%. Nineteen percent of older adults ages 65–69 have hearing impairments. By ages 80–84 the rate has risen to 33%. Six percent of older adults ages 65–69 have experienced injurious falls. Using the geriatric conditions listed above, almost 50% of all adults 65–69 have one or more geriatric conditions that if counted as a disability would indicate that one in two adults experience troubling or debilitating disabilities before age 70.

Finn (1999) reports that "There are many caretakers of disabled and elderly people who are essentially homebound as a result of their responsibilities at home" (p. 220). Finn goes on to say that a number of social and emotional problems develop from being "alienated" or "socially quarantined" from the larger society, including depression, loneliness, alienation, lack of social interaction, lack of information, and lack of access to employment (Braithwaite, 1996; Coleman, 1997; Shworles, 1983). In a study of the impact of physical and emotional disabilities, Druss et al. (2000) write that:

> Combined mental and general medical disabilities were associated with high levels of difficulty across a variety of functional domains: bed days, perceived stigma, employment status, disability payments, and reported discrimination. These findings may best be understood by the fact that co-morbid conditions, unlike either mental or general medical conditions alone, are most commonly associated with deficits spanning several domains of function. In turn, respondents with deficits across multiple domains have few areas of intact function available to make up for their existing deficits. The uniquely high levels of functional impairment associated with combined conditions speak to the potential importance of integrated programs that can simultaneously address an individual's medical and psychiatric needs. (p. 1489)

Finn (1999) studied the content of messages sent by people with disabilities using the Internet as a form of group therapy. He found that most correspondents wanted to talk about their health and about specific issues of treatment and quality of care but that overall, the correspondents acted as a support group helping others cope with emotional, medical, and social issues. These issues included "highly technical descriptions of medications, procedures, and equipment to subjective accounts of treatment experiences. There also was considerable discussion of interpersonal relationship issues such as marital relationships, dating, and sexuality" (p. 228). Finn (1999) reminds us that many disabled people are home bound and that the Internet becomes an important part of the communicating they do each day. This is particularly true for homebound people who may also have difficulty speaking or hearing.

Pain is often related to health problems that can be disabling. Not to diminish the real pain many people experience who suffer from serious disabilities and other incapacitating conditions, Bruner (1990) argued that pain is essentially experienced subjectively. Despite attempts to objectively describe pain, the subjective reality includes the individual's physical condition and his or her psychological, socio-cultural, and spiritual self. While medicine may categorize pain according to biological, psychological, or idiopathic sources, most pain sufferers become focused on relief from pain. Organizing one's life around pain can affect families so pervasively that by the time patients come for comprehensive pain management, new patterns of communication, roles, and structures have replaced the family environment that existed before pain became the central organizing feature.

Pain becomes "chronic" when it has been in existence for six months, and is recognized for its debilitating psychological and social effects (Snelling, 1990). Pain sufferers have very concrete needs, but their lives have been characterized by "a sense of loss of self" (Kelley et al., 1997). Just as pain becomes primary in its sufferer's world, it also becomes central in the family's world. There are significant personal and social costs associated with pain: loneliness, isolation, withdrawal and avoidance, anxiety, depression, fear, lack of trust, impaired sexual relationships, loss of productivity, strained marital and family relationships, overuse or misuse of medical care, addiction, and the development of a pain identity (Kelley et al., 1997).

Pain research based on principles from ego psychology has identified a number of significant contributing factors to the perception and experience of chronic pain, including a history of childhood abuse and family dysfunction (Mersky et al., 1978); physical and emotional abuse (Engel, 1959a,b); increased dependency and the resulting attitudes of caregivers (Berry et al., 1995). Effective interventions focus on helping the patient understand the pain experience, and providing short-term, ego supportive counseling (Roy, 1981a). The behavioral approach, for example, assumes that when pain responses, such as grimacing, complaining, sighing, and moaning, are systematically followed by favorable consequences, such as sympathy, attention, and avoidance of unpleasant tasks, the pain behavior is reinforced and maintained (Roy, 1981a,b). The negative role of the spouse and other loved ones in maintaining and perpetuating chronic pain receives considerable focus in this model.

The contingency management approach (Bonica, 1990; Fordyce, 1990) to pain management is widely accepted, and many distinguished pain management programs are derived from this model. Approaches address the patient's self-talk, reframing the situation to promote cognitive restructuring, changing reinforcers within the family, and enlisting loved ones as part of the treatment strategy. The goal of treatment is to help the patient return to normal functioning without pain medications, or with reduced reliance on medication. Pain behaviors are ignored; appropriate activity and interactions are reinforced with attention and praise. The approach may result in the patient learning to live a normal life by ignoring the pain. Changing family interactions and responses to pain are reframed as constructive caring, and the role of the worker in this model is to teach pain patients and their families to eliminate the subject of chronic pain from their family system interactions (Roy, 1981a).

Success in this model is dependent on several factors: (1) a supportive family amenable to retraining; (2) a patient able to learn new skills; and (3) available community supports to maintain changes (Roy, 1981a; Snelling, 1990). The behavioral model acknowledges the impact of knowledge and attitudes on pain (Brockopp et al., 1996) and may include effective non-pharmacological strategies such as relaxation, imagery, and distraction (Korcz, 2003). "Family oriented" treatment in this model places a significant focus on modifying the family response behaviors to pain, as an aspect of contingency management.

Crook et al. (1984) estimated that 25% to 50% of community dwelling elderly suffer from chronic pain, with rates of 45% to 80% for elderly who live in nursing homes (Roy and Michael, 1986). Chronic pain is associated with rheumatoid arthritis and delayed healing from injuries. While medication is frequently indicated to help relieve pain in older adults, Cook (1998) reports that outcome studies have shown that cognitive and behavioral techniques are also effective in helping clients manage pain. Cook (1998) studied a treatment group of 22 nursing home residents who received cognitive behavioral pain management training. The participants reported less pain and less pain-related disability than those in an attention/supportive control group. Participants with serious cognitive impairment were not included in the study. Treatment gains in the cognitive behavioral group were maintained at a four-month follow-up. Widner and Zeichner (1993) note that cognitive pain management methods include distracting oneself from the pain, reinterpreting pain sensations, using pleasant imagery, using calming self-statements, and increasing daily pleasurable activities. Parmalee et al. (1991) found that cognitive and behavioral techniques help clients reduce dependence on medication for pain management. Morley et al. (1999) and van Tulder et al. (2000) have found cognitive therapy to be effective in reducing a patient's level of pain and his or her use of pain medications. Flor et al. (1992) found that multidisciplinary pain treatment programs that incorporated cognitive-behavioral therapy and behavioral therapy approaches were significantly more successful than programs that used only one treatment or programs with no other treatments.

An interesting aspect of pain is the controversy over the existence of "fibromyalgia," a disease that primarily affects middle-aged and older women and is characterized by chronic, widespread pain of unknown origin. Many of its sufferers are afflicted by other similarly nebulous conditions such as irritable bowel syndrome. As many as 10 million people may suffer from the disorder (Berenson, 2008), but these figures are sharply disputed by doctors who do not consider fibromyalgia a medically recognizable illness and who say that diagnosing the condition actually worsens suffering by causing patients to obsess over aches and pains that other people simply tolerate. The diagnosis of fibromyalgia itself worsens the condition by encouraging people to think of themselves as sick and to overly obsess about their pain. In general, fibromyalgia patients complain not just of chronic pain, but of many other symptoms including back pain, chronic fatigue syndrome, and ringing in the ears, among other conditions. Many also report that fibromyalgia interferes with their daily lives, and with activities such as walking or climbing stairs. However, according to Berenson (2008), who interviewed a number of doctors who are skeptical about the disorder and was told that most people have aches and pains but go through their lives managing their pain without obsessing about it.

As an example of how people cope with pain, one older adult client in severe pain from back problems said that in the morning when the pain was its most severe he tried to immediately remove himself from awareness of the pain by doing his daily routine of making coffee and then going to the computer to work. He says he isn't aware at all of the pain when he works. He told the author, "I went for physical therapy, did epidurals for pain management, and saw a pain psychologist. It didn't help at all and I was becoming an insufferable pain in the ass to my wife and family, who were getting tired of listening to me complain about my back pain. So after undergoing those treatments and using medication that just made me groggy and clouded my thinking, I started doing some reading on the Internet about managing pain without medication. As a result, I think I developed a pretty common sense way of dealing with it. My wife gave me back rubs at night, I slept on a heating pad that helped loosen the tight muscles in my back, and I'd get up and at 'em in the morning. I'd get lost in the work I did on the computer and the pain went away, or at least my awareness of the pain.

"I have a serious back problem. It's not in my head. I had a benign growth removed from my spinal cord and I have damage from that plus I have a vertebra that moves. Tennis kills me, but I play through the pain. One doctor said I'd need spinal fusion surgery, but looking at the results I found on the Internet that the pain doesn't go away for most people who have the surgery, I've stuck to my approach. When the old guys I play with compare notes, they all suffer from pain but they don't let it get the best of them. You can learn to ignore pain. That's what I've done, and that's what a lot of older people I know have done. Depending on medications or surgery makes you lose control and most pain is something we can all learn to control."

16.3 ASSISTED LIVING

Older adults who can no longer live at home because of disabilities or lack of suffcient health sometimes transition to assisted living facilities (AFLs). ALFs vary from small residential houses for three residents, to very large facilities providing services to hundreds of residents. Most states have enacted laws governing these facilities, and have also recognized that these facilities play an important role in caring for the elderly that may not filled by traditional nursing or retirement homes. People who live in newer assisted living facilities usually have their own private apartment. There is generally no special medical monitoring equipment or the 24-hour nursing staff that one would find in a nursing home. However, trained staff are usually on-site around the clock to provide other needed services. Where provided, private apartments have their own small kitchens, bathrooms, living areas, and bedrooms. Alternatively, individual living spaces may resemble a dormitory or hotel room consisting of a private or semi-private sleeping area and a shared bathroom. There are usually common areas for socializing, as well as a central kitchen and dining room for preparing and eating meals. More recently-built facilities are designed with an emphasis on ease of use by disabled people. Bathrooms and kitchens are designed with wheelchairs and walkers in mind. Hallways and doors are extra-wide to accommodate wheelchairs. These facilities are by necessity fully compliant with the Americans with Disabilities Act (2008) or similar legislation elsewhere.

While the range in quality is substantial and not all ALFs offer all of the the following services, residents of assisted living facilities usually have meals provided, some health care management and monitoring, help with activities of daily living such as bathing, dressing, and eating, housekeeping and laundry, medication reminders and/or help with medications, recreational activities, and security and transportation (Eldercare Locator, 2008).

Although assisted living is less expensive than nursing home care, it is still fairly expensive. Depending on the kind of assisted living facility and type of services an older person chooses, the cost can range from less than $10,000 a year to more than $50,000 a year. Across the United States, monthly rates average $1,800 per month. Because there can be extra fees for additional services, it is very important for older persons and their families to find out what is included in the basic rate and how much other services will cost (Eldercare Locator, 2008).

16.4 TERMINAL ILLNESS

Christakis (2007) reports that physicians often fail to give terminally ill patients a prognosis and writes, "In one study of nearly 5,000 hospitalized adults who had roughly six months to live, only 15% were given clear prognoses. In a smaller study of 326 cancer patients in Chicago hospices, all of whom had about a month to live, only 37% of the doctors interviewed said they would share an accurate prognosis with their patients, and only if patients or their families pushed them to do so" (p. 1). The result, according to Christakis, is that doctors can make the end of life more difficult because "patients are given no chance to draft wills, see distant loved ones, make peace with estranged relatives or even discuss with their families their wishes about how to live the end of their lives. And they are denied the chance to make decisions about what kind of medical care they want to receive" (p. 1). Because doctors overestimate the time a patient has left to live by tripling it, patients are often encouraged to have needlessly painful and expensive medical procedures that complicate the late stages of life.

The CDC (2007) reports that "More than one-third of US deaths are preventable. Three behaviors – smoking, poor diet, and physical inactivity – were the root causes of almost 35% of US deaths in 2000. These behaviors are risk factors that often underlie the development of the nation's leading chronic disease killers: heart disease, cancer, stroke, and diabetes" (p. 5).

Hardwig (2000) notes that people with terminal illnesses often suffer from an inability to find meaning in the last moments of their lives and are unable to deal with significant issues related to family and other loved ones. Often they feel "cast out" because they are no longer healthy or productive and feel as if they are a burden to others because they are unable to care for themselves, in even very basic ways. Hardwig suggests that people with terminal illnesses often feel isolated and angry about their lives and frequently feel abandoned by friends, family, and by God. Most of all, they feel betrayed by their own bodies and often have no way of dealing with the physical and emotional changes they are experiencing. Hardwig (2000) believes that "[f]acing death brings to the surface questions about what life is all about. Long-buried assumptions and commitments are revealed. And many find that the beliefs and values they have lived by no longer seem valid or do not sustain them. These are the ingredients of a spiritual crisis, the stuff of spiritual suffering" (p. 29).

Hardwig (2000) indicates that the following problems facing people with terminal illness frequently create difficulty in finding meaning in the last moments of life: (1) the medical care system often takes important treatment decisions out of the hands of terminally ill patients; (2) use of pain killing drugs leaves dying patients unable to think clearly and distorts the days and weeks before death occurs; (3) no one listens to terminally ill patients or helps them resolve unfinished business; (4) in a death-denying society, families may not allow terminally ill patients to discuss issues that often help the terminally ill person find important life messages and also help the family with bereavement; (5) family members may not want to "let go" of a loved one and thereby ignore the terminally ill patient's desire to end life naturally without intrusive life supports or treatments.

Caffrey (2000) confirms the role of psychotherapy in work with terminal illness. He believes that "palliative" care alone – the reduction of anxiety and depression related to dying, is short-sighted. In discussing his experiences with terminal patients, Caffrey writes, "end-of-life psychotherapy can go well beyond conventionally understood palliative care. I hope that [my experiences working with terminally patients] will inspire therapists working with terminally ill persons to keep their sights high, feel confident that major growth is possible, and communicate that confidence to their patients" (p. 529).

McClain et al. (2003, p. 1606) studied the spiritual well being of terminally ill patients and found that low levels of spirituality correlated highly with "end-of-life despair, providing a unique contribution to the prediction of hopelessness, desire for hastened death, and suicidal ideation even after controlling for the effect of depressive symptoms and other relevant variables" (p. 1606). The authors believe the most important single dynamic of spirituality is faith, since it provides hopefulness even during the end stages of terminal illness. The existence of hopefulness translates into cooperative relations with the treatment staff, better resolution of interpersonal and family problems, and a desire to live longer.

16.5 BEST EVIDENCE FOR WORK WITH TERMINAL ILLNESS

Just as the approaching end of a therapy session often stimulates candor and disclosure in a patient, so the approach of death can focus and stimulate life forces in a dying person. Kubler-Ross (1969, 1997) identified the "unfinished business" that so often keeps dying persons temporarily alive. The unfinished business can be simple or complex, but it usually has deep personal roots. The dying person is concerned, not so much about death per se, but about death as a constraint on life matters that need attending to. A student at Kubler-Ross's Death and Dying Seminar expressed amazement that the dying patients and hospital staff at her seminar "talked so little about death itself." In a summary remark, Kubler-Ross (1969, 1997) counseled, "We can help them die by trying to help them alive" (Caffrey, 2000, p. 519).

Greenstein and Breitbart (2000) write that Existentialist thinkers such as Frankl see suffering in those who are experiencing life-threatening illness as a catalyst for finding meaning in their experience. Terminal illness offers a patient the opportunity for personal growth in the process of learning to cope with pain and the possibility of death. Fromm et al. (1993) and Andrykowski et al.

(1993) have found positive emotional and social changes as well as an increased sense of meaning in life when people are diagnosed with malignancies and following bone-marrow transplantations. Greenstein and Breitbart (2000) write that "patients report reordering their priorities, spending more time with family, and experiencing personal growth through the very fact of having had to cope with their traumatic loss or illness" (p. 486).

Suffering may lead to empathy and the willingness to reach out to others. Morris Schwartz, the subject of *Tuesdays with Morrie* (Albom, 1997), used his illness to teach his student important lessons about life, and as Greenstein and Breitbart (2000) write, "Frankl felt that one of the things that helped him to cope with and ultimately survive his concentration-camp experience was his responsibility to publish the manuscript that was destroyed upon his arrival there, and to lecture at universities about the psychology of the concentration camp experience" (p. 486).

One of the curative functions of treating clients with serious or terminal illnesses and disabilities in a group context is that the sense of connectedness among people often becomes an overriding positive experience that helps group members cope with painful and distressing conditions in ways that prolong life and add to its meaning.

In describing the shift clinicians must make in order to use the strengths perspective with clients in crisis, Blundo (2001) believes that we must "de-center" ourselves from old traditions that assume "that 'truth' is discovered only by looking at underlying and often hidden meanings, making causal links in some sequential order leading to the 'cause' of it all" (p. 302). Instead, Blundo believes that we need to engage clients in crisis in a highly collaborative dialog, which may result in surprising outcomes for the client and the worker. He also thinks that a strengths-oriented approach to clients, without preconceived ideas of underlying pathology, will yield the most positive and meaningful results. When applied to the client with serious or terminal illness, this means that the process of a truly client-centered dialog may achieve startling information that moves clients into new areas of understanding of their situation and its relevance to their lives.

Lloyd-Williams (2001) reports that depression is apparent in a fourth of the terminally ill patients he has screened. Because depression may seriously interfere with medical treatment, comfort at the end stages of life, and psychological well being, the author suggests that treating depression is an important aspect of our work with the terminally ill. Another reason for treating depression in end-stage terminal illness is that symptoms of the illness may be increased by depression and physical distress may improve as the depression lifts. Lloyd-Williams (2001, p. 35) proposed the following strategies for the management of depression in patients with advanced cancer:

1. The establishment of good rapport.
2. Thorough psychiatric assessment and relief of poorly controlled symptoms.
3. Underlying organic factors detected and treated where possible.
4. Normal sadness and grief at the end of life differentiated from those indicating a depressive disorder.
5. Supportive psychotherapy for the patients in order to reduce sense of isolation.
6. Family intervention to support relatives.
7. Use of selective antidepressants.

In summarizing successful coping strategies used by seriously and/or terminally ill patients, Livneh (2000) suggests the following strategies:

1. **Problem-focused/solving coping and information seeking:** These strategies refer to resolution of the stress and anxiety of illness through information gathering, focused planning and direct action taking. These approaches have had positive effects on global mental health (Chen et al., 1996), have lead to decreased levels of depression and anxiety (Mishel and Sorenson, 1993), and have increased vigor (Mishel and Sorenson, 1993).
2. **Fighting spirit and confrontation:** These strategies are described as accepting a serious and perhaps life-threatening diagnosis while optimistically challenging, tackling, confronting, and recovering from the illness and have been linked to longer survival among people diagnosed with cancer (Greer, 1991) and to decreased scores on anxiety and depression (Burgess et al., 1988) and to decreased emotional or psychological distress (Classen et al., 1996).
3. **Focusing on positives:** This group of coping strategies (which includes positive restructuring and positive reframing) has been associated with psychological well-being (Ell et al., 1989) lower emotional distress (Carver et al., 1993) and increased vigor (Schnoll et al., 1995).

4. **Self-restraint:** This stratgey refers to personal control to cope with the stresses of a serious or terminal disease and is a predictor of lower emotional distress (Morris, 1986) but may also lead to a reduction of quality-of-life among survivors of such illnesses as cancer (Wagner et al., 1995).

5. **Seeking social support:** Seeking support and assitance from others has been linked to decreased emotional/psychological distress (Stanton and Snider, 1993), better psychosocial adaptation (Heim et al., 1997), and greater perceptions of well-being (Filipp et al., 1990).

6. **Expressing feelings or venting:** While the evidence is mixed, two studies show decreased depression (Chen et al., 1996) and better emotional control (Classen et al., 1996) when venting of feelings takes place. The negative aspect of this coping strategy is that angry patients sometimes allienate loved ones and the professional staff, which may lead to increased feelings of depression and loss of social supports in patients.

7. **Using humor:** Carver et al. (1993) found that the use of humor resulted in decreased emotional distress among people with cancer.

8. **Finding increased life meaning:** Many writers discuss the potential for increased meaning of life as a result of serious or terminal illnesses. McClain et al. (2003) found that high levels of spirituality in dying patients lead to hopefulness that resulted in a more cooperative relationship with the treatment team, improved resolution of long-standing emotional problems, and the desire to live longer. Finn (1999) believes that spirituality leads to "an unfolding consciousness about the meaning of human existence. Life crises influence this unfolding by stimulating questions about the meaning of existence" (p. 487). Balk (1999) suggests that three issues must be present for a life crisis to result in spiritual changes: "The situation must create a psychological imbalance or disequilibrium that resists readily being stabilized; there must be time for reflection; and the person's life must forever afterwards be colored by the crisis" (p. 485). Kubler-Ross (1969, 1997) believes that terminal illness often leads to life-changing growth and new and more complex behaviors which focus on meaning- of-life issues, while Greenstein and Breitbart (2000)write, "Existentialist thinkers, such as Frankl, view suffering as a potential springboard, both for having a need for meaning and for finding it" (p. 486).

16.6 NURSING HOMES

As illness and disabilities become incapacitating, older adults may move from independent living to assisted living, and eventually, to nursing homes. Fewer older adults live in nursing homes today than ever before. In 2006 about 7.4% of Americans aged 75 and older lived in nursing homes as compared to 8.1% in 2000 and 10.2% in 1990. Even so, almost two million older adults live in nursing homes, at an annual cost of $65,000–100,000 according to the 2006 MetLife Market Survey of Nursing Home and Home Care Costs (2006). The percentage of the oldest age group of seniors living in nursing homes has declined from more than 21% of the 85-plus population in 1985 to less than 16% of the 85-plus population in 2006 according to the National Nursing Home Survey (2008), a government study. Fifty-three percent of nursing home admissions stay less than a month. Several reasons for the decline include better older adult health that makes independent living possible for a longer period of time, the increased use of assisted living facilities, children caring for older parents at home often with outside help, and the fact that many older adults cannot afford a long-term nursing home stay even they need it for health reasons or the options are not good ones.

One of the reasons older adults unnecessarily go to nursing homes is the lack of after-care help provided in acute care facilities. Landefeld et al. (1995) matched 651 patients over 70 years of age, with confounding factors taken into consideration, and randomly assigned them to a special unit treating older adults or to general adult hospital unit. The patients who were treated in a special older adult unit significantly improved their ability to perform daily living activities on discharge and had a reduction in admissions to nursing homes over patients treated in a general hospital unit. Kleinpell (2004) found that a greater emphasis on discharge planning from acute facilities reduced the length of hospitalization and readmissions. Kleinpell also found that early comprehensive discharge planning resulted in older adult patients reporting that they experienced less concern about managing their care at home, knew their medicines, and knew danger signals indicating potential complications.

Hickman et al. (2007) reviewed 26 controlled studies related to older adults in acute care and their health and mental health following discharge. The researchers concluded that patients experienced a lower probability of going to a nursing home when, (1) a team approach to care delivery was used in a designated unit for older patients; (2) the team used targeted assessment techniques to prevent complications following discharge; (3) the acute care facility increased its emphasis on discharge planning; and (4) there was better communication between care providers, families, and referring physicians.

Many elderly residents of nursing homes experience mental health problems, particularly depression. Yet Bruhl et al. (2007) found that staff was accurately able to recognize depression in only 55% of the cases. Focused interventions, however, have been shown to improve mood and behavior among nursing home residents (Williams, 2007; Li and Carwell, 2007), and increasingly studies indicate that specific interventions that increase physical activity and strength contribute to overall improvement in health status and reduction in falls.

Haggstrom et al. (2007) indicate that the research evidence suggests that allowing choice, flexibility, and a variety of activities suited to diverse interests can mitigate the negative impact of institutionalization. In addition, the physical environment of the nursing home has an impact. Findings suggest that quality of life and safety are impacted by the physical layout, supportive features and finishes, reduced noise, and access to outdoor spaces. These improved environmental characteristics are linked to better outcomes for residents including improved sleep, way finding, orientation, reduced aggression and disruptive behavior, improved social interaction, and overall satisfaction and well-being. Nursing homes which focus on opportunities for residents to be physically active and healthy can increase resident safety as well as staff morale.

16.7 HELPING OLDER ADULTS MAKE AN INFORMED DECISION ABOUT NURSING HOMES

Baum (1999) suggests the following steps in helping an older adult choose and properly use nursing home services:

1. It is always a good idea for family members or professionals to do some research well in advance of a nursing home stay. When older adults are placed, there often isn't time to do an immediate search for the best nursing home.
2. Before choosing a nursing home, check on the alternatives. If the care needed is at the custodial level, an assisted living facility might be a better choice. If skilled nursing is needed, narrow the selection down to facilities located near family and friends, to make visits easier.

3. Meet aides, visitors, and the two most important staff in the facility – the administrator and director of nursing, who together set the tone for quality of care. A copy of the most recent Department of Health Services annual survey inspection report should be available in a main area. Check to see if deficiencies and citations are cited in the report and read the "plan of correction." Ask what steps the facility has taken to prevent recurrence of problems.

4. Request copies of the admittance agreement and Patient/Resident Bill of Rights. Observe patient care during different staff shifts, and visit the dining room during meal times. Notice if there are pleasant, accessible outdoor areas and if residents are well groomed and treated with dignity.

5. If skilled nursing care is physician-recommended, and if the prospective resident has been in the hospital for three days, Medicare will pay the costs for the first 20 days and part of the costs for the next 80 days. Get a written statement from the physician. This statement is very important if an insurer disputes the need for skilled care.

6. Make certain older adults are visited often and that roommates are at the same level of functioning. Don't let the older adult take valuable items with him or her because of the possibility of theft or loss.

7. Make sure that family and other loved ones walk with a relative during visits and that daily walking is included in the care plan to help them stay in good physical condition. A nursing home resident who is not walked often may soon lose the ability to walk.

8. Nursing home staff are not allowed to physically or chemically restrain a resident. A doctor may not order restraints without the permission of the resident or responsible party. That includes the use of anti-anxiety or tranquilizing drugs.

9. Both the resident and the responsible parties have access to the patient/resident record book, which should be reviewed periodically. It contains doctors' notes and orders, nurses' progress notes, incident reports, medications, and various documentation. The resident's Durable Power of Attorney for Health Care and Advance Directive documents should be included in the patient record book. Check medications and dosages listed, and don't hesitate to ask why a medication is given and what its potential side effects are.

10. If the resident is not bed-bound, avoid separating him or her from the world outside. A car trip, picnic or something not overly

taxing is good therapy. Nursing home staff should help transfer the resident to and from the car. If that isn't possible because of the patient's condition, fresh flowers, recent photos and family and friends often lift the spirits of nursing home patients.

A CASE STUDY: EVIDENCE-BASED PRACTICE WITH TERMINAL ILLNESS

Benjamin Lytle is a 62-year-old professor of chemistry who has been diagnosed with advanced prostate cancer. Ben had been experiencing discomfort and pain for over a year but did not seek medical help until he began noticing blood in his urine. The cancer metastasized quickly and had moved into a number of organs in his body. The doctors gave him less than a year to live. He has had surgery to remove his prostate and is on chemotherapy, which doesn't seem to be helping. Ben is depressed and ill from the chemotherapy treatments. He is seriously thinking of suicide and has consulted a physician who performs assisted suicides. His physician has recommended that Ben seek help for the depression, but Ben has been too depressed and weak to even consider it. A hospital social worker dropped by his room during one of his reactions to chemo when he was too ill to return home. The social worker sat and listened to Ben talk about the "mess" he'd made of his life and how his early death was just another example of "what a loser I am."

Talking to the social worker seemed strangely comforting so when she suggested that they continue talking, uncharacteristically, Ben agreed. Ben hates the feminizing way helping professionals make him feel and described what it felt like going to a marital counselor when his marriage fell apart. "I felt like someone lobbed off my balls, which is funny because that's exactly what's happening to me now." The social worker was much more understanding than the marital counselor and Ben felt she wasn't going to make him feel weak.

As Ben continued seeing the worker on a bi-weekly basis, he shared with her his life disappointments. She listened and observed that he was being very hard on himself because she felt that Ben had done amazing things in his life. Ben wasn't so sure he agreed and wondered if the worker was just trying to placate him as he moved toward death. The worker assured him that she didn't believe placating ever worked, but it certainly wouldn't work with a highly intelligent person like Ben. As Ben thought about their conversations, he began to realize that he'd been successful in many small and large ways but that an inner voice, the voice of his father, kept insisting that he'd been a failure. Gradually, the inner voice changed and Ben felt that he was beginning to see what the worker meant. He also felt better physically, although his health was declining and death was imminent.

Ben decided that he would return to teaching even if he didn't make it through the semester. He felt he would be a much more considerate teacher than he'd been. He also decided to talk to everyone with whom he'd stopped talking because of real or imagined conflicts. This included many colleagues and family members who, he thought, had hurt him over the years. As Ben began to talk to old friends and members of his family, he felt elation at being able to try and resolve old hurts before he died. The people he spoke to felt the same way and said that they'd missed Ben and were happy to have him back in their lives.

Ben made it through the semester and, with a good deal of help from his doctors, through the next semester. By the time death was only days away, Ben had developed a support network that consisted of estranged friends, family, former students, and the people he'd met in the hospital during his treatment. Before he passed away, Ben told the worker, "You saved my life. I was full of bile before we started talking and now I feel a strange sort of happiness and contentment. I think I've made a difference in people's lives the past year. I think I lived longer because I was able to get rid of a lot of the toxic feelings I had inside. You always treated me with respect, and you acknowledged my intelligence. It made me want to do as much for myself and for others as possible. I'll leave the world, but a lot of who I am will stay on. I owe a lot to you for helping me put my anger to constructive use. And sure, nobody wants to die while they're still young, but if it happens, you make the best of it and you try and touch other people in some way. Getting my life in order made me live six months longer and it gave me more time to make up with people I love. Thank you for the gift of life. Every day I live beyond what the doctors said is a gift from God."

In describing her work with Ben, the worker said that, "Like many dying patients, Ben was angry over dying. He had his mind set on suicide because of the pain he was in, but also because he felt so helpless. He'd always thought that he had control over his life and now, for once, he had no control at all. Helping him see his strengths, respecting his anger, encouraging his need to finish unfinished business, and watching his transformation from an angry and hateful person to a loving and kind person has been a very special experience for me. I see it so often that when people search for endings that include resolving old conflicts, they live longer, happier, and more pain-free lives. While death isn't pleasant, I think people like Ben die peacefully. One of the patients I worked with about the time Ben was in his last few days shared something he'd written with me and with the other patients on his hospital ward. It gave meaning to many of us."

I will go to the river and I will lie in peace.

And when the sun sets, I will sleep the peaceful sleep of a child.

And when it is dark and night comes,

I will go from this place to the next,

And I will be with God, and I will know

His tender mercies.

16.8 A PERSONAL STORY: RECONNECTING WITH AN ABSENT TERMINALLY ILL PARENT

"My husband's parents divorced when Jack was 17; his father was an alcoholic, and Jack saw little of his father after the divorce. When Jack was in his thirties, he reconnected briefly with his father, but saw him intermittently. Ten years later, Jack's father contacted him once more. He was dying, and wanted to see his son. Jack and his sister Letty drove 75 miles to visit their father. Letty had been in touch with her father, but as his health began to fail, he was often talking about seeing Jack again. Letty knew that Jack was reluctant to talk to his father, having many old feelings which were painful. 'Better to let sleeping dogs lie,' was his usual saying. It was a strangely calm meeting. Their father, Joe, had been recently diagnosed with pancreatic cancer, was given a terminal diagnosis of an expected life of only 30 days remaining. Joe had opted to have hospice care and remain at the nursing home, where he had lived for the past three months.

"Jack and Letty were quickly able to set aside old resentments, recognizing that his father did not have long to live. Joe had obviously been thinking a lot about this reunion. 'I know I haven't been much of a father to either of you,' he told Jack, 'but I don't have much time left. I figured we might spend some of it on the important things.'

"They spent some time talking to their father before he became quite tired, and needed to rest. Letty and Ben spoke to the nurse at the nursing home, who filled them in on Joe's care. They made an appointment to meet with the hospice social worker the next day.

"Over the course of the next several weeks, Jack and Letty spent hours with their father. The nursing home had a courtyard, and so they pushed their father's wheelchair outside in the afternoons, so he could enjoy the flowers and the sunshine. They talked over past times, good and bad, and had the opportunity to make amends for a number of issues from the past.

"Jack said, 'good, bad, or ugly, you're my father, and I'm grateful for this last chance to set some things right.' Joe said he wasn't in much pain, and his hospice nurse took good care of him. The social worker helped them talk about funeral plans, what to expect, and opened the door for many conversations they had never expected to have.

"On the day Joe died, Letty and Jack had just come back from lunch. Joe was only briefly awake that day, and opened his eyes to say, 'it isn't so bad now. Thank you.' Later, Jack and Letty recalled that moment many times, and felt, for them, and in their situation, it summed up a lifetime. Jack said, 'That was the best gift my father could have given us. Hospice helped us have that time with our father. He wasn't much of a father when he was alive, but we felt we owed each other something, nevertheless.' And there was peace in that." – SYB.

16.9 SUMMARY

This chapter discusses disabilities, serious illness, pain, assisted living and nursing homes. As older adults live healthier lives and alternative living and care giving arrangements become more common, decreasing numbers of older adults use nursing homes. When nursing homes are used, it's often for a short period of time. A case study and a personal story illustrate the positive changes that often take place when terminally ill patients are allowed to finish unfinished business.

16.10 QUESTIONS FROM THE CHAPTER

1. Some people with terminal illness find great strength in resolving unfinished personal business. Can you think of unfinished business that might be important to resolve for anyone with a terminal illness?

2. Many people choose assisted living facilities when they could easily live by themselves. Why do you think that is? Should we make the standards for getting into an assisted living facility more difficult to encourage more independence in older adults who may be able to do for themselves but choose not to?

3. Viktor Frankl survived the Holocaust and wrote about his experiences as a survivor. Do you think people who have survived genocide do so because they find meaning in the experience or because they have a tremendous will to live and do whatever it takes to survive?
4. The idea of treating depression in terminally ill people seems a little unrealistic. Isn't terminal illness a good reason to be depressed and shouldn't our treatment focus on patient comfort and an opportunity to live the last part of their lives with dignity, honor and as little discomfort as possible?

REFERENCES

Albom, M. (1997). Tuesdays with Morrie: An old man, a young man, and life's greatest lesson. New York: Doubleday Press.

Americans with Disabilities Act of 1990, (2008), ADA Home Page. <http://www.ada.gov/>

Andrykowski, M. A., Brady, M. J., & Hunt, J. W. (1993). Positive psychosocial adjustment in potential bone marrow transplant recipients: Cancer as a psychosocial transition. *Psycho-oncology, 2*, 261–276.

Balk, D. E. (1999). Bereavement and spiritual change. *Death Studies, 23*(6), 485–493.

Baum, R. (1999). No need to worry, just be informed. Foresight can make a big difference with planning for a nursing home (July 7). <http://www.community-newspapers.com/archives/campbellreporter/07.07.99/seniors-9927.html/>

Berenson, A. (2008). Drug approved. Is disease real? (Jan. 14). Nytimes.com. <http://www.nytimes.com/2008/01/14/health/14pain.html?pagewanted=1&_r=2/>

Berry, P., & Ward, S. (1995). Barriers to pain management in hospice: A study of family caregivers. *The Hospice Journal, 10*(4), 19–33.

Blundo, R. (2001). Learning strengths-based practice: Challenging our personal and professional frames. *Families in Society, 82*(3), 296–304.

Bonica, J. J. (1990). Multidisciplinary/interdisciplinary pain programs. In J. J. Bonica (Ed.), *The management of pain* (pp. 197–208). Philadelphia, PA: Lea & Febiger.

Braithwaite, D. O. (1996). Exploring different perspectives on the communication of persons with disabilities. In E. B. Ray (Ed.), *Communication and disenfranchisement: Social health issues and implications* (pp. 449–464). Hillsdale, NJ: Lawrence Erlbaum.

Brockopp, D., Warden, S., Colclough, G., & Brockopp, G. (1996). Elderly hospice patients' perspective on pain management. *The Hospice Journal, 11*(3), 41–53.

Bruhl, K., Luijendijik, H., & Muller, M. (2007). Nursing and nursing assistants' recognition of depression in elderly who depend on long term care. *Journal of American Medical Directors Association, 8*(7), 441–445.

Bruner, J. (1990). *Acts of meaning.* Cambridge, MA: Harvard University Press p. 24.

Burgess, C., Morris, T., & Pettingale, K. W. (1988). Psychological response to cancer diagnosis – II. Evidence for coping styles. *Journal of Psychosomatic Research, 32,* 263–272.

Caffrey, T. A. (2000). The whisper of death: Psychotherapy with a dying Vietnam veteran. *American Journal of Psychotherapy, 54*(4), 519–530.

Carver, C. S., Pozo, C., Harris, S. D., Noriega, V., Scheier, M. F., & Robinson, D. S. (1993). How coping mediates the effect of optimism on distress: A study of women with early stage breast cancer. *Journal of Personality and Social Psychology, 65,* 375–390.

CDC and Merck (2007). *The State of Aging and Health in America.*

Chen, C. C., David, A., Thompson, K., Smith, C., Lea, S., & Fahy, T. (1996). Coping strategies and psychiatric morbidity in women attending breast assessment clinics. *Journal of Psychosomatic Research, 40,* 265–270.

Christakis, N.A. (2007). The bad news first (Aug. 24). <http://www.nytimes.com/ 2007/08/24/opinion/24christakis.html?th=&emc=th&pagewanted=print/>

Cigolle, C. T., Langa, K. M., Kabeto, M. U., Tian, Z., & Blaum, C. S. (2007). Geriatric conditions and disability: The health and retirement study. *Annals of Intern Med., 147,* 156–164.

Classen, C., Koopman, C., Angell, K., & Spiegel, D. (1996). Coping styles associated with psychological adjustment to advanced breast cancer. *Health Psychology, 15,* 434–437.

Coleman, L. M. (1997). Stigma: An enigma demystified. In L. J. David (Ed.), *The disability studies reader* (pp. 216–231). New York: Routledge.

Cook, A. J. (1998). Cognitive-behavioral pain management for elderly nursing home residents. *Journal of Gerontology: Psychological Sciences, 53B,* P51–P59.

Crook, H., Ridout, E., & Browne, G. (1984). The prevalence of pain complaints among a general population. *Pain, 18,* 299–314.

Druss, B. G., Marcus, S. C., Rosenheck, R. A., Olfson, M., et al. (2000). Understanding disability in mental and general medical conditions. *American Journal of Psychiatry, 157*(9), 1485–1491.

Eldercare Locator: Assisted Living (2008) <http://www.eldercare.gov/eldercare/Public/ resources/fact_sheets/assisted_living.asp/>

Elderly hospice patients' perspective on pain management. *The Hospice Journal, 11* (3), 41–53.

Ell, K. O., Mantell, J. E., Hamovitch, M. B., & Nishimoto, R. H. (1989). Social support, sense of control, and coping among patients with breast, lung, or colorectal cancer. *Journal of Psychosocial Oncology, 7,* 63–89.

Engel, G. (1959a). Psychogenic pain and the pain prone patient. *American Journal of Medicine, 26,* 899–918.

Engel, G. (1959b). The onset of facial pain: A psychological study. *Psychotherapy and Psychosomatics, 34*, 11–16.

Filipp, S. H., Klauer, T., Freudenberg, E., & Ferring, D. (1990). The regulation of subjective well-being in cancer patients: An analysis of coping effectiveness. *Psychology and Health, 4*, 305–317.

Finn, J. (1999). An exploration of helping processes in an online self-help group focusing on issues of disability. *Health & Social Work, 24*(3), 220–231.

Flor, H., Fydrich, T., & Turk, D. (1992). Efficacy of multidisciplinary pain treatment centers: A meta-analytic review. *Pain, 49*, 221–230.

Fordyce, W. (1990). Contingency management. In J. Bonica (Ed.), *The managment of pain* (pp. 1702–1709). Philadelphia, PA: Lea & Febiger.

Frankl, V. E. (1978). Psychotherapy and existentialism: Selected papers on logotherapy. New York: Touchstone Books.

Fromm, K., Andrykowski, M. A., & Hunt, J. W. (1993). Positive and negative psycho-social sequelae of bone marrow transplantation: Implications for quality of life assessment. *Journal of Behavioral Medicine, 19*, 221–240.

Greenstein, M., & Breitbart, W. (2000). Cancer and the experience of meaning: A group psychotherapy program for people with cancer. *American Journal of Psychotherapy, 54*(4), 486–500.

Greer, S. (1991). Psychological response to cancer and survival. *Psychological Medicine, 21*, 43–49.

Haggstrom, E., & Kihlgren, A. (2007). Experiences of caregivers and relatives in public nursing homes. *Nursing Ethics, 14*(5), 691–701.

Heim, E., Valach, L., & Schaffner, L. (1997). Coping and psychosocial adaptation: Longitudinal effects over time and stages in breast cancer. *Psychosomatic Medicine, 59*, 408–418.

Hickman, L., Newton, P., Halcomb, E. J., Chang, E., & Davison, P. (2007). Best practice interventions to improve the management of older people in acute care settings: A literature review. *Journal of Advanced Nursing, 60*(2), 113–126.

Kelley, P., & Clifford, P. (1997). Coping with chronic pain: Assessing narrative approaches. *Social Work, 42*, 266–277.

Kleinpell, R. M. (2004). Randomized trial of an intensive care unit based early discharge planning intervention for critically ill elderly patients. *American Journal of Critical Care, 13*(4), 335–345.

Korcz, I. R. (2003). Oncology social workers perceived barriers to cancer pain and the relationship to the functional assessment of pain and non-pharmacological strategies. *851. Social Work Abstracts, 39*(2).

Kubler-Ross, E. (1969, 1997). *On Death and Dying.* New York: Touchstone.

Landefeld, C., Palmer, R., Kresevic, D., Fortinsky, R., & Kowal, J. (1995). A randomized trial of care in a hospital medical unit especially designed to improve the functional outcomes of acutely ill older patients. *New England Journal of Medicine, 332*(20), 1338–1344.

Li, L., & Conwell, Y. (2007). Mental health status of home care elders. *Gerontologist, 47*(4), 528–534.

Livneh, H. (2000). Psychosocial Adaptation to Cancer: The Role of Coping Strategies. *Journal of Rehabilitation* (April 1). Found on the Internet 14.04.2005 <http://www.findarticles.com/p/articles/mi_m0825/is_2_66/ai_62980227/print/>

Lloyd-Williams, M. (2001). Screening for depression in palliative care patients: A review. *European Journal of Cancer Care, 10*(1), 31–36.

McClain, C. S, Rosenfeld, B., & Breitbart, W. (2003). Effect of spiritual well-being on end-of-life despair in terminally-ill cancer patients. *Lancet, 361*(9369), 603–1608.

Mersky, H. & Boyd, D. (1978). Emotional adjustment and chronic pain. *Pain* (5), 173–178.

Metlife Survey of Nursing Home and Home Care Costs (2006, September). <http://209.85.173.104/search?q=cache:ybv4XP1CgNQJ/> : <www.metlife.com/WPSAssets/18756958281159455975V1F2006NHHCMarketSurvey.pdf+metlife+survey+of+nursing+home+costs&hl=en&ct=clnk&cd=1&gl=us&client=firefox-a/>

Merriam-Webster, (1991). *Ninth new collegiate dictionary*. Springfield, MA: Merriam-Webster, Inc pp. 846, 1179.

Mishel, M. H., & Sorenson, D. S. (1993). Revision of the Ways of Coping Checklist for a clinical population. *Western Journal of Nursing Research, 15*, 59–76.

Morley, S., Eccleston, C., & Williams, A. (1999). Systematic review and meta-analysis of randomized controlled trials of cognitive behaviour therapy and behaviour therapy for chronic pain in adults, excluding headache. *Pain, 80*, 1–13.

Morris, T. (1986). Coping with cancer: The positive approach. In M. Watson & S. Greer (Eds.), *Psychosocial issues in malignant disease* (pp. 79–85). New York: Pergamon Press.

National Nursing Home Survey: Next-of-Kin Component and Followup (NNHSF) Public-Use Data Files (2008, September). National Center for Health Statistics. <http://www.cdc.gov/nchs/products/elec_prods/subject/nnhsf.htm/>

New York Times (2007). Editorial: World's best medical care? (August 12). <http://www.nytimes.com/2007/08/12/opinion/12sun1.html/>

Older Americans Update 2006: Key indicators of well-being (2007). Federal Interagency Forum on aging related statistics. National Center for Health statistics. <www.agingstats.gov/>.

Parmalee, P. A., Katz, I. R., & Lawton, M. P. (1991). The relation of pain to depression among institutionalized aged. *Journals of Gerontology, 46*, 15–21.

Rand Corporation (2004). The Quality of health care received by older adults. Retrieved on the Internet 23.01.2007 <http://www.rand.org/pubs/research_briefs/2005/RB9051.pdf/>

Roy, R. (1981a). The social worker's role in a behavioral management approach to chronic pain. *Social Work in Health Care, 3*(2), 149–157.

Roy, R. (1981b). Chronic pain: A social work view. *The Social Worker-Travailleur Social, 54*(2), 60–63.

Roy, R. (1981c). Social work and chronic pain. *Health and Social Work, 6*(3), 61–65.

Roy, R., & Michael, T. (1986). A survey of chronic pain in an elderly population. *Canadian Family Physician, 32*, 513–516.

Schnoll, R. A., Mackinnon, J. R., Stolbach, L., & Lorman, C. (1995). The relationship between emotional adjustment and two factor structures of the Mental Adjustment to Cancer Scale. *Psycho-Oncology, 4*, 265–272.

Shworles, T. R. (1983). The person with disability and the benefits of the microcomputer revolution: To have or to have not. *Rehabilitation Literature, 44*(11/12), 322–330.

Snelling, J. (1990). The role of the family in relation to chronic pain. *Journal of Advanced Nursing, 15*(7), 771–776.

Stanton, A. L., & Snider, P. R. (1993). Coping with a breast cancer diagnosis: A prospective study. *Health Psychology, 12*, 16–23.

van Tulder, M., Ostelo, R., Vlaeyen, J., Linton, S., Morley, S., & Assendelft, W. (2000). Behavioral treatment for chronic low back pain. *Spine, 26*, 270–281.

Wagner, M. K., Armstrong, D., & Laughlin, J. E. (1995). Cognitive determinants of quality of life after onset of cancer. *Psychological Reports, 77*, 147–154.

Widner, S., & Zeichner, A. (1993). Psychologic interventions for the elderly chronic pain patient. *Clinical Gerontologist, 13*, 3–18.

Chapter seventeen

Hospice and Bereavement

17.1 INTRODUCTION

The author wishes to thank Ms. Rebecca Hampton, MSW for the use of material she developed on hospice care for an advanced social policy class the author taught, and for her perceptive insights into the workings of the Medicare-supported hospice program.

This chapter discusses two end-of-life issues human service workers frequently deal with at some point in their career: hospice and bereavement. Hospice is a program provided through Medicare to ease the suffering of dying patients in the last six months to a year of life. Bereavement refers to the process of grieving for a loved one. When bereavement is unresolved or very long lasting we refer to it as prolonged or traumatic grief. It is one of the more difficult-to-treat problems we encounter because, unlike depression, prolonged grief is often unresponsive to therapy unless we first understand the many complex reasons for the traumatic nature of the grief. A case study explains how prolonged grief can be triggered by unresolved anger at a lost loved one.

17.2 HOSPICE

Hospice provides a team of skilled professionals working together to provide palliative care for terminally ill patients facing life-threatening illness. While under hospice care, terminally ill patients and their caregivers receive medical attention, counseling, bereavement services, volunteer help, symptom management, grief counseling, and supportive services.

Under Medicare regulations patients who receive hospice care are not permitted to seek aggressive treatment. In its place they receive treatment that provides symptom and pain management provided by a medical director, nurse, and a certified nursing assistant (CNA) working together with the patient and their family to provide case management. The medical director is responsible for regulating medications, nutrition, and overall case management. The nurse is responsible for overseeing the medications, nutrition, and case management on a more daily basis. Nurses also monitor and dress wounds, ensure that the patient has the right durable medical equipment (DME), and advocate for any other needs to the doctor, facility, family, and hospice. The certified nursing assistant provides hygiene care and delivers medical supplies and other daily needs.

To receive hospice benefits covered by Medicare, a person must meet all of the following criteria:

1. They must be eligible for Medicare Part A.
2. A physician or medical director must certify that the patient has a terminal prognosis of six months or less to live.
3. The patient must sign a statement choosing hospice care instead of Medicare-covered medical care, which might be much more aggressive than the care provided by hospice.
4. The patient must choose a Medicare-approved hospice program.
5. Once they are admitted to hospice, the terminally ill patient may receive two ninety-day election periods of service, followed by an unlimited amount of sixty-day periods.
6. A person must show a decline in health during each certification period in order to be recertified for continued hospice care.
7. A physician must deem the patient eligible and appropriate to remain on service after each certification period.

Hospice care can be provided at home or in an assisted living facility or nursing home but patients often choose to live at home because it is more comfortable than a nursing home and family can be involved in the patient's care. When living at home isn't possible the hospice team works with the staff of the facility to provide the extra care given when a patient is in hospice. A third way patients can receive hospice services is in a hospice inpatient unit. Some hospices provide long-term care in their facility for their patients, while others restrict full-time care to a brief stay in the unit. The benefits of long-term care include constant monitoring and close supervision of symptoms with a palliative care perspective.

According to the National Hospice and Palliative Care Organization (NHPCO) nearly 1.3 million people received hospice care in 2006, a 162% increase in 10 years. Thirty-six percent of all deaths in the USA were under a hospice program (NHPCO, 2007, p. 1). A large majority of hospice patients are age 65 or older, with only 18% under 65. Most hospice patients are Caucasian (NHPCO, 2007, p.4).

Minority patients often under utilize hospice care. Rhodes (2006) suggests the following reasons: lack of knowledge about hospice programs; mistrust of the health care system; conflicts between an individual's spiritual and cultural beliefs and the goals of hospice care; the preferences for aggressive life-sustaining therapies; racial bias by care providers; and cultural insensitivity to the ways various racial and ethnic groups view terminal illness. Welch et al. (2006) found that African-American family members were less likely to rate the care their family members received at the end of life as "excellent" or "very good." They were also more likely to have concerns about being told what to expect when their loved one died, and more likely to be distressed about the amount of emotional support they received from the health care team during their loved one's last days.

NHPCO (2007) reports that hospice care may prolong the lives of some terminally ill patients. Among the patient populations studied, the mean survival was on average 29 days longer for hospice patients than for non-hospice patients. The largest difference in survival between the hospice and non-hospice cohorts was observed in congestive heart failure patients where the mean survival period increased from 321 days to 402 days.

Although hospice care can provide superb symptom management and comfort and dignity in death, hospice services are underutilized by the dying population. "Fewer than one-third of patients receive hospice care near the end of life and one-third of patients enroll in the last week of life" (Casarett et al., 2006, p. 472). Underutilization of hospice can result in increased costs in end-of-life care, increased hospitalization, unmanaged symptoms, and increased pain in death.

There are a number of reasons why the Medicare Hospice Benefit is underutilized. Among them is a person's desire for life-sustaining treatment, lack of access to services, non-referral by the family or physician, lack of knowledge of the program, and hospice admission practices. A desire to seek life-sustaining treatment is often a barrier to receiving hospice services. Persons receiving hospice services are restricted from obtaining aggressive treatments for their hospice diagnosis. As an example, an older adult suffering from cancer is unable to have radiation treatment to cure the cancer. Zimmermann (2004) suggests that denial of impending death may be an additional reason patients and family members reject hospice care and instead seek aggressive treatment when additional medical help may either result in death or leave the patient in additional discomfort and pain.

In urban areas with large elderly populations there are often many competing hospice organizations. This ensures that every person who is eligible and desires hospice services can receive them. However, those living in rural areas may not be able receive the same benefits because there are fewer hospice organizations and fewer people being served.

Although hospice has great appeal, Winter et al. (2007) asked a sample of terminally ill patients about dying without active treatment. In general they felt it would be a lonely experience. The study supported the notion that social interaction is one of the most important features of a "good death." Given a choice between, "life-prolonging treatment versus comfort care may in fact represent a choice between being surrounded by others (perhaps including medical personnel) versus being alone. If so, the choice in favor of life-prolonging treatment may indicate a preference for social interaction rather than for the active treatment itself" (Winter et al., 2007, p. 626). Decisions about palliative care may then be delayed because aggressive treatment represents the possibility of increased medical care, which in the minds of those sampled, could protect them against the loneliness of dying alone.

The authors believe that these findings have significance for a number of issues related to terminal illness and note,

> Healthcare providers should be cognizant of the diversity of beliefs about dying and the possibility that patients may be ignorant about the relevant options. They should take time to inquire about what patients (or surrogate decision makers) believe and take care to inform them fully about treatments, both active and palliative, rather than assume adequate knowledge. Similarly, advance care documents should provide much more complete information about treatment options. Adequate knowledge is essential for informed decision-making and true patient autonomy. (Winter et al., 2007, p. 628)

17.2.1 Best evidence for the effectiveness of hospice

Miceli and Mylod (2003) examined the satisfaction of family members with the end-of-life care their loved ones received. Data were collected from 1,839 individuals receiving care from 17 different care agencies nationwide. Although family satisfaction with hospice care was generally quite high, situational factors played a role. The timing of the referral was critical, with families rating services lower, almost across the board when the referral to hospice was deemed "too late." Additionally, families expressed greater satisfaction when the patient's care was overseen by the hospice director, rather than a personal physician. Each of these findings has important implications for physicians, patients, and families as they begin to plan for end-of-life care.

An NHPCO (2004) report noted that more than 70% of family members of patients who received hospice care at home rated the care as "excellent." The report indicated that bereaved family members of patients with home hospice services (in contrast to the other settings of care) reported higher satisfaction, fewer concerns with the care, and fewer unmet needs. Major findings of the report indicate the following:

- One in four patients who died did not receive enough pain medication. This was 1.6 times more likely to be a concern in a nursing home than in hospice at home.
- One in two patients did not receive enough emotional support. This was 1.3 times more likely to be the case in an institution than hospice.
- Twenty-one percent of family members complained that the dying patient was not always treated with respect. Compared with hospice, this was 2.6 times higher in a nursing home and 3 times higher in a hospital.
- One in four respondents expressed concern over physician communication and treatment decisions.
- One in three respondents said family members did not receive enough emotional support.
- Respondents whose loved ones received hospice in a home setting were the most satisfied. More than 70 percent rated hospice care as excellent. Fewer than 50 percent gave that grade to nursing homes or home health services (p. 1).

In a randomized, controlled trial of terminally ill cancer patients and their primary care givers, Kane et al. (1984) found that patients enrolled in a hospice program experienced significantly less depression and expressed more satisfaction with the care their loved ones received. Additionally, caregivers of hospice patients showed somewhat more satisfaction and less anxiety than those in the control group. Teno et al. (2004) found that loved ones who died at home with hospice services reported fewer unmet needs and greater satisfaction with their experience. Miller et al. (2003) observed that hospice enrollment improved pain assessment and management for nursing home residents.

Gazelle (2007, p. 322) reports that a reason hospice tends to be underutilized (the median length of hospice service is only 26 days, with one-third of patients referred to hospice care during the last week of life) is the lack of knowledge by physicians about hospice, concerns that the physician will lose control of the medical care, and a desire to aggressively treat the terminal illness. Gazelle believes that "many oncologists and other physicians regard the death of a patient as a professional failure. Many also fear that they will destroy their patients' hope, which physicians may believe lies only in efforts to increase the quantity rather than quality of life. Furthermore, physicians receive little training in the compassionate discussion of bad news" (p. 322). Nonetheless, Gazelle reports that

> Hospice care can successfully address the critical end-of-life concerns that have been identified in numerous studies: dying with dignity, dying at home and without unnecessary pain, and reducing the burden placed on family caregivers. Evaluation studies reveal consistently high family satisfaction, with 98% of family members willing to recommend hospice care to others in need. And the extensive expertise of physicians specializing in hospice and palliative medicine was recognized in 2006, when the field was accredited as a fully independent medical subspecialty. (p. 323)

17.3 BEREAVEMENT

Balk (1999) indicates that bereavement, the loss of a significant person in ones life, can result in physical and emotional problems, the most significant of which may include:

> [I]ntense and long-lasting reactions such as fear, anger, and sorrow. Bereavement affects cognitive functioning (e.g., memory distortions, attention deficits, and ongoing vigilance for danger) and behavior (e.g., sleep disturbances, excessive drinking, increased cigarette smoking, and reckless risk taking). It impacts social relationships as outsiders to the grief become noticeably uncomfortable when around the bereaved. And bereavement affects spirituality by challenging the griever's very assumptions about the meaning of human existence. (Balk, 1999, p. 486)

Jacobs and Prigerson (2000) suggest that while symptoms of bereavement may include all of those noted by Balk, bereavement sometimes develops into a very long-term problem which the researchers describe as "complicated or prolonged grief" lasting more than a year. The symptoms associated with complicated grief include highly intrusive thoughts about the deceased, numbness, disbelief, feeling dazed, and a loss of a sense of security. Complicated grief seems unresponsive to the usual treatments for bereavement, including interpersonal therapy alone or with tricyclic antidepressants. Finally, complicated bereavement results in longer duration and strength than normal symptoms of depression following the loss of a loved one.

Balk (1999) believes that bereavement is a catalyst for spiritual change because it triggers a life-threatening crisis that, in turn, threatens "well-being, challenges established coping repertoire, and over time, produces harmful and/or beneficial outcomes" (p. 486). While agreeing that loss of a loved one creates a life-changing crisis, Stroebe (2001) points out a number of problems with grief work. First, she reports that there is little empirical evidence that working through grief is a more effective process than not working it through. Second, there are very different ways of working through grief prescribed not only by cultures, but also by religion, by gender, and by socio-economic groups. She writes, "There is no convincing evidence that other cultural prescriptions are less conducive to adaptation than those of our own" (p. 654). Third, grief work limits itself to dysfunctional adaptations and has symptom removal rather than a broader understanding as its end goal. Finally, grief work lacks a precise definition and is poorly operationalized in research studies. This results in Stroebe (2001) asking, "What is being worked through? In what way?" (p. 655).

In answering these questions, Stroebe (2001) identifies the following major issues related to our understanding of bereavement:

1. How do people who have suffered the loss of a loved one cope with their loss?
2. How do we differentiate between normal and what Stroebe calls "complicated" or dysfunctional grief?
3. What are the defining causes of traumatic and non-traumatic bereavement?
4. Can people who cope with the death of a loved one do so in ways that are unrelated to meaning-of-life issues and focus primarily on coping with the removal of typical grief-related symptoms (depressions, sleep problems, inability to take over functions formerly performed by a loved one, grief that lasts a very long time, etc.)?
5. Does non-traumatic grief with no underlying symptoms following the loss of a loved one suggest denial or other behaviors that may result in later and, perhaps, more severe grief?

17.3.1 Best evidence for grief work

Piper et al. (2002) studied the relationship between the expression of positive affect in group therapy and favorable treatment outcomes for complicated (long-lasting) grief. The authors found a strong positive correlation between these two variables in a number of therapy groups studied. The authors believe that positive affect (smiles, nods in agreement, sympathetic looks) conveys optimism in the person and has a positive effect on others in the group. The authors also found positive affect to correlate well with a cooperative attitude and a desire to do the work necessary to resolve the complicated and traumatic grief they were experiencing. This was true regardless of the type of treatment that was offered, and no difference was seen in the effectiveness of cognitive-behavioral approaches or interpersonal approaches. Affect rather than the approach was the overriding factor in successful resolution of prolonged grief.

Kendall (1994) found cognitive-behavioral therapy effective with children suffering from separation anxiety after the death of a loved one. The authors report that treated children had reduced fears, less anxiety, better social skills, and lower scores on depression inventories. These gains continued in follow up a year after the end of treatment. The authors are uncertain if this same finding would be applicable to adults suffering prolonged grief. Jacobs and Prigerson (2000) note that self-help groups have been effective, to some extent, as adjuncts to professional therapy by "offering the inculcation of hope, the development of understanding, social supports, a source of normalization or universalization, and a setting to learn and practice new coping skills" (p. 487). Raphael (1977) studied a three-month psychodynamically oriented intervention for high-risk, acutely traumatized widows during the first stages of grief. The author defined high risk as the lack of support by a social network, the suddenness or unexpected nature of the death, high levels of anger and guilt, ambivalent feelings about the marital relationship, and the presence of other life crises related to or predating the death of a spouse. The predating life crises were often financial, work-related, involved children, substance abuse in the spouse of widow, or marital infidelity. When compared to the control group, the treatment group had better general health, was less anxious and depressed, and had fewer somatic symptoms.

Because of their concern that traumatic grief should be considered a separate diagnostic category due to its unique set of symptoms, Jacobs and Prigerson (2000) call for the development of a specific therapy for the treatment of grief. By specific therapy, they suggest one that "focuses on separation distress and relevant elements of traumatic distress that addresses several tasks (such as educating about the nature of these types of distress), helps individuals to cope with the distress, and mitigates the distress using variety of strategies" (p. 491).

CASE STUDY: EVIDENCE-BASED PRACTICE WITH PROLONGED GRIEF

Ellen Steward is a 63-year-old mother of three adult children whose husband suddenly passed away following a major heart attack. Ellen's husband was a health fanatic who worked out daily, often in preference to spending time with her. Jonathan, Ellen's 67-year-old husband, thought he was experiencing chest pains in the middle of the night but, as is the case with some heart victims in extreme denial, he went to the gym at 4:00 a.m. and began working out until he passed out and was pronounced dead at the scene. Ellen was left with a large number of debts, no insurance, and few benefits beyond social security.

Jonathan passed away over a year ago but Ellen has traumatic grief as noted by severe depression, high levels of anxiety, very angry and intrusive thoughts about Jonathan and the financial condition he left her in, and obsessive thoughts about what she wished she'd said to him before he died – uncomplimentary and angry remarks that conveyed her depth of despair over her current situation. Her physician referred Ellen to a therapist when she continued to complain of prolonged grief more than a year after Jonathan's death.

Ellen's therapist met with her and they immediately began a discussion of what was keeping Ellen from resolving her feelings of grief. Ellen was stymied, so the therapist suggested that she make a list of everything that came to mind and that she also do a literature search into the typical causes of prolonged grief and the best evidence of how to treat it so that they might continue the discussion at the next session. Ellen was initially angry that she was asked to do work that the therapist should be doing for her, and complained to her referring physician who encouraged her to give it a little more time. She half-heartedly did what the therapist had asked of her and returned only slightly prepared for further discussions at the next meeting.

When asked why she wasn't better prepared, Ellen became angry and confrontational. "You haven't even said you're sorry about my predicament," she said, and angrily confronted the therapist for doing what her husband always did: leaving decisions up to her. The therapist said she appreciated the feedback and did feel badly about Ellen's predicament. Still, she wondered why Ellen was unprepared and explained that only by working together could they resolve Ellen's painful and extended grief. Ellen promised to do more for the next session and, with the help of her precocious 10-year-old granddaughter, she was able to find Internet articles that seemed to very clearly explain why her grief wasn't going away and what she might do about it.

The next session with the therapist was very business-like and purposeful. Ellen was excited about what she'd read, described it to her therapist, and together they planned the following strategy to treat Ellen's symptoms of prolonged grief:

1. Ellen needed to discuss all the reasons for her anger at Jonathan. The therapist urged her to write them down and to bring the list with her the next session. Before she could resolve her anger with Jonathan, she had to be clear about *all* the reasons for her anger, even if they seemed illogical or suggested that Ellen's anger was unfounded.

2. If there was anything she could directly do about her anger, she would do it. Examples included trying to develop a strategy to help with finances, including a return to work.

3. She would join a self-help group for prolonged grief begun by a remarkable woman who had also gone through prolonged grief after the death of her 15-year-old son in a car crash.

4. Ellen would be seen by a psychiatrist to evaluate the use of anti-depressive medications and to supervise the medical treatment of her depression.

5. She would start a daily regimen of exercise and diet supervised by a nutritionist provided through her health care plan.

6. Her spiritual and religious ties had been broken after Jonathan's death. She missed both and planned to reestablish them.

7. She had distanced herself from Jonathan's family. While she had been close to them when Jonathan was alive, she felt irrationally angry and blamed them for Jonathan's obsessive worry about his physical condition. Jonathan's father began having heart attacks in his mid-forties. Ellen felt they had done too little to moderate Jonathan's anxiety about his health and subtly encouraged his over-indulgence in exercise. Ellen decided that it was important for her to reestablish her contact with the family because she and her children missed them.

8. She would continue on in treatment for at least 12 sessions.

Ellen's prolonged grief began to moderate itself after two months of treatment. By the third month she was back to her old self, although she still attended the self-help group and saw the therapist once a month to monitor her depression. She no longer took antidepressants, has maintained her exercise regimen and diet, and sees her in-laws regularly. She still has difficulty reestablishing her religious ties and continues to blame God for taking her husband. "Maybe I'll never feel the same way," she said, "but you never know. I keep hoping and, of course, I go to synagogue on the High Holy Days, but most of it just makes me mad, and I think that maybe I'm a spiritual person but not a religious one."

The Therapist's Comments

In commenting on Ellen's grief the therapist said: "I don't know that I would call her depression prolonged. It seems to me that people experience grief in their own unique way and Ellen's quick recovery, once she was in therapy, is a good example of how people respond to death and how therapy can be a helping process. Giving people assignments to help in their own recovery is energizing, and encouraging their own involvement in treatment can be very empowering. Ellen needed a little push and then she was better. She'll have moments of sorrow and despair. When you love someone and they pass on before their time, you expect that to happen. But on every measure of social functioning, Ellen is doing a great deal better. From the paucity of good sound evidence on the treatment of prolonged grief, one can't help but think that even at a professional level, we are still a death-denying society. One last thought. Grief and depression are two separate issues. Yes, people in grief feel depressed but you have to treat the grief as a separate issue. Many people find it hard to talk about death but you can't really help people cope with the death of a loved one without talking about the impact it's had. And you have to talk to people about their own notions of death because that's what drives their grief. In Ellen's case, she had begun losing her religious faith even before her husband died. The reasons are complex but she had a very confused relationship with her faith and yet was obligated to give her husband a religious funeral. It was very confusing to her. She says she hasn't been able to reconnect with her religious beliefs, and while I've encouraged that she try, it doesn't feel right to her and she's begun attending a group that discusses spirituality. It suits her needs now but at some point it time it may be important for her to have further discussions about her faith and why it's left her."

17.4 SUMMARY

This chapter discusses end of life issues including the use of hospice in the late stages of a terminal illness and EBP with bereavement and prolonged grief. The chapter also discusses the rules that apply to the use of Medicare-sponsored hospice programs and why hospice isn't used more. The most significant reasons for the under utilization of hospice appears to be concerns about dying alone and lack of referrals to hospice by physicians. A case study identifies the use of EBP with an older adult woman experiencing prolonged grief over the death of her husband.

17.5 QUESTIONS FROM THE CHAPTER

1. Giving up on life and choosing death by selecting hospice is contrary to the way most people think. Do you think you'd choose death if you had a terminal illness, or would you continue seeking medical solutions to maintain life?
2. Coping with the loss of a loved one may never be possible for some people. Can you imagine the death of a loved one that might be terribly difficult to cope with and that might have traumatic repercussions?
3. Although there were interesting reasons why some minority groups fail to use hospice care, don't you think it's a sign of a loving and caring attitude to want loved ones to live as long as humanly and medically possible?
4. Everyone reacts to the death of a loved one in different ways. Why do you think it's necessary for us to distinguish between normal and prolonged grief?

REFERENCES

Balk, D. E. (1999). Bereavement and spiritual change. *Death Studies, 23*(6), 485–493.

Casarett, D., Van Ness, P. H., O'Leary, J. R., & Fried, T. R. (2006). Are patient preferences for life-sustaining treatment really a barrier to hospice enrollment for older adults with serious illness? *Journal of the American Geriatrics Society, 54*(3), 472–478.

Gazelle, G. (2007, July 26). Understanding hospital – An underutilized option for life's final chapter. *New England Journal of Medicine, 357*(4), 321–324.

Jacobs, S., & Prigerson, H. (2000). Psychotherapy of traumatic grief: A review of evidence for psychotherapeutic treatments. *Death Studies, 2*(6), 479–496.

Kane, R. L., Wales, J., Bernstein, L., Leibowitz, A., & Kaplan, S. A. (1984). Randomized controlled trial of hospice care. *Lancet*, 890–892.

Kendall, P. C. (1994). Treating anxiety disorders in children: Results of a randomized clinical trial. *Journal of Consulting and Clinical Psychology*, *62*, 100–110.

Medicare. (2004). *Medicare benefit policy manual*. Retrieved 1.12.2007, from <http://www.cms.hhs.gov/manuals/Downloads/bp102c09.pdf/>

Miceli, P. J., & Mylod, D. E. (2003, September–October). *Am J Hosp Palliat Care*, *20*(5), 360–370.

Miller, S. C., Mor, V., & Teno, J. (2003). Hospice enrollment and pain assessment and management in nursing homes. *J Pain Symptom Manage*, *26*, 791–799.

National Hospice and Palliative Care Organization: NHPCO Facts and Figures: Hospice Care in America. (2007, November) Edition <http://www.nhpco.org/files/public/Statistics_Research/NHPCO_facts-and-figures_Nov2007.pdf/>

Piper, W. E., Ogrodniczuk, J. S., Joyce, A. S., & McCallum, M. R. (2002). Relationships among affect, work, and outcome in group therapy for patients with complicated grief. *American Journal of Psychotherapy*, *56*(6), 347–362.

Raphael, B. (1977). Preventive intervention with the recently bereaved. *Archives of General Psychiatry*, *34*, 1450–1454.

Rhodes, R. L. (2006, September). Racial disparities in hospice: Moving from analysis to intervention. *Virtual Mentor*, *6*(9), 612–616.

Stroebe, M. S. (2001). Bereavement research and theory: Retrospective and prospective. *American Behavioral Scientist*, *44*(5), 854–865.

Teno, J. M., Clarridge, B. R., Casey, V., et al. (2004). Family perspectives on end-of-life care at the last place of care. *JAMA*, *291*, 88–93.

US Department of Health and Human Services. (2005). *Medicare hospice benefits*. Retrieved 1.12.2007, from <http://www.medicare.gov/publications/pubs/pdf/02154.pdf/>

Welch, L. C., Teno, . J. M., & Mor, V. (2006). End-of-life care in black and white: Race matters for medical care of dying patients and their families. *J Am Geriatr Soc.*, *53*, 1145–1153.

Winter, L., Parker, B., & Schneider, M. (2007). Imagining the alternatives to life prolonging treatments: Elders' beliefs about the dying experience'. *Death Studies*, *31*(7), 619–631.

Zimmermann, C. (2004). Denial of impending death: A discourse analysis of the palliative care literature. *Social Science & Medicine*, *59*(8), 1769–1780.

Part six

Policy Issues and the Future of Care for Older Adults

Chapter eighteen

Final Words: Some Concerns about the Future of Older Adults

Although this book has focused on clinical issues, there are many policy implications for successful aging, which one must mention because they impact successful aging. Clearly, with Americans' increasing lifespan coupled with economic problems and the need to work longer, many older adults face a very different life after 65 than previous generations of older Americans who were financially able to retire early. The following are some of the issues that appear likely to affect aging in the future.

18.1 A LOOMING FINANCIAL CRISIS FOR OLDER AMERICANS CAUSED BY THE LACK OF SAVINGS AND SIGNIFICANT INCREASES IN THE COST OF LIVING, PARTICULARLY HEALTH CARE COSTS

Because Americans are not saving enough for retirement and only half of all employers sponsor retirement plans, Powell (2008) predicts that 150–200 million Americans will not have enough income to retire in a meaningful way, or at all. According to Powell, the average retirement income for a couple 65 and older is $25,610, with the median a meager $16,451. This is a far cry from the 70% to 80% of before-retirement income needed to maintain a similar standard of living on a mean American income of $48,451 and a median American income of

$65,527. Retirees in the bottom fifth of income – those with less than $8,261 in 2006 – get almost 90% of their money from social security with little to defray the significant increased cost of living Americans are currently experiencing. Powell wonders how Americans 65 and over will be able to afford health care, which is estimated to be $215,000 just to pay for medical expenses not covered by Medicare for 20 years following the start of Medicare benefits. If a couple lives to an average age of 92, the health care expenses rise to over $500,000 in today's dollars. This does not factor in the average cost of a year for a semiprivate nursing home room ($69,000), a year for a unit in an assisted living facility ($35,628), $19 an hour for home health aides, or $61 a day at an adult daycare center. These are estimates based on current costs that are expected to rise beyond the cost of living in future years.

These data come at a time when many people are concerned about changes in Medicare because the fund to keep Medicare afloat is quickly being depleted. What will large numbers of older Americans do if Medicare decreases its medical payments to retirees, and supplementary insurances follow suit? Medicare is already trying to reduce costs. PSA tests, which are so important in screening for prostate cancer, are currently limited by Medicare to one test a year even though prostate cancer can spread rapidly, and any older male with a higher than normal PSA will want to be tested repeatedly and frequently.

An attempt to lower Medicare costs by frequently contacting Medicare recipients by phone not only failed to prevent costly hospitalizations by helping older adults take better care of themselves to prevent more serious illness, but it found that many older adults had very limited knowledge about their conditions. Even with prompting from nurses the older adults who were contacted often failed to take necessary preventative actions (Abelson, 2008), a finding that bodes badly for the health of older Americans in an era of concern for the ability of Medicare to maintain itself financially. According to nurses making the calls, patients with diabetes often had never heard of an endocrinologist.

18.2 THE LACK OF AVAILABLE MEDICAL CARE

A critical medical problem for older adults is the lack of available primary care doctors. In Massachusetts, which recently increased availability of medical care through a universal health program, newly insured patients in rural and urban areas are finding a shortage of primary care doctors. If we move toward universal health care, and one hopes we do, there will clearly not only be a doctor shortage but an increase in the numbers of patients doctors will feel obligated to take. Sack (2008) describes how doctors in parts of Massachusetts have increased the numbers of patients seen from 18–20 a day to 25–30, eliminating or reducing the number of physical examinations, which take 45 minutes each, thus creating concerns about quality of care and the possibility of increased medical errors so often criticized in managed care. Sack (2008) reports that the number of primary care doctors has decreased by 50% since 1998 and that by 2020 there will be a need for 40% more primary care doctors, numbers unlikely to be reached without significant incentives for more doctors to choose primary care as their specialty over more lucrative specializations. Sack also reports that the country will need 85,000 new doctors by 2020 just to care for the expanding population and attrition in the medical profession. A looming doctor shortage will see a large increase in foreign-born and trained doctors with potential language barriers which could make communicating with older adults more difficult.

18.3 MORE PRESSURE ON OLDER ADULTS TO CARE FOR THEIR CHILDREN AND THEIR CHILDREN'S CHILDREN

Kleiner et al. (1998) report that the number of grandchildren living with their grandparents increased from 2.3 million to 4 million between 1980 and 1996. Over a third of those children were being raised solely by grandparents without the presence of either parent. Half of the grandparents raising grandchildren were ages 50–64, while 20% were over 65. Many grandparents in this situation suffer from economic difficulties or need to make job-related changes to accommodate child-caring responsibilities. According to Kleiner et al. (1998), many grandparents are denied benefits provided to foster parents because of their blood relation to the child, even though they may be in just as much need.

Kleiner et al. (1998) also report that older grandparents who may be coping with serious and frequent health issues experience problems with stamina and often feel emotionally and physically drained from their caretaking roles. As a result, they wonder if older grandparents may be unable to continue their parenting role and worry about what will happen to their grandchildren if something happens to them. The new responsibilities of caring for grandchildren often prevent grandparents from taking part in social activities with friends who may not want to include young children in their activities. Further, grandparents must often help children deal with the traumas that precipitated their role as caregivers. Those traumas may include the death of a parent, parents in prison, neglect or abuse of children by their parents, war, teenaged pregnancies, or any number of reasons a child can no longer live with a parent. Added to the stress of grandchildren living with older grandparents is the stress of their children and their grandchildren living together with older parents, and one can see how these arrangements may create serious problems for older adults.

Although there are positives that can occur when grandparents take caretaking responsibilities for grandchildren, including a more stable and supportive environment and protection from abuse and neglect (Burton et al., 1995), Shore and Hayslip (1994) found that custodial grandparents, when compared to traditional grandparents, report increased rates of behavioral problems among the children for whom they care. This may be explained in part by children coming to live with grandparents at a time of increased stress in the child's family of origin. Nonetheless, it does point out another area of increased stress for older adults caring for their grandchildren. However, as Kleiner et al. (1998) conclude, there has been too little research conducted on the impact of children raised by grandparents to know with certainty how children fare when they live with their grandparents, and whether it's a good idea for the children or for the older grandparents caring for them.

18.4 OLDER MEN AND THEIR SPECIAL NEEDS

As more and more men live longer lives, they will be prone to the same emotional problems affecting all older adults, but often without the belief that talking helps resolve inner turmoil. It is therefore very important for the human services to develop helping approaches that require a different approach to older men than those currently in use with clients who have been socialized into the benefits of counseling and psychotherapy. In discussing male socialization and the assumptions of counseling and psychotherapy, Robertson and Fitzgerald (1992) argue that traditional notions of psychotherapy are often ill suited for men for the following reasons: (1) while psychotherapy and counseling require self-awareness, men are encouraged to hide their feelings; (2) counseling and psychotherapy often require clients to admit that they have a problem, but men have been taught to deny that they have problems; (3) therapists often encourage clients to share their vulnerabilities, but men have been taught to hide their vulnerabilities so they can maintain a competitive edge; and, (4) counseling and psychotherapy ask clients to openly explore their problems with another person, but men have often been socialized to distrust others, to maintain rational control over their lives, and that "self-exploration should be done independently and on an intellectual level" (Robertson et al. 1992). In further explaining male resistance to therapy, the authors write:

> Many approaches to personal counseling require that clients bring a sense of self-awareness to the counseling room (client-centered, humanistic, gestalt, existential, and others); yet men appear to be socialized away from self-awareness and encouraged to control (or hide) their feelings. In addition, personal counseling is designed for people who admit they have problems, but men are generally taught to compete on their own and not admit that they need help. Many counselors further invite clients to disclose their vulnerabilities; men, however, are taught to hide their vulnerabilities to maintain a competitive edge. Finally, counseling asks clients to explore their lives openly with another person, whereas men are socialized to be in rational control of their lives, implying that any self-exploration should be done independently and on an intellectual level. Given these considerations, it seems reasonable that men avoid a process that requires them to consider failure instead of success, cooperation instead of competition, and vulnerability instead of power. (Robertson et al., 1992, p. 241)

These concerns about men and the use of treatment suggest a different approach to working with older men. In a study of how men view therapy, Robertson et al. (1992) devised two brochures; one which described counseling in a traditional way, while the other described therapy using terms such as classes, workshops, and seminars. Both brochures discussed reasons for coming for counseling (depression, academic failure, relationship problems, etc.) and described staff competence, waiting periods, and cost. Both brochures looked alike. The study found that men with traditional attitudes toward masculinity reacted more positively to descriptions of counseling which were consistent with male socialization processes. The authors concluded that men are more likely to stay in treatment when the service offered is supportive, reinforcing, instructional (advice giving), and non-confrontational, and write:

> [C]ounseling psychologists need to offer programs that emphasize self-help and problem-solving approaches, rather than offering solely counseling for deeper insight into self-development and personal emotions. Our findings are consistent with the tradition in counseling psychology

that encourages the use of culturally sensitive formats for providing services to clients representing ethnic minorities and those designated as "special populations." Although it is not usual to think of men in this fashion, it is also true that the masculine mystique generates a unique assumptive world that appears to function as a barrier to men in many areas (e.g., emotional, psychological). (Robertson et al., 1992, p. 245)

The special needs of older men are particularly important when it comes to the way men approach their health. Gupta (2003) reports that women are twice as likely as men to visit their doctors once a year and are more likely to explore broad-based preventative health plans with their physicians than are men. Men are less likely to schedule check-ups or to follow up when symptoms arise. Men also tend to internal-ize their emotions and self-medicate their psychological problems, while women tend to seek professional help. Virtually all stress-related diseases – from hypertension to heart disease – are more common in men.

American men between the ages of 45 and 64 suffer an estimated 218,000 heart attacks a year, compared with 74,000 a year for women in the same age group, one of the many reasons women live more than seven years longer than men (Drug Store News, 1998). Epperly and Moore (2000) report that men are at much greater risk of alcohol abuse than women, with the highest rates of alcoholism occurring in men between 25 and 39 years of age. However, age is not a deterrent for risk factors in men, and 14% of men over 65 are alcohol dependent as compared to 1.5% of women in the same age group. Male suicides in men over 65 are six times the rate of the general population, according to Reuben et al. (1996).

These findings of greater health problems among men are not explained by biological differences related to gender. Harrison et al. (1988) write that "Research suggests that it is not so much biological gender that is potentially hazardous to men's health but rather specific behaviors that are traditionally associated with male sex roles which can be (but in the case of women are not) taken on by either gender."

Saunders (2000) reports that a poll by Louis Harris and associates in May and November 1998 indicated that 28% of the men as compared to 8% of the women had not visited a physician in the prior year. While 19% of the women didn't have a regular physician, 33% of men didn't have one either. More than half of the men surveyed had not been tested for cholesterol or had a physical examination in the prior year. Waiting as long as possible to receive needed medical care was a strategy used by a fourth of the men studied, and only 18% of the men surveyed sought medical care immediately when a medical problem arose.

Additional health data paint an equally troubling picture of male health. *Drug Store News* (1998) reported the following information for American pharmacists: (1) women still outlive men by an average of six to seven years, despite advances in medical technology; (2) the death rate from prostate cancer has increased by 23% since 1973; (3) oral cancer, related to smoking, occurs more than twice as often in men; (4) three times as many men as women suffer heart attacks before age 65. Nearly three in four coronary artery bypasses in 1995 were performed on men; (5) bladder cancer occurs five times more often in men than women; (6) nearly 95% of all DWI cases involve men; (7) in 2001, suicide rates for all men had increased from 9.4 per 100,000 in 1970 to 19.3 per 100,000, while suicide rates for men over 60 were from 10 to 12 times higher than suicide rates for older women, with men over 85 having an astonishing suicide rate of 54 per 100,000 as compared to women in the same age group of 5 per 100,000 (CDC, Found on Internet May 2004).

These serious health and mental health problems suggest that special approaches are required in both medicine and the human services to help men take better care of their physical and emotional health, and that deteriorating health problems for men will escalate as more men enter the last third of their lives.

18.5 MAKING BETTER USE OF OLDER ADULTS

Many states have shortages of trained and experienced human service workers, teachers, physicians, and other professionals. In the small town in which the author lives, there are a number of retired clinical social workers, psychologists, and counselors from other states who want to work or volunteer a day or two a week, but either receive little interest from social agencies because of their ages, or aren't permitted to work because they lack a state license and don't want to go through the extended time and trouble of becoming licensed in a new state.

The licensing laws, which were originally developed to raise the level of practice, have so many unnecessary hoops to jump through that many older semi-retired professionals would rather not go through steps that seem irrational and, frankly, biased against older people. Writing about the employer view of older workers, Fein (1994) writes:

> Despite a decade-long push by private and government organizations to market older people as reliable and mature workers, advocates for people 55 and older say their efforts have largely failed.

They say that employers continue to view age not in terms of experience or stability but as deterioration and staleness. (p. 1)

It's shameful, that when older professionals ask to volunteer for agency work they are offered tasks so beneath them that out of a feeling of humiliation they withdraw their offers to volunteer. When you've been a high-level social worker, counselor or psychologist much of your life, answering phones or filing paper just doesn't excite most of us. A number of retired human service workers have been writing to their legislators urging the repeal of unnecessary requirements for older adults who can prove they are trained, have worked in the human services, and would like to help reduce the national shortage of human service professionals. It's too soon to know if change will take place but one hears that many younger workers are unhappy with licensing laws and the rigid ways they are administered. If 80 is the new 60, as we so often hear, then there are many years of help left that retired human service workers can offer social agencies in America, and which older adults in many fields can offer organizations facing labor shortages or shortages of trained workers.

18.6 CONCLUDING WORDS

Growing old in America is not the gentle process we so often hear and read about in the media. Many older adults face hard times ahead as medical costs spiral out of sight and reductions in coverage threaten the economic security of many lower- and middle-income older men and women. With increasing recognition of the need to stay healthy by living a successful aging lifestyle, many older adults are likely to live another 30 years past the age of retirement. What they do with their time and how organizations use their talents will define the way many older adults approach aging. To do nothing more than participate in leisure activities and travel is not what most older adults want when they retire. They want to feel valued, appreciated, and utilized in ways that help the community. They want to leave a legacy for their children and for their extended families and friends.

One worries that, for many older adults, the thrill of not working will be replaced by growing boredom and lethargy, and that anxiety about health issues will dominate their lives. The growing numbers of retirement communities that are detached from the larger community adds to this concern. Much as one can see that retirement communities offer fellowship and a richness of activities in a community of older people, they can also be rigid and dogmatic places to live where older adults are worried about breaking rules and being ostracized. And surprisingly, they can be places where people live very lonely lives, often forgotten and uncared for when they experience a crisis. One hears of communities without doctors close by and administrators who don't think the health and well-being of residents is their concern.

One wonders about the vitality of our society and whether we have grown complacent and politically detached, and whether older adults will give up on social progress, believing there is too little for them to do to matter, so why even try. I worry that older adults will be forced to work well beyond a point of burnout because the economic safety nets in savings, pension plans, and social security are quickly disappearing, and that the ability to gradually cycle off full-time work will be replaced by work well beyond the point of being physically and emotionally exhausted. One sees an increasing number of tired and frail older adults working in stores and restaurants. Their fatigue is palpable.

We live in a society of the moment and in this moment the worries, the desires and the dreams of older adults have been replaced by concerns that our youth aren't up to the task of maintaining and growing a vital and progressive society. Where the wisdom of age is often valued in other societies, in America age is often a sign of deterioration and a lack of productivity.

Finally, I worry about the health of the human services. We are not the respected, appreciated frontline people we were several generations ago. And yes, the conservative nature of our politics hasn't helped, but one sees serious problems in the way the human services function. Few men enter the human services and one can see that it bodes badly for developing treatment approaches for men, particularly older traditional men. The quality of the people entering the human services must be maintained, but after 40 years as an educator I see a decline in the ability of students entering social work. Many are acutely aware that they have writing problems or have trouble thinking critically and want to do something about it, but many others ride by on a cushion of mediocrity acceptable to the overworked academics training human service professionals. When you have graduate students who cannot write a simple term paper and ache at their lack of writing ability because in four years as undergraduates no one asked them to do extended writing assignments, you know we are letting down the clients who need the very best we can offer.

This moment in time is a turning point in the lives of older adults. I hope we put much more energy into helping the growing numbers of older adults who face the grim prospect of growing old without close family ties or good friends, and who live lonely and isolated lives. Loneliness is everything it's cracked up to be, and we should ache for the lonely older men and women of America and set our shoulders to the grindstone to make certain that every American who reaches that point in time when they no longer want to or are able to work, that every single one of them will have a loving, caring, and sympathetic world to live in where their only concern should be trying to make the very best of their lives and continuing to dream the dreams that keep us all young and vital.

18.7 PERSONAL STORY: ON THE JOYS OF BEING AN OLDER PUBLISHED AUTHOR

I recently attended a lecture by my fellow writer Christopher Hitchens about the war in Iraq. I count Mr Hitchens as a colleague because I've published nine books in the past four years, although my students think the bad jokes I include in all my books are the best part of them.

Mr Hitchens was brilliant and entertaining. I could probably learn a lot from him about being a successful writer, like wearing a white suit, drinking wine during the lecture, using words that would make my sainted mother blush, and fingering a cigarette so longingly that even though I don't smoke, I wanted to grab it out of his hand and smoke it for him.

The truth is that I put my heart and soul into my books even though they haven't sold enough copies to buy me a cup of coffee. You write to please yourself. I have a book coming out next year about children that makes me proud when I read it. I'm almost done with a mystery novel set in my hometown of Grand Forks, North Dakota, with descriptions of the weather that no one believes, and stories about my friends and teachers that make me choke back tears in the early morning when I write.

One of my books is about men, but it's really about my father and the tough and tender immigrant people I grew up with in North Dakota. Another book is about psychological resilience, but it's really about my daughter and members of my family who struggle with illness and every imaginable setback, and yet come out of that struggle stronger than ever. Another book is about positive psychology, an approach to helping others that focuses on what's right about people. I wrote it in the mountains of Utah where, everyday, deer and moose would come to my door and watch me write. No one can ever put a money value on that special experience.

My daughter Amy has contributed to many of my books. This is what she wrote about her juvenile onset diabetes: "After having diabetes for fourteen years, it has become more than a chronic disease for me, more than a steady companion; diabetes is very much a part of who I am. Diabetes is not a burden, nor is it a crutch. It is just a disease that I, and millions of others, live with every moment of every day. I live with diabetes as though it were my troubled child – a lot of work and occasionally painful, but in the end, oddly beautiful and uniquely mine." Who wouldn't want to write books when you can include such beauty?

This morning on my 68th birthday I got up at 6:00 a.m. and wrote the end of my book on aging. It is sunny and cool in the Arizona mountains, and the birds and squirrels are scampering around taking drinks from the pond, which my office faces in the back of our home. The scrub jays fly in, one after another, to pick up the peanuts in the shell we leave out for them and which they bury all over our property to retrieve when the spirit moves them. They are very picky and often snatch up five or six and discard them before they find the right one. I can tell that the raccoons have somehow gotten into the bird feeder and sprinkled birdseed on the ground where more varieties of birds are eating the leftovers than I can describe. A family of doves and quail parade by the pond at one point and sing a happy birthday song.

This place I live in with my life partner Patricia and my magical dog Maxie in the mountains of Arizona near Sedona is my dream of paradise. How like my life that my dog is a rescue dog and my life partner is someone I met so late in life. You can never give up on the dream. In this magical place we have mesquite trees, huge boulders with lush desert vegetation, and a waterfall and pond in our backyard. Deer, owls, coyotes, hawks, javelinas, eagles, and birds of every variety come to the pond to drink.

As I look out this morning before I begin to write, the one thing I know for certain is that I feel blessed to be able to do what I've always wanted to do; to be a published writer and to understand, in my daughter's words, that our task "is simply to discern what our gifts are and to utilize them. Because, in the end, we are each our own Tooth Fairies, taking what has been lost and giving gold in return." – MDG.

REFERENCES

Abelson, R. (2008, April 7). Medicare Finds How Hard it is to Save Money. NYTimes .com Retrieved May 4, 2008 at: http://www.nytimes.com/2008/04/07/business/ 07medicare.html?_r=1&th=&oref=slogin&emc=th&pagewanted=all

Burton, L., Dilworth-Anderson, P., & Merriwether-de-Vries, C. (1995). Context of surrogate parenting among contemporary grandparents. *Marriage and Family Review, 20*, 349–366.

Drug Store News. (1998). Men's health at a glance: A fact sheet for pharmacists (July 20). Found on the Internet 17.05.2004 (http://www.findarticles.com/cf_0/m3374/n11_v20/20969541/p1/article.jhtml?term=men+%2B+health (No author listed or volume/issue or page)

Epperly, T.D. & Moore, K.E. (2000). Health issues in men: Part II. Common psychosocial disorders. *American Family Physician* (July 1). Found on the Internet <http://www.findarticles.com/cf_0/m3225/1_62/65864000/print.jhtml/>

Fein, E.B. (1994). Frustrating fight for acceptance; for older job seekers, a sad refrain: "I'd love to hire you, but you just won't fit in" (January 4). ntimes.com. <http://query.nytimes.com/gst/fullpage.html?res=9902E0DA103EF937A35752C0A962958260&sec=&spon=&pagewanted=all/>

Gupta, S. (2003, May 12). Why men die young. *Time, 161*(19), 84.

Harrison, J., Chin, J., & Ficarrotto, T. (1988). Warning: Masculinity may be dangerous to your health. In M. S. Kimmel & M. A. Messner (Eds.), *Men's lives* (pp. 271–285). New York: Macmillan.

Kleiner, H.S., Hertzog, J. & Targ, D.G. (1998). Grandparents acting as parents. Purdue University Cooperative Extension Service (January). <http://www.uwex.edu/ces/gprg/article.html/>

Powell, R. (2008). Bleak Retirements for 150 Million? *Marketwatch* (March 28). <http://articles.moneycentral.msn.com/RetirementandWills/InvestForRetirement/BleakRetirementsFor150Million.aspx?page=all/>

Reuben, D. B., Yoshikawa, T. T., & Besdine, R. W. (Eds.), (1996). *Geriatrics review syllabus; A core curriculum in geriatric medicine* (3rd edn). New York: American Geriatric Society (pp. 207–210).

Robertson, J., & Fitzgerald, L. (1992). *Journal of Counseling Psychology, 39*(2), 240–246.

Sack, K. (2008). In Massachusetts, Universal Coverage Strains Care (April 5). <http://www.nytimes.com/2008/04/05/us/05doctors.html?_r=1&th=&oref=slogin&emc=th&pagewanted=print/>

Saunders, C. S. (2000). Where are all the men? Retrieved 15.05.2003 http://www.findarticles.com/cf_0/m3233/11_34/63602907/print.jhtm. *Patient Care, 16*(4), 12–18.

Shore, J. R., & Hayslip, B. (1994). Custodial grandparenting: Implications for children's development. In A. E. Gottfried & A. W. Gottfried (Eds.), *Redefining families: Implications for children's development*. New York: Plenum Press.

Index